p 157.

Current
Psychiatric
Therapies
VOL. III — 1963

Current

Psychiatric

Therapies

AN ANNUAL PUBLICATION

VOL. III – 1963

Edited by

Jules H. Masserman, M.D.

Professor of Psychiatry and Neurology, Northwestern University, Chicago, Illinois

GRUNE & STRATTON   **NEW YORK · LONDON**

Contents

PART V: CHILDHOOD AND ADOLESCENCE

PART VI: THE FAMILY

PART VII: GROUP THERAPY

PART VIII: INSTITUTIONAL AND COMMUNITY

PART IX: FORENSIC CONSIDERATIONS

INDEX

Preface

SINCE this is the third volume in a series begun as recently as 1960, it is perhaps a bit early to talk about traditions; however, the following characteristics of all the issues to date may be noted:

New principles of psychiatric therapy, better ways of applying old ones, and more comprehensive integrations of both theory and practice continue to appear.

As psychiatric therapists gain greater grasp and confidence, they tend to discard cultist jargon, elision and obscurity in favor of clarity and precision of operational presentation.

Consequently, suitable contributions to this series perennially become more numerous; indeed, some excellent offerings had to be postponed for future publication to keep Volume III within reasonable size. Nevertheless, one pleasant custom has been retained: i.e., every current President of the American Psychiatric Association (this year, Jack R. Ewalt), contributes a leading article; and in this volume one of the Association's immediate past presidents, Francis Braceland, has extended this custom retrospectively.

Finally, the editor feels he has again served only one humble function: to mediate the clinical wisdom and expository skill of his contributors to the rapidly growing readership of this series. To the authors and their audience, therefore, once more his sincere thanks.

JULES H. MASSERMAN, M.D.
EDITOR

Northwestern University
Chicago, January 1, 1963

Roster of Contributors

Nathan W. Ackerman, M.D., Clinical Director, Family Mental Health Service, Jewish Family Service Association of New York, New York, New York.

Dominick A. Barbara, M.D., Psychoanalyst in Charge, Speech Department, Karen Horney Clinic, New York, New York.

Francis J. Braceland, M.D., Psychiatrist-in-Chief, Institute of Living, Hartford, Connecticut. President, American Psychiatric Association, 1957-58.

Selwyn Brody, M.D., Chief Psychiatrist, Children's Village, Dobbs Ferry, New York.

Arthur P. Burdon, M.D., Associate Clinical Professor of Psychiatry, Louisiana State University School of Medicine, New Orleans, Louisiana.

Richard L. Cohen, M.D., Director of Training, Philadelphia Child Guidance Clinic and Oakbourne Hospital, Philadelphia, Pennsylvania.

R. Cooper, Ph.D., Burden Neurological Institute and Frenchay Hospital, Bristol, England.

H. J. Crow, M.A., M.B., Ch.B., Burden Neurological Institute and Frenchay Hospital, Bristol, England.

Charles Clay Dahlberg, M.D., William Alanson White Psychoanalytic Institute, New York, New York.

Jack R. Ewalt, M.D., Bullard Professor of Psychiatry, Harvard Medical School and Superintendent, Massachusetts Mental Health Center, Boston, Massachusetts. President, American Psychiatric Association, 1963-64.

Dana L. Farnsworth, M.D., Professor of Hygiene and Director, University Health Services, Harvard University, Cambridge, Massachusetts.

Barbara Fish, M.D., Associate Clinical Professor of Psychiatry, New York University School of Medicine, Psychiatrist-in-Charge, Children's Service, Bellevue Hospital, Psychiatric Division, New York, New York.

Stephen Fleck, M.D., Psychiatrist-in-Chief, Yale Psychiatric Institute, New Haven, Connecticut.

Jacob H. Friedman, M.D., Director, Neuropsychiatric Service, Fordham Hospital, Bronx, New York.

Nicholas G. Frignito, M.D., Medical Director, County Court of Philadelphia, Philadelphia, Pennsylvania.

H. H. Garner, M.D., Professor and Chairman, Department of Psychiatry and Neurology, Chicago Medical School, Chicago, Illinois.

J. J. Geller, M.D., Consultant, Bergen County Mental Health Center, New Jersey. Faculty, W. A. White Institute of Psychiatry, Psychology and Psychoanalysis, New York, New York.

Elizabeth Jacob, M.A., Jewish Family and Community Service, Chicago, Illinois.

Mordecai Kaffman, M.D., Director, Child Clinic of the Kibbutzim, Oranim, Kiriath Tivon, Israel.

Harold Koenig, M.D., Department of Neurology and Psychiatry, Northwestern University Medical School, Chicago, Illinois.

Ruth Koenig, M.D., Chicago Psychoanalytic Institute, Chicago, Illinois.

Lawrence C. Kolb, M.D., Professor and Chairman of Psychiatry, College of Physicians and Surgeons, Columbia University, New York, New York.

Ogden R. Lindsley, Ph.D., Director, Behavior Research Laboratory, Harvard Medical School and Metropolitan State Hospital, Waltham, Massachusetts.

Sandor Lorand, M.D., Professor of Clinical Psychiatry, Downstate Medical Center, State University of New York, Brooklyn, New York.

Rollo May, Ph.D., Training Analyst, William Alanson White Institute of Psychiatry, Psychoanalysis and Psychology, New York, New York.

Warren G. McPherson, M.D., Chicago Psychoanalytic Institute, Chicago, Illinois.

Arthur A. Miller, M.D., Chicago Psychoanalytic Institute, Chicago, Illinois.

Hugh Mullan, M.D., Director, New York Alcoholism Vocational Rehabilitation Project, New York, New York.

Carlton W. Orchinik, Ph.D., Mental Health Psychologist, County Court of Philadelphia, Philadelphia, Pennsylvania.

D. G. Phillips, F.R.C.S., Burden Neurological Institute and Frenchay Hospital, Bristol, England.

Robert N. Rapaport, Ph.D., Lecturer in Social Anthropology, Harvard University, Cambridge, Massachusetts.

Harold Rosen, M.D., Associate Professor of Psychiatry, Johns Hopkins University School of Medicine, Baltimore, Maryland.

William Ryan, Ph.D., Chief Psychologist, Mount Auburn Hospital, Cambridge, Massachusetts.

Albert E. Scheflen, M.D., Associate Professor of Research Psychiatry, Temple University Medical Center, Philadelphia, Pennsylvania.

Philip F. D. Seitz, M.D., Chicago Psychoanalytic Institute, Chicago, Illinois.

Harley C. Shands, M.D., Professor of Psychiatry, College of Medicine, State University of New York, Brooklyn, New York.

Ralph Slovenko, LI.B., Associate Professor of Law, Tulane University, New Orleans, Louisiana.

Edward Stainbrook, M.D., Professor and Chairman, Department of Psychiatry, School of Medicine, University of Southern California, Los Angeles, California.

Robert L. Stewart, M.D., Department of Psychiatry, University of Cincinnati College of Medicine, Cincinnati, Ohio.

Dorothy Stock, Ph.D., Department of Psychiatry, University of Chicago, Chicago, Illinois.

Gene L. Usdin, M.D., Chief of the Department of Neurology and Psychiatry, Touro Infirmary and Associate Professor of Clinical Psychiatry, Tulane School of Medicine, New Orleans, Louisiana.

Adrian Van Kaam, Ph.D., Associate Professor of Psychology, Duquesne University, Pittsburgh, Pennsylvania.

A. Earl Walker, M.D., Professor of Neurological Surgery, Johns Hopkins University School of Medicine, Baltimore, Maryland.

Lewis R. Wolberg, M.D., Medical Director, Postgraduate Center for Psychotherapy, New York, New York.

PART 1

PRINCIPLES OF PSYCHIATRIC THERAPY

The Art of Psychotherapy

by FRANCIS J. BRACELAND, M.D.

> God opens one book to physicians that a good many of you
> don't know about—The Book of Life. That is none of your
> dusty folios with black letters between pasteboard and leather
> but it is printed in bright type and the binding of it is warm
> and tender to every touch. They reverence that book as one
> of the Almighty's infallible revelations.
>
> *—Oliver Wendell Holmes—Elsie Venner*

THE ART OF MEDICINE is based on the skillful use of human relationships as well as the skillful application of scientific knowledge. Evidence abounds that while the emotions, attitudes and expectations of patients are of great importance in their response to treatment, the emotions, attitudes and expectations of the physician are equally important. It has been suggested that the practice of medicine flourishes best when doctors think most highly of their functions. There is truth in this statement if we assume that objectivity and scientific perspective are not lost in the process. Therapeutic optimism is a powerful force for good, despite the occasional occupational hazard known as *furor therapeuticus*. To believe that we can help our patients in some manner, no matter what their condition may be, and that it is our obligation to try is an indispensable professional attitude for the true physician.

The observant doctor hardly needs a scientific treatise to know that it is not always *what* he does that helps the patient, but rather *how* he does it. Nor can he help noticing that now and then a patient recovers when he, the doctor, has been at a complete loss as to what to try next. Psychotherapists observe the same phenomenon and have sometimes

1

referred to it as the sudden transference cure. They have also noted that inadvertent breaks in technique seem to facilitate more constructive work with certain patients. They are even witnesses to spontaneous recoveries. Here, presumably, the patient has an experience which makes something fall into place for him and he is able to make sense of something that had eluded him before.

The understanding and manipulation of social forces is a major ingredient of the art of medicine. Not only do the ideas that people have about illness in general, or about a particular illness, influence their manifestations; such ideas also influence the course and outcome and even the response to etiological treatment. What the patient ascribes the illness to and believes it to mean, his notions of treatment, his cooperation or lack of it, his will to recovery or the reverse, the confidence or lack of confidence he has in the physician and in physicians in general—all of these factors make their contribution to the presenting problem. Some patients need symptoms. If they are unable to keep the ones they have, they may summon up others far worse. For patients with serious personality disorders, physical symptoms may channel off anxiety that would otherwise be dealt with more drastically.

Psychiatrists deal with many of the people who have resorted to the more drastic solutions. Psychiatric problems are many and complex, and so are the possible causes. However, disturbed human relationships are usually important in the chain of causation as well as in the persistence of a psychiatric disorder, and corrective experience in the doctor-patient relationship is necessary. All forms of psychotherapy stress the quality of this relationship. The therapist himself is a therapeutic force. His use of himself matters more than the doctrine or method he follows. In this relationship there must be something akin to faith. Jerome Frank reminds us that faith, hope, eagerness and joy are healing emotions and that the therapist should never underestimate their importance.

The art of psychotherapy involves the creation of the proper atmosphere from the start. The therapist seeks to mobilize the patient's expectation of help, even though the patient may deny that he needs it. To gain the patient's trust often calls for great resourcefulness and even a large degree of self-sacrifice. Unquestionably it is easier to help patients who seek psychotherapy on their own than it is to help those who come unwillingly. But the real test of the therapist is to overcome the distrust and estrangement of the patient he is privileged to treat.

The doctor's attitude will be as important as any verbal communication. He must have the courage to be himself and be prepared to accept the patient as he is. He needs to be relaxed and quiet and at ease with the patient and never lose sight of the fact that there is more to understand than is first apparent. It is a commonplace to say that a great part of the medical art is in knowing how to listen. There are many individuals who need little more than the opportunity to talk and to verbalize their thoughts and feelings. Ideas and feelings which cannot be discussed are extremely threatening to many people. Once spoken, however, they can be examined and reduced to their proper proportions. For others, the problem is essentially that they have not had any opportunity to express themselves before and no one has had time to listen. Relief follows swiftly when these persons encounter a trained and sympathetic listener.

In too many cases, unfortunately, matters are not as simple as noted. Patients require an extended period of therapy before the experience becomes corrective. The therapist must arrive at emotional as well as intellectual understanding. Emotional understanding presupposes mutuality, an appreciation of what the emotions under observation mean to the patient, an identification. Identification is the basis of all emotional understanding, and it depends less on conscious effort than on a desire to understand and an ability to sympathize. To identify, the therapist must be able to feel, if only briefly, that he is the other person. To do this, he must be able to dispense with his awareness of himself. In this way, there arises a mutual experience. Michael and Enid Balint describe this aspect of psychotherapy as biphasic. The psychotherapist must first identify, and then withdraw from the identification and become an objective professional person again. They submit that this is one of the ways a professional relationship differs from a private relationship.

Another major difference is the expert knowledge of the physician. In addition to having the ability to identify in the right setting while having only a limited involvement with his patient, the doctor has at his fingertips special knowledge and skill as the result of his training and experience. He uses this knowledge as he listens and observes. He uses it with discrimination, not rigidly or automatically as the untrained person coversant with theoretical knowledge would tend to do.

The art of psychotherapy is concerned with the dynamics of communication, including all the nuances, allusions and non-verbal cues which may be of significance. The therapist needs to be in command of himself at all times, remaining alert not only to changes in the patient's tensions, feelings and behavior but also to the changes being produced in himself. Self-understanding is of major importance. The therapist must not act out his own immature impulses and needs in the treatment situation. He must not reject the patient because he is difficult or not easy to love or because he is hostile and uncooperative. He has to endure frustration, to remain cool under personal attack, and to master fear, however formidable the patient happens to be.

There are levels of communication. Even silence can be communication. The confidence which grows out of companionable silence may pay important dividends later. If the therapist is free from anxiety he will more readily determine the proper form of contact with the patient. Such a consideration is of great importance in dealing with psychotic patients.

The psychiatrist's ability to help a patient depends in part on his training and on the image the patient has of him as a physician, but it also has something to do with his really caring about the patient's welfare and the physician's ability to bear a great burden of responsibility on the patient's behalf. To be therapeutic, he may have to change himself, to sacrifice certain feelings and attitudes which bring him satisfaction. He will have to guard against the rise of unwonted zeal— the need to imbue the patient with the doctor's own philosophy of proprieties in feeling and behavior, against the need to cure quickly and completely, against the need to prescribe and instruct and interfere in ways that do more harm than good. The inexperienced therapist may be tempted to do these busy things. Although the therapist must maintain his own identity and his own privacy, he can never be a stranger to his patient. He cannot help revealing what he is and what he believes in. He shows this in countless ways. He must therefore believe in the methods he uses, for if he believes in them, the patient is more likely to accept them. It is also incumbent upon him to believe in the inherent capacity of even the most regressed patient to attain, with help, a better solution of his difficulties. There can be no giving up in the face of apparent failure or of painfully slow progress interspersed with relapses. The long-term view is required. Even an imperfect result is a source of satisfaction to the dedicated psychotherapist.

What the doctor has to do, as the Balints see it, is to accept the whole of the muddle presented by the patient. In some treatments, what he has to do is "to accept the illogical, irrational parts of his patients, take them seriously, and even though they are only fairy-tale-like wishes or fears, not deny their importance and power." The therapist himself must accept the fantasies of the patient before he can ask the latter to test and accept reality.

Today the deteriorating patients common in the past are much less in evidence in psychiatric hospitals. This happy situation is due to drug therapy, to vastly improved hospital atmosphere, to improved psychotherapeutic programs and other factors. Certainly there has been encouraging progress in treating psychotic patients by psychotherapeutic means. Intensive psychotherapeutic work with psychotic patients has brought new insights. For the psychotic patient, the essential factor in his response to psychotherapy is the feeling of having been understood by the therapist.

C. Mueller notes that the literature over the years reveals the diversity of paths by which the therapist may be able to establish contact with the patient and provide the stimulation necessary for a return to reality. The decisive element of success is always difficult to establish and it varies from patient to patient. The particular school of psychiatric thought to which the therapist adheres seems to be less important than his ability to be creative, to use himself as a therapeutic tool, to respond to the patient's requirements in the here and now and to change his approach as the situation warrants. There can be no absolute positions in psychotherapy. Flexibility is indispensable. This is especially the case when we are dealing with psychotic patients. The method of approach will depend on the condition of the patient. Some therapists address themselves to the non-psychotic portions of the personality in an effort to establish a working relationship. Others meet the patient on his own ground, entering into his psychotic world in order to reach him. Some therapists become adept in paraverbal or non-verbal communication with psychotic patients. They do so on the basis that ordinary language has little if any communicative value in working with some of these patients. According to Mueller even when language is intact, the therapist may be unable to bridge the gap between himself and the patient by verbal means for nothing he can say has as much impact on the patient as the patient's own thoughts and images, his cosmic experiences and his whole allegorical world. To reach him, the therapist has to learn his language and understand the fascination of his internal experience. The doctor-patient relationship may then afford the patient the opportunity of recapturing the lost "thou" and the "we" within the threatening "you" and "they" of his own distorted universe.

More gratification must be afforded the psychotic than the neurotic patient. The psychotic patient cannot tolerate much frustration. When it is necessary to impose a limit on aggressiveness, the therapist should attempt to do so by his own person rather than by restraints or by retaliation. The rational, objective attitude is unbearable to the patient, and so is the passive attitude of benevolent neutrality. The belief that the psychotic patient is incapable of transference is no longer tenable. However, the transference is likely to be on a very archaic and undifferentiated level. In the schizophrenic, for example, it is intense, stormy and rapidly fluctuating, demanding much and accompanied by violent rages and aggressive behavior. In his delusional ideas the patient moves constantly from one extreme to the other. He himself incarnates both good and evil, and the same ambivalence is apparent in the transference. As the therapist emerges increasingly from his non-existence for the patient, the more ambivalent the transference becomes.

At the same time, appearances may be deceiving. The patient may be insulting, rejecting or physically abusive because he is afraid. The therapist has assumed for the patient the evil, perhaps seductive aspects of the patient's own personality. This is a role which the therapist must accept before the patient may come to recognize and to accept as his own these repressed, distorted aspects of himself. It is important that the psychotherapeutic experience provide a relationship different from the patient's expectations, different indeed from the relationship he has tried to provoke by his usual maneuvers.

Countertransference is more difficult with psychotics than with neurotics. Yet it is an extremely important factor in their treatment. Savage calls it the therapist's biggest asset and his biggest stumbling block. Countertransference is more massive, chaotic and fragile with psychotic than with neurotic patients. There is an element of fear to be dealt with, along with any narcissistic tendencies disturbing to the relationship. While an element of magical omnipotence is almost indispensable, as Savage puts it, it can lead to serious errors. If the patient's progress is slow, the therapist may lose interest, or he may put more pressure on the patient than the patient can tolerate, or he may overestimate the patient's progress. If the therapist wishes to prove something by his treatment, if he is looking for something to verify some pet theory, the patient may be lost forever, at least to him. If he needs to be successful, to be a healer against all odds, the result may be disastrous for all concerned.

In sum, the processes of recovery in psychotic patients take place in the dynamic framework of transference and countertransference. Progress during therapy depends in a certain sense on the self-discipline of the therapist, indeed on self-sacrifice. Sometimes the patient recaptures his forces and profits from therapy at the very moment the physician is enduring almost unbearable frustration or sense of failure. It is as if he had to part with something himself before the patient could even start on the road to recovery.

In clinical medicine, cure usually means to return the patient to the status quo ante. To say that the patient "is as good as he ever was" is a cause for universal rejoicing. This criterion is not valid in psychiatry. The premorbid state represented by this anterior status is the source of the patient's difficulties; if he is simply returned to this condition, he remains vulnerable. The personality is still weak and fragile; the disturbance may recur with the advent of the slightest frustration or temptation. The goal in psychiatry is to improve the status quo ante, hence to reinforce and strengthen the personality. It is not easy. There is much more to learn of the art of using the human personality in an infinite number of ways to create different psychological effects and to make the bond between patient and therapist a surer instrument of healing.

There is no universal blueprint for the psychotherapist. There is only a task. Of this task the Balints have this to say: "The therapist must never forget that he is a professional and that his task is not to love or to be strict or to make good the deprivations in the patient's past or present, but to listen attentively to what is said and to understand it in a professional capacity, and in particular never to forget that there is always something new to understand. What he must be on the lookout for are not faults in the patient's environment or history, but misunderstandings, exaggerations, painful contradictions, and omissions, which characterize and color the patient's present wishes, hopes and vision."

All of this constitutes the fusion of the scientist and the healer and this constitutes the true art of medicine. Like all great art, the art of psychotherapy is the skillful and creative application of scientific knowledge to a human problem. Ruskin wrote, "Fine art is that in which the hand, the head and the heart of man go together."

REFERENCES

BALINT, M., AND BALINT, E.: Psychotherapeutic Techniques in Medicine. Springfield, Ill., Charles C Thomas, 1962.

MUELLER, C.: Les therapeutiques analytiques des psychoses. Rev. franc. psychan., 22:575, 1958.

SAVAGE, C.: Countertransference in therapy of schizophrenics. Psychiatry, 24:53, 1961.

FRANK, J. D.: The dynamics of the psychotherapeutic relationship; determinants and effects of the therapist's influence. Psychiatry, 22:17, 1959.

Intercurrent Factors in Psychotherapy

by Lewis R. Wolberg, M.D.

W E ARE OFTEN confronted with the confounding phenomenon of marked improvement in patients who, frustrated by an inability to get well under the care of reputable psychiatrists, turn in desperation to quacks whose off-beat methods seem to turn the tide.

These contradictions, difficult as they are to explain, contaminate the climate in which we must evaluate our results in psychotherapy. They would seem to indicate that, in some cases, patients benefit more from bizarre treatment methods rendered by inexperienced and even untrained individuals than from traditionally tested procedures executed by mature and skilled specialists. On the surface, it would appear that something must be amiss. However, when we look closely at the phenomenon of emotional improvement, we can see that factors other than method or experience are involved in the complex course of happenings that constitute therapeutic gains. Unless we pay heed to these extra-therapeutic dimensions, we are prone to credit to our specific treatment process the healing effects of extraneous agents. While this may be of no importance from a practical point of view, it is of vital significance in any attempt to evaluate the role of our therapeutic methods which have seemingly helped in getting the patient to feel better and function better. Let us then consider the most important of the coincidental factors involved in psychological change.

The Spontaneous Remission or Cure

There is, unfortunately, a tendency to minimize the healing forces that are residual in the individual that enable him to recover from a considerable degree of psychological disruption without benefit of formal treatment. Fluctuations in the course of any emotional illness are quite characteristic, periods of remission developing which are followed by periods of exacerbation. It is quite likely that there is nothing haphazard in this cycle, emotional mechanisms in the psyche being as important as healing elements that operate during physical illness and tending to

8

bring the individual to psychological homeostasis. The human being is constantly evolving defenses to external stress and inner tensions which, if successful, restore his functional equilibrium. He may, for example, buttress his failing repressions, and, by sealing off noxious conflicts, restore to himself his shattered sense of mastery. He may coordinately bolster his depleted defenses and even evolve more constructive ways of dealing with his current difficulties. The means by which this is accomplished will vary with the circumstances which plague him and with the opportunities at his disposal. The repertoire of available modes are legion. Not only may these restore the old neurotic balances of power; sometimes surprisingly they may, without design, promote enduring personality growth.

No matter how victimized the individual may be by past unfortunate conditionings, he is always capable of some determinate learning under propitious circumstances. His expectation of failure, his misinterpretation of the reality situation, his transferential projections, his repetitive compulsive re-enactments of self-defeating behavior will tend, of course, to sabotage his successes. Inferential discoveries are nevertheless going on around the matrix of his neurotic responses, reconditioning at least some neurotically structured reactions.

Instances of reconditioning in even severe neurotic and psychotic disorders have been recorded in persons who have by chance come under the guidance of a well-disposed and intelligent authority or group, or who have found a congenial environment that differs from the characteristic milieu. These changes are not fortuitous; they follow certain laws of learning. Where the individual finds an environment that does not actively repeat the punitive, frustrating conditions of his past; where it provides him with a modicum of security and some means of gratifying vital psychological needs; where it gives him a feeling of knowing what is expected of him and some ability of living up to these expectations; where it nurtures in him a sense of belonging and of being wanted; where it provides him with opportunities to expand his capacities and skills—there will be optimal conditions for learning. Obviously those individuals whose emotional problems have undergone minimal structuralization in the form of neurotic and character disorders will learn best in a favorable environment. Where extensive organization has occurred, conflictual strivings will tend to be perpetuated even in a good setting. There still may be spontaneous periods of improvement, particularly where the environment absorbs and deals in a tolerant and constructive way with the individual's neurotic impulses and behavior without excessive punishment or withdrawal of love.

It will be seen, therefore, that the so-called spontaneous remission or cure does not take place in a vacuum. It results from the operation of forces which exert a healing influence on neurotic patterns. Even though these processes are not deliberately designed, but obtrude themselves through what appears to be chance under the impact of a "spontaneous" need to heal oneself, the individual takes advantage of the healthful elements in his environment in order to fulfill himself and to grow.

During psychotherapy, spontaneous forces nurture constructive learning in situations outside of the psychotherapeutic setting. The relief of symptoms and the reconditioning of neurotic patterns may be the product of these external agencies. It is, therefore, essential to assay the relative impact of these informal spontaneous therapeutic experiences on the individual when we attempt to evaluate the specific role that psychotherapeutic techniques have played.

The Placebo Dimension

In a considerable number of persons the yearning for health is so intense that exposure to any kind of psychotherapy seems to sponsor symptomatic improvement on the basis of a "placebo influence." Because relief may be credited to the psychotherapeutic techniques that are being employed, it is necessary to keep the placebo dimension in mind when appraising the value of a particular kind of psychotherapy.

Placebo action has long been recognized by the medical profession as a potent healing force. Indeed the prescription of inert substances was a standard parcel of medical practice for many years, being embodied in the tradition of giving pink sugar pills and injecting sterile water for their suggestive effects. These may be quite powerful even to the point where direct statements regarding a presumed drug action, or suggested innuendoes, induce a psychological reaction diametrically opposed to the true pharmacological effects of the drug. Research explorations on medicaments in the form of double-blind studies, pay respect to the adventitious placebo factor, recognizing that a mental influence may contaminate the impartial appraisal of a substance.

What holds true for drugs probably also holds true for systems of psychotherapy. The individual projects into these systems his expectations of cure, and he may react quite remarkably to techniques and agencies that he enshrines with powers they may not really possess. During the heyday of orgone therapy, many intelligent people were benefitted by interludes in an orgone box. An acquaintance of the author claimed that he had gotten more out of three months of periodic insertions inside a box than out of three years of intensive psychotherapy with a well-known and skilled psychiatrist. In fact he was so impressed by the results that he bought a "his" and "her" box for himself and his wife. He also built a small orgone box for his cat. These boxes, he insisted, reduced his psychiatric, medical and veterinary bills to insignificant proportions.

Psychiatric therapies which in the mind of the patient possess esoteric or mystical qualities are most likely to induce a placebo effect. Thus hypnosis and psychoanalysis, charged as they are with supposed meta-psychological powers, are apt to instill in the patient a feeling of magical influence. This instrumentality although an artefact may promote confidence in the treatment method. By the same token, a negative placebo effect may obtain, if, by virtue of what he imagines will take place, the patient has lack of faith in, or fears being hurt by, a special kind of therapy. The chances are then that his attitude will inhibit the effectiveness of treatment.

During the past few years, I have had an opportunity tentatively to test this hypothesis. Due to the intensive publicity given to hypnosis as a treatment method, I have been consulted by a considerable number of persons whose sole motivation for therapy was to control obnoxious habits and symptoms. Chief among these have been obese persons who have wanted to reduce, but were unable to stop overeating, chain smokers whose physical well-being was being threatened by their intake of nicotine and coal-tar, and impotent men whose lack of functioning threatened their marriages and general opinion of themselves. A universal question was: "Can hypnosis cure me?" In roughly one-third of cases I replied: "It is impossible to say. Generally problems such as yours require deeper psychotherapy over a long-term period, since the basis of the trouble is in personality difficulties and insecurities that originated in childhood. However, there is a fifty-fifty chance that you might feel better with hypnosis if you turn out to be a good subject." In one-third of cases, I have replied enthusiastically: "Yes, hypnosis can definitely help symptoms such as yours. If you keep at it, it is bound to work. You can't keep yourself from responding." In one-third, my pessimistic response has been: "Probably not. Hypnosis is no cure-all. It can help some problems but not all. In your case, the difficulty seems to be too deep-rooted and the habit too firmly entrenched to respond to any other than long-term psychotherapy. However, if you want to try hypnosis first, we can." Symptomatic responses to hypnosis have been directly in proportion to my positiveness and enthusiasm. Apparently the hope that I inspired, and the patient's conviction that the method could work acted as a potent agent in mobilizing curative forces.

Tigani el Mahi,[1] the well-known psychiatrist from the Anglo-Egyptian Sudan, has commented on the powerful factor of confidence in the treatment method as an ingredient in cure. Among native groups who are imbedded in magic and witchcraft, the most adroit application of dynamic psychotherapy produces meager results, principally because the victim of an emotional problem is convinced that his suffering is the consequence of a curse or other evil magic from an offended spirit. The adroit use of a fetish, or the exorcism of the force responsible for the bewitchery will, in a surprising number of instances, bring about the improvement of cure of even long-standing neurotic and psychotic illnesses.

We need not go to primitive tribes to detect evidences of magical thinking in psychological cures. Thus civilized patients hospitalized with bleeding peptic ulcers were given hypodermic injections of distilled water accompanied by the statement that this was a new remedy for bleeding ulcers.[2] Seventy per cent were remarkably helped over a long-term period. In a number of studies of psychiatric outpatients in whom the sole therapy was the administration of inert placebo substances, 55 per cent showed a marked improvement.[3]

Placebo effects are usually, but not always, temporary. In many instances the improvement acts, like in the "spontaneous cure," as a vehicle for the reorientation of the individual to his total adjustment. How the placebo influence operates to exert a more than temporary effect will vary with the underlying problems. In some instances, the idea of being protected brings about a security feeling with greater self-confidence and a heightened capacity to handle challenging relationships with people. The placebo may thus act as a basis for reorganization of attitudes which may become entrenched in a favorable milieu.

The operation of the placebo element gives us insight into the fact that patients may be helped by psychotherapies which seem scientifically unsound, provided that there is faith and trust in their validity and power.

THE RELATIONSHIP DIMENSION

Every helping situation is characterized by a special kind of relationship that develops between client, patient and counselor-therapist. In this relationship the individual invests the authority with benevolent protective powers, and he relates to the latter with expectant trust. Implicit, if not explicit, is the understanding that the authority has the knowledge, the skill and the desire to help the person overcome the problem for which professional services have been sought. The more bewildered and helpless the person, the greater the reliance he places on expert individuals. This is certainly the case in the sick patient afflicted with a physical ailment who seeks from a physician surcease from pain and suffering. It is a most important factor in the psycho-therapeutic situation particularly at the beginning of treatment.

The relief the patient experiences as he starts psychotherapy is generally the product of the relationship dimension. No matter how non-directive the therapist may imagine himself to be, and irrespective of how much he discourages any dependency intent on the part of the patient, the latter will project his need for solace and comfort onto the therapist and the therapeutic situation. The importance of this relation-ship factor is too often minimized, and credit for the modification is falsely extended to the special techniques and maneuvers executed by the therapist. It is important to realize that, irrespective of the brand, the depth and the real worth of the psychotherapy that is being employed, improvement may be sustained in some instances for an indefinite period as a pure product of the relationship. It must be remembered, however, that benefits accruing from the relationship are the forerunners of therapy, not the end-all. Unless there is a correction of stress sources, and/or a restructuring of personality, the amelioration may cease upon termination of treatment.

The Factor of Emotional Catharsis

The sheer act of talking can provide an individual with considerable emotional palliation. It furnishes a motor outlet for the release of tension. It softens inhibitions and liberates conscious and unconscious conflicts that have been held in check. It exposes suppressed attitudes and ideas that the person has been keeping from himself, and it encourages him to subject these to the rationale of critical reasoning. It brings to the surface repudiated and fearsome impulses, with their attendant feeling of shame. In this way it takes the strain off automatic channels which have been used to unload accumulated neurotic energy.

In the unburdening process, there is often a relief of guilt feelings in relation to past experiences, particularly sexual acting-out, anal activities, hostile or aggressive outbursts, and competitive strivings. Guilt is appeased as one examines sexual phantasies as well as antisocial and unethical impulses. Discussing these gives reassurance that one is not a helpless victim of uncontrollable strivings, that he has not been irrepar-ably damaged by his past. Reviewing incidents in which one has been hurt, humiliated or exploited also tends to put these into proper perspective. Sharing one's fears of disease and mutilation robs them of their frightening quality. Relinquished are conscious restraints which rob the person of his spontaneity. In short, the putting into words of diffuse and terrorizing feelings, and the acceptance of the pronouncements without condemnation and rejection, enables the person to gain greater control over his emotions.

These developments may occur in the presence of any listener, whether this be a sympathetic friend, a respected authority such as a physician, teacher, lawyer, minister, or a psychotherapist. It is consequently necessary to keep this in mind when we estimate the differential effects of a psychotherapeutic system, so as to discount the non-specific relief gained by verbalization. It is, of course, scarcely necessary to mention that the agency of emotional catharsis, like the other factors previously mentioned, operates in all psychotherapies and is technically encouraged by the activities of the therapist.

RATIONALISTIC, ESCAPE AND CONTROL DEVICES

Frequently an emotionally disturbed individual may engage in activities which are designed toward, and result in, an alleviation of his symptoms. Devices are employed which generally have widespread sanction and are incorporated in established institutions of society. These activities in themselves may promote improvement which must be isolated from the effects of coordinate psychotherapy.

In the course of his existence, every individual evolves a philosophy which serves to give substance to his being, and provides a design around which he patterns himself and his life goals. Codes of behavior and ethics are organized to bolster his conscience, and values are incorporated to justify non-fulfillment of needs. In the face of failure in adaptation with ensuing anxiety, the individual may attempt to deal with his turmoil by developing new philosophical ways of looking at things. He may thus assume as a virtue the maintenance of a stoical attitude, accepting his plight as unavoidable, the endurance of which tests his competence as a person. In this way he makes capital out of his disasters, and he secures equinimity through martyrdom. Many of the present-day mystical philosophies stress the unimportance of personal affliction and external hardship, focusing the individual's attention on establishing contact with his inner self, the essence of being. In this way the individual detaches himself from his suffering and seeks joy in meditation and self-contemplation.

The patient may also evolve the tactic of pushing out of his mind sensations of pain, substituting for them thoughts of health and pleasure, thereby eliminating customary preoccupations with suffering. He may convince himself that his symptoms are actually an escape from responsibilities in life. To resume sensible living, he must banish thoughts of illness, paying little attention to his symptoms since solicitude merely tends to aggravate them. The patient may then embark on what he considers "proper thinking habits." By engaging in thoughts of happiness and health, he attempts to side-step his calamities and illnesses. By obliterating suffering from his mind, he hopes to feel no distress. He may rationalize his trouble by assuming that he is not alone in strife, that there are those more disabled, more unfortunate than himself. He may dedicate himself then to bringing other persons to his new-found optimisms. He may decide that striving for success and perfection are false objectives that can bring only exhaustion and disappointment. He may therefore scale down his ambitions and content himself with modest goals that are within the range of immediate fulfillment. He may make an inventory of his good qualities and recognize that there is much for him to be thankful. He may rule himself to live in the spirit of forebearance, tolerance, sympathy, and altruism, reviving, in the course, his religious convictions.

By turning to religion, many persons are able to help themselves to tolerate the destructive effects of their neuroses. Putting oneself in the hands of a power stronger than man who can lead one to paths of safety and glory can be extremely reassuring if one's faith is sufficiently strong to accept kinship with the Divine Being. In union with God, the individual does not have to struggle alone; he is helped to endure his travail, to conquer evil thoughts and impulses, and to achieve confidence and strength in living.

In addition to philosophic and religious aids to suffering, the individual may indulge other modes of gaining relief. He may rectify environmental distortions that serve to exaggerate his tension. For instance, he may move into a residential area that is not so riddled with quarreling and disturbed neighbors. Or some difficulties may spontaneously cease to exist, as where a destructive supervisor or foreman is replaced with a kindly genial one. A hostile member of his family may regain control over his emotions, or may be drafted into the army, or may move to another city, thereby removing a potential stress source. The patient may also find relief from his symptomatic preoccupation by externalizing his interests in arts, crafts, hobbies, music, games, physical exercise, sports and recreation. Diverting his energies into useful channels of activity may have a most salubrious effect upon him. In this reference, engagement in social activities, joining clubs and dancing groups, may invoke a most constructive influence not the least of which is the sharing of experiences with others.

The patient may also gain relief from his problems by running away from trouble sources. He may rightfully decide that his difficulty is stirred up by a destructive home environment, or an impossible work situation, or a relationship problem with which he cannot cope. He may consequently remove himself bodily from his predicament by going on a long vacation, or he may permanently attempt to rupture his contacts. Thus, he may seek a divorce, or quit his job, or abandon his girl friend; and these disengagements may, if auxiliary problems do not intervene, temporarily, at least, relieve his distress. He may indulge in excessive drinking which deadens his sensations; or he may take tranquilizers which ameliorates them; or imbibe sleeping potions which submerge them.

It is essential, therefore, that we alert ourselves to the contingencies of rationalistic, escape and control devices in evaluating a psychotherapy, making appropriate allowances for worthy happenings that have little to do with the actual techniques that are being employed.

The Role of Resistance

So far the elements that have been described have operated in the service of symptom relief and the sponsorship of a productive therapeutic experience. There are some negative processes, however, that can sabotage all psychotherapies that may interfere with an impartial appraisal of their worth. We may subserve these under the heading of "resistance."

It is not remarkable that resistance comes into evidence because therapy constitutes an attack on the patient's way of life as well as on his cherished value systems. It threatens to upset the delicate balance between repressed elements of the personality and the repressing forces. To give up his defenses, however, maladaptive as they may be, is to expose himself to dangers that he considers far greater than the inconveniences already suffered as a result of his symptoms.

Resistance may take myriad forms limited only by the repertoire of defenses the individual has at his disposal. The patient may spend his time on evasive and aggressive tactics, fighting the therapist, or proving he is wrong, or winning him over with gestures of helplessness, praise or devotion, or seeking vicarious means of escaping or evading treatment. Fatigue, listlessness, inhibitions in thinking, lapses in memory, prolonged silences, intensification of complaints, pervasive self-devaluation, resentment, suspiciousness, aggression, forced flight into health, spurious insight, indulgence in superficial talk, engagement in irrational acts and behavior (acting out), and expressed contempt for normality may occupy the patient to the detriment of his progress.

Among the most treacherous of resistances are those that issue out of the relationship between therapist and patient, described by Freud as transference manifestations. Here the smoldering embers of the past, unconscious needs, demands, impulses and fears, are fanned into a conflagration in the crucible of the therapeutic relationship. The ideas, sentiments, feelings and action tendencies residual in formative conditionings with early parental and sibling figures are mobilized and projected toward the therapist who becomes a virtual reincarnation of the objects which originally inspired them. There is in this reconstructed mirage a distortion of reality, albeit a distortion that is vigorously denied by the patient. The patient acts toward the therapist as if the latter were the embodiment of total good or total evil. There may be a veering back and forth from idealization to deprecation. The therapist may be regarded as loving, nourishing, opulent protector who has the wisdom and power of a demigod. Cloaked in this mantle of omnipotence, the therapist must then display his magical skills which will disintegrate the patient's troubles, and lead into paths of health, success and glory. The patient may, for a while, actually become convinced that this is being accomplished, particularly where the therapist shares with the patient lofty sentiments about himself. The patient will then feel singularly protected and his symptoms will abate. Soon, however, there are frightening but exciting phantasies of an erotic nature. There may be desires for complete amalgamation with the therapist. There may be fears of mutilation and disintegration. Feelings toward the therapist will then change and the patient will be outraged at what he considers a deception practiced by the therapist. Fury or fear may then explode the benefits derived from treatment, and the patient may then abandon the therapist and go off in quest of new and infallible Gods. There are many other strange and interesting kinds of interferences that emerge from the transference which are peculiar to the inner psychological needs and specific past experiences of the patient.

Resistance may consume the total energy of the patient leaving little zeal for positive therapeutic work. Sometimes a skilled therapist may bypass resistance by prodding reality into the face of the patient. Sometimes it may be worked through by analytic interpretations. Often it operates despite attempts to dissipate it, bringing the best efforts of the therapist to a halt.

Because resistance is so often concealed and rationalized, it may be difficult to expose. Even an experienced therapist may be deceived by its subtleties. What is perplexing is how to differentiate forces that operate to destroy the effectiveness of therapy from those that are inherent in a poor therapeutic system. An interview with both patient and therapist may not always reveal what has been happening. A factor that must be considered is that the therapist may be unadept in detecting and dealing with resistance which is, as has been pointed out, to a greater or small degree, an inevitable part of any treatment process. On the other hand, the most talented and capable therapists will be confronted with some patients who cling doggedly to their resistance despite skillful handling. Quite unfairly, then, a special therapy may be branded as intrinsically worthless, whereas it has really become marooned on the reefs of resistance.

Summary

Adventitious elements enter into all psychotherapies, influencing the process for the good or bad. These elements may enhance or neutralize the activities of the therapist, bringing progress to a halt or expediting it beyond reasonable expectancy. The most common coincidental forces contaminating therapeutic results are those of spontaneous remission, placebo effect, the relationship dimension, emotional catharsis, resistance to cure, and a variety of rationalistic, escape and control devices. It is doubtful if the therapist can avoid these contaminations; he must instead accept them as inevitable. His skill is related to the advantage he takes of their positive virtues, while reducing the negative influences they may wield.

REFERENCES

1. Tigani el Mahi: Personal communication.
2. Volgyesi, F. A.: "School for patients," hypnosis-therapy and psychoprophylaxia. Brit. J. M. Hypnotism., 5: 8-17, 1954.
3. Gliedman, L. H., Nash, E. H., Imber, S. D., Stone, A. R., and Frank, J. D. Reduction of symptoms by pharmacologically inert substances and by short-term psychotherapy. Arch. Neurol. & Psychiat., 79: 345-351, 1958.

Model and Goal in Psychotherapy

by HARLEY C. SHANDS, M.D.

WHEN SOME PSYCHIATRISTS use the term "psychotherapy," they generally refer to a procedure derived from psychoanalysis and ostensibly oriented toward the "cure" of "illness." They often ignore that in so doing they are using only one of many possible models and selecting only one of many possible goals. There are other models, each with its appropriate goal, which may be used to describe a psychotherapeutic relationship and the events internal to it. The procedure followed in any case depends upon the (explicit or implicit) selection of a model, and the termination of the process is a function of the decision that the goal implicit in the model has either been reached or that it is unreachable.

The situation existing in the United States for the last twenty years is worthy of comment. American psychotherapy derives mainly from a technique developed in the late nineteenth century in a middle-European middle-class Jewish culture, and it has been exhibited in a highly industrialized, relatively young nation of diverse racial strains welded into a tradition of strongly Calvinist protestant derivations. It must be considered at the beginning of any discussion, therefore, that we are not talking about a phenomenon which we can expect to find widely reproduced. Psychotherapy in this sense is not only culture-bound but also class-bound; within these limitations, there appear to be alternative descriptive models which can be used to illuminate the events taking place.

As a tendency to "believe in" psychotherapy as a panacea has declined, a concomitant tendency to examine it has increased. An indication of this change is that where once psychoanalysts could confidently assert that the therapist was doing research and therapy at the same time, it has by now become quite generally accepted that a commitment to influence the patient in any relationship makes the therapist an unreliable reporter.

The change in attitude can be described as a shift from subjectivity toward objectivity; the psychotherapist is coming increasingly to be aware of the need for an objective examination of himself as well as of the patient. This is "sauce for the gander" added by the force of circumstances to the "sauce for the goose" traditionally offered to the patient. Prior to the recent past, the self-examination of the therapist was thought to have been completed by his experience in his training analysis. Although it was often repeated within the group that one's self-analysis should never cease, it was tacitly assumed that the therapist could be trusted to keep himself corrected. By contrast, psychotherapists recently have shown a greater tendency to accept the likelihood that distortions are likely to continue to be a problem.

We find psychotherapy in its various versions becoming a movement to be studied in its geographic, historical, and social contexts. Psycho*therapy* becomes not the approach to all forms of mental *illness*, but rather one way of approaching complex human problems which have traditionally been (and which remain) difficult of solution. Instead of devoting ourselves to questions of how to cure the previously incurable, we ask questions about psychotherapy of a much more general nature. What are its origins? What are its functions? What other procedures does it resemble, and in what ways? Why are there great differences in its popularity in different social and geographical contexts?

From the historical point of view, these questions tend to return the problem toward the position taken by Freud. The American preoccupation with the exclusively medical applications of psychoanalytic theory has never been thoroughly shared by psychoanalysts in other parts of the world. Within the medical orientation in American ways, it has never been possible to demonstrate the therapeutic value of psychotherapy on an objective, or even on a widely shared consensual, basis. Critics have tended to be either excessively destructive or excessively kind, with rarely a disinterested observer to be found.

It is in the United States that psychotherapy has reached its greatest popularity, and it is also here that the field has been more intimately a part of medicine than anywhere else.[1] Along with this there has grown a tendency to conceptualize problems of "emotion" and of "behavior" as those of health and disease, to a point where it has almost seemed subversive to question whether or not the medical model was the one most appropriate as an approach to the understanding of discorded behavior.

This persistent trend in this country is at variance with the reverence in which Freud is held, because his opinions are contradicted by his followers. It is of some interest to look at the record. In the first place, Freud denied that psychoanalysis was primarily concerned with relieving suffering or curing disease; he commented that its function was to replace "neurotic misery" by "human unhappiness." Secondly, he denied that he himself participated in the medical point of view; he says in 1927,[2] "After forty-one years of medical activity, my self-knowledge tells me that I have never really been a doctor in the proper sense." About psychoanalysis, he says, ". . . I have assumed as axiomatic something that is still violently disputed. . . . that psychoanalysis is not a specialized branch of medicine. I cannot see how it is possible to dispute this." And, in describing what a psychoanalyst appears to him to be, he says, ". . . these words, 'a secular spiritual guide,' might well serve as a general formula for describing the function which the analyst, whether he is a doctor or a layman, has to perform in his relation to the public."

In this same paper, on the other hand, Freud also underlines some facts which are still prominently true, to the effect that many of the prominent practitioners in this field are of medical origin, and that a medical training is a good beginning for the psychotherapist. It would appear, therefore, that psychotherapy appeals to tendencies found in persons who choose medical training; but it might also appear that perhaps it is most appealing to those who do not find in medicine as more traditionally defined the kinds of satisfactions they seek.

The newer developing interest in research in psychotherapy follows a medical tradition in that it tends toward a separation of the practitioner from the investigator, and also in that the investigator has tended to collaborate with persons trained in specialized and more basic areas of the scientific field. Modern medicine in general tends to regard the practitioner as a skillful person, as an artisan or even perhaps an artist, but to assign the investigative role to someone having (at least for the time being) a commitment of a different sort.

A consistent trend in medical investigation has been that of joining forces with workers in the physical sciences. The novel implication of modern psychiatry is the collaboration in investigation with persons trained in the social sciences. With this association the opportunity is available to look at psychotherapy as one of many possible types of institutionalized human relationship, and to seek to understand it further by using other such relationships as models or analogies.

With the broader outlook implicit in this new approach, it becomes possible to look at problems of psychotherapy with a less rigid "set." When, as in the older medical tradition, we look for the appropriate "prescription," we limit ourselves; but when we begin primarily to try to understand, unexpected potentialities and resemblances offer themselves on every hand.

We may now examine the implications of the idea that psychotherapy as a "dyadic," institutionalized, human relationship can be construed in many different ways, and that in every different method of construing, the goals and techniques are relevant to the "model" used. A different model requires a different approach, and, as in other forms of human dyads, there appear to be a large number of ways of arriving at mutually satisfactory (or unsatisfactory) solutions. What appears to me the most interesting of the implications of this way of looking at the problem is that in psychotherapy we have a simplified human relationship allowing intensive investigation.[3] By the intensive examination of many pairs of participants it becomes possible to examine the permutations of human relatedness in a relatively small field.

Some of the possible analogies may be briefly reviewed. Practical psychotherapy is an art, analogous to other artistic procedures, perhaps most specifically to the *drama,* placing it thus in a category emphasizing the feeling content of the experience. But it has also been suggested that psychotherapy can be seen as a *game,* in the modern sense of game theory, a classification which emphasizes the development of skills. Structured human relationships can be grouped as *roles* in a socio-logical sense, and there are many who emphasize that the principal task of psychotherapy is that of socializing or "adjusting" deviant human beings. In still a different setting, it is apparent that psychotherapy involves learning, and learning theorists have also claimed it as in their area of interest. An even more limited version would emphasize that psychotherapy has the principal intellectual function of the derivation of a *self-concept,* and that therefore it can most importantly be seen in a cognitive context; to my own particular predisposition, the psycho-logical system of Piaget[4] has much to say about this aspect of the procedure.

This partial list may indicate that psychotherapy is seen by various observers as almost as complex as human life itself; for this reason it appears of some importance to attempt to clarify in at least a superficial way some of these various attitudes toward the procedure and to point out how the implicit ("unconscious") model held by the therapist governs both his procedures and goals.

ALTERNATIVE MODELS

Cure

The commonest model employed by medical psychotherapists is that psychotherapy is a medical procedure, directed toward the resolution of disease. In this model the goal is apparent, as in the case of other medical procedures: it is to "cure" the patient, or, if it is decided that cure is impossible for any reason, so to help the patient as to relieve distress or to restore a disturbed physiological balance.

Spiritual Guidance

In Freud's own model, that of the psychoanalyst as a "secular spiritual guide," he suggests the resemblance of the function of the psychotherapist and the religious counsellor. In the famous *Varieties of Religious Experience,* William James[5] explored in detail the reports of many persons who underwent a dramatic conversion experience. In most of these reports, there are evidences that the conversion of a sinner is regularly attended by a dramatic relief in various symptoms. In discussing these reports, James spoke of a "schism in the soul" which was repaired or healed by the acceptance of a different view of the world.

Adjustment

Many writers have emphasized that psychotherapy resembles acculturation. The idea of "adjustment" implies fitting oneself into a group which offers to the newcomer certain differences in rules and values from those held prior to his entry into the group. In human life the newborn must accommodate himself to the family group, and after the first five or six years of life, to the peer group and the authority system which he encounters in school. Psychotherapy is often seen as a way of compensating for an inadequate group learning experience in early life. The task of the "novice" is to learn the role assigned to him by the group and to play it in a way which is consistent with the occupancy of the same role by other members of the group.

Drama

In an alternative description using the same term and somewhat the same idea, we can see the psychotherapeutic session as a drama, in which the patient has to learn to play the role of the patient and the therapist that of the therapist. Many of the curious and "abnormal" attitudes demonstrated by a psychotherapist become much easier to understand when we think of him as forbidden to "be himself," just as an actor is forbidden to be himself. Instead he has to learn to play a role, with the specific purpose of helping the patient to learn to play the reciprocal role. In this model, the importance of the didactic analysis in the training of the psychotherapist becomes much clearer; it would be absurd to suggest, in the medical model, that every surgeon undergo the operations which he proposes to carry out upon his patients. When the problem is formulated in terms of the social group or the drama model, the goal is again quite clear, by definition: the patient finishes psychotherapy when he has learned well enough to take his proper role. If one sees acculturation as a human drama, it is implied that learning a role is a part of learning the whole "play"; therefore, if one learns a role well, he learns by implication at the same time the role of the partner. Hanns Sachs once said that the end of an analysis was the point at which the patient realized there was no end, meaning in general that the patient has to take the responsibility of self-analysis after the termination of the formal analysis. Here the patient ends the formal procedure by taking both roles and applying the therapeutic techniques to himself, as an experienced actor can sometimes succeed in being both the leading actor and the director in the same play.

Game

In relatively recent years, the idea has been suggested that psychotherapy can be seen as a very complex "game" played by two participants over a long period of time. The goal is implicit in this definition: the patient has to learn the rules of the game in order to play it successfully, and if he is to be maximally successful, he must attempt, by applying the rules he has learned, to get the better of his therapist. When the therapist admits that he can teach the patient no more, and when the patient begins to demonstrate that in certain crucial areas in the situation he has learned how to best the therapist, it can be considered that the training has finished. It is a curious paradox in this model, and widely in life, that the novice must learn early in his training to put up with consistent losing during the training period; if he insists upon winning too soon, before the whole game is appreciated by him, he may lose in the long run.

The "game" idea has something to offer about the over-all strategy of the patient's life in determining certain of his decisions. In game theory, one type of strategy is called "minimax" since the effort is to minimize loss while maximizing gain. In persons with emotional disorders, one sees a distorted version of this strategy. The psychoneurotic patient often is so much oriented toward minimizing losses that he never risks enough (money, or effort, or "libido") to make it at all likely that he will gain anything. On the other hand, in compulsive gamblers, it can often be found that the gambler will risk much more than he can afford in the vain hope of maximizing his gain. Thus, at both ends of the distribution, there is a distortion: the timid psychoneurotic patient plays a "minimin," and the gambler a "maximax" game. In the psycho-therapeutic situation, one often attempts to help the patient learn that if he is to benefit from a relationship, he must "invest" as much of himself as he can afford to lose, but no more: the young lover must not be faint-hearted, but on the other hand, it is pointless to continue to try to wrest approval from a parent who has not given it for twenty years. In the therapeutic situation, it is important that the patient make a valiant effort to solve his problem, but it is vital that he not continue year after year in a relationship which is not yielding the desired results.

IDENTITY

Another central idea, principally developed by Erikson[8] in recent years, has been that psychotherapy has to do with the formation of an identity, with the answer to the question, "Who am I?" This line of inquiry derives from one of the earliest of sociological studies, that of Durkheim.[6] In his book on suicide, Durkheim paid attention to the problem of *anomie*, of "namelessness," as a factor predisposing to suicide.

Problems of identity formation are especially characteristic of ado-lescents, moving from childhood onto the broader field of experience of adult life. If we use the model of identity-seeking, again we find the goal of psychotherapy built into the definition; it is the finding or the estab-lishment of an identity, upon whatever terms the subject finds possible.

This formulation allows us to see the problem of psychotherapy in two importantly different contexts. First, any available role allows one to participate in human experience, and, by virtue of this participation, to avoid the painful experience of anomie. The psychotherapist in a supportive relationship often offers to the patient the opportunity of participation in a way offered by no other person in the patient's field. At the opposite extreme, training in psychotherapy may also offer the possibility of learning a view of the self so abstract and durable as to allow one a considerable amount of independence from the necessity of immediate participation. The human being who has adequately learned to "conserve" the self can tolerate alienation from others without developing the manifestations of anomie.

MODES OF ACTION

In this list we find that just as the goal is implicit in the model, so to a considerable extent are the procedures. Using the medical model, the therapist tends to understand himself as oriented toward *helping*, toward the relief of symptoms. In general, the medical model implies the use of active agents which the therapist can prescribe to a patient who has the primary responsibility of taking the medicine prescribed on the schedule outlined by the doctor. The activity of the psychiatrist prescribing tranquilizing agents fits the model precisely. However, most psychotherapists, medical or otherwise, emphasize the importance of the active participation of the patient in the process, with "motivation for therapy" occupying a very prominent place in the list of characteristics of the desirable patient. In a modern development in medicine, that of the specialty of rehabilitation, the procedures of the rehabilitationist much more closely approximate those of the psychotherapist in this regard; but the rehabilitationist to a much greater extent that other physicians takes for granted the impossibility of "cure." He deals in situations in which the emphasis by and large is upon *compensation* rather than final cure.

"Spiritual Influences"

"Spiritual guidance" can be discussed both from the standpoint of the religious and that of the secular spiritual guide. In the religious context, the guidance involved is explicitly toward the acceptance of a certain religious system. In this model, the emphasis in the procedure is clearly upon *persuasion* as the principal operation of the guide or therapist.[7] He seeks to convince the prospective member of the group; Christ invited his fisherman disciples to come be "fishers of men." The motivation of the spiritual guide in this version is usually that of a deeply held conviction that his way is the only way to salvation.

In Freud's comments about the function of the analyst as a "secular spiritual guide," he carefully differentiates "analysis" as a special category; he says,[2] "We [analysts] do not seek to bring [the patient] relief by receiving him into the catholic, protestant, or socialist community. We seek rather to enrich him from his own internal sources. . . ." In this kind of statement, Freud demonstrates the egocentricity of the enthusiast; many an evangelist has said essentially the same thing, denying that the goal was that of an "adjustment" to a group and asserting that it is the goal of "finding the truth" or "being illuminated" or freed. Many modern authorities would feel that the burden of proof is upon anyone who differentiates his own system from the effect which he sees other systems as utilizing; certainly it would be almost impossible to find a more passionately devoted in-group than the Freudian analysts.

Cultural

When the central model employed is that of acculturation into a social group, then the goal is clearly that of adjustment. The activity of the therapist in such a situation involves a thorough participation by him in the values of the culture, with his activity emphasizing the importance of the values consensually held; he is to a considerable extent the spokesman of the culture, and the outcome of the therapeutic process will be measurable in terms of how closely the patient emerges the "creature of the culture." This kind of formulation is likely to arouse protest from psychotherapists who pride themselves upon "liberating" patients from constraints, including cultural ones; but the whole emphasis upon "adjustment" implies the acceptance of consensual values and modes of behavior.

The emphasis in an "identity" model is upon the development of a sense of historical continuity in the life history of the individual, and upon the definition of the self in terms of one's own background and experience, with a tendency toward the minimization of the influence of random factors upon future decisions. In this model, the goal of psychotherapy would seem to be that of having the patient understand current problems not only in relation to the demands of the moment but also in terms of his whole previous experience with problems in the same category, with a realistic assessment of his assets and liabilities in relation to the immediate problem. Such a goal might be formulated the other way around by saying that the attempt is to help the patient be less a "function of the immediate situation," or, in still another way, less "other-directed" in relation to the immediately present others.

CONSERVATION

When we speak of the establishment of an identity, we use terms the character of which implies a value judgment; it is obviously better to have an identity than not to have one. But it would appear that, given the appropriate kind of social system, many people get along very well without the kind of western democratic egalitarian identity of which Erikson speaks. In many cultures, the possession of such an identity would probably be a severe embarrassment. In avoiding some of these implications, it is of interest to look at some possibilities offered by Piaget in his use of the term "conservation" to refer to one of the principal intellectual goals of the western world, and to apply the term to the specific problem of the "conservation of the self." This use of the term, "conservation" is analogous to that of the use in physics, i.e., in "conservation of matter" or "conservation of energy." He is concerned with the manner in which children come to be able to see the same basic material in very different forms.

According to Piaget, in interpretation of some very imaginative experiments, children learn sequentially to "conserve" different aspects of objects during the period of preadolescence. At about the age of 7 or 8, they learn that a given amount of plasticine remains the same despite changes in shape; around 10 or 11 they learn that the weight of a given amount of substance remains the same despite differences in shape, and at about 12 or 13 they learn that a given volume remains constant in different vessels. In all of these developments we find the same trend: that of learning to look for the "object" in different contexts. A somewhat similar line of investigation has been pursued by Witkin[9] in his "embedded figures" test, where the subject is given the task of finding in a confusing total picture a form identical to that of a simple figure. In linguistic terms, this process is similar to that of discovering denotative identity in different connotational settings.

In these studies Piaget deals with inanimate objects, and the development takes the child up to the threshold of adolescence. Throughout the period of adolescence, the human being is predominantly concerned with the problem of the conservation of other human beings and of the self. That is, in this stressful period, the human being must learn his own specific sexual identity in actual relationship with members of the opposite sex, and he also must begin to learn how to take care of himself outside the shelter of the family. In both instances, the problems are similar in form to the specifically cognitive problems of dealing with inanimate objects (although very much different in context and in intensity).

In this view the objectification of the self becomes a problem in the same series as the objectification of other objects; the differences become primarily quantitative and methodological. The self is always more various than any other "object" because one has such a variety of data about it; and, on the other hand, the methods of learning to depend upon one's own self-concept have to be quite different from methods of dealing with others because the distance receptors (sight and hearing) by means of which we apprehend others are never immediately applicable to self-observation.

Self-Examination

Since the self cannot be investigated by the primary sensory devices through which we objectify others, the method of objectification has to be through the technique of a *vicarious* examination. One has to examine oneself by proxy, through the eyes and ears of another. We have to learn to objectify the self through the sampling of the other's reaction. Two historically important trends in the Western world can be seen in the earlier history of this development. First, the idea of the self as a unit has obvious relations to the Judaic tradition of monotheism, and second, the emphasis placed upon a direct and personal relation to the deity in the protestant reformation finds a lineal descendant in the technique of intimate personal self-examination in the psychotherapeutic situation. These two influences appear to have a good deal to do with an understanding of the fact that psychotherapy in the analytic sense, of Jewish origin, has found its principal place of influence in those countries in which the influence of ascetic (i.e., Calvinistic) protestant-ism has been most pronounced. The technique in general is one of individualizing (i.e., objectifying) oneself through a prolonged and intimate relation in which one participates vicariously with another whose distance from the self remains remote throughout.

In societies in which the degree of possible diversity is small, or in those in which the roles available to the developing youth of the culture are rigidly and strictly defined and enforced, there is very little oppor-tunity for the person to be much concerned with the problem of "individuation" or conservation. He remains, we would assume with many kinds of gratifications, a "creature of the culture" or a "function of the situation." It is only when the tolerance of the social system is very greatly increased through the possession of material excess, and where a premium is placed upon successful "differentness" that we can find much evidence of a preoccupation with individuating oneself. Even during the period of time in which the Catholic Church dominated all western civilization, the emphasis was upon the "imitation of Christ," the merging of oneself into the deity, and the loss of individuality. The rigid stamping out of dissidence and deviance remains to this day a central part of monastic life.

Particularly in the United States, we find that the adolescent has to learn how he can be the "same individual" as a student in class, a competitor in sports, a lover in an automobile, a member of a youth group in church, a member of a fraternity, and so on. Each of these different roles calls upon quite different aspects of his being, and his task is to learn how he can be so many people and at the same time always be the same one. Where as a young infant he was preoccupied in part with the problem of how his mother could at times be so loving and at others so stern and punishing, in adolescence he has to deal with a similar diversity of roles in which he finds himself performing various activities. Many of these roles often appear to an adolescent quite incompatible with the "instructions" implicitly and explicitly given to him by parents, teachers, and other authorities; but no one other than himself can finally come to the point of making the essential decisions and instituting the behavioral sequences which he learns to see as characterizing himself and no other person in just this way.

TRANSFERENCE

Techniques utilizing one or another form of analysis of the transference make it possible for the patient in psychotherapy to see, first the therapist, and then reciprocally himself, as occupying a number of roles. The psychotherapeutic situation remains ambiguous enough for the patient to allow himself to participate in it in many different ways, just as a child can play many different games to amuse himself over a period of time. In each such event, the therapist insists upon having the patient express his feelings and thoughts about the therapist. In Piaget's term, this amounts to an exaggerated "centering" of the therapist in the field. With repetition, the feeling of astonishment tends to wear off, and the patient comes to be able to see that he is, for instance, angry with the therapist, or unreasonably affectionate toward him, in a way which resembles a previous occurrence of the same sort. As the events come to be strung together in a series, the patient can see himself increasingly as the agent responsible for the series, and as this happens, his self-awareness comes to take the place of the other-awareness immediately apparent in transference manifestations. Through the successive centering and decentering of the therapist, the patient comes reciprocally to understand his own participation. It is paradoxically necessary for the patient to have the capacity to over-react to an aspect of the therapist when it first appears if he is eventually to be able to integrate this apparently novel event into a series. Shakow[10] has pointed to the inability of schizophrenic patients first to develop high arousal (or centering, in Piaget's term) in a new situation and second to demonstrate reduced arousal (decentering) as the situation becomes familiar; this dual difficulty correlates well with the well-known resistance to transference analysis.

In the psychotherapeutic situation, as the various manifestations of the "transference" appear, the patient finds himself from time to time, frightened, angry, affectionate, grateful, and outraged; in each of these attitudes he is likely first to understand the situation as being attributable to the therapist, who therefore appears remarkably different from one period to another. In the process of first participating in the intense emotional experience of the transference relationship, and then subsequently (after a period of "working through") detaching himself from the situation, in company with the therapist, and looking back upon it by means of interpretation, the patient tends to improve his capacity to understand the therapist, and then (reciprocally) himself, as an "object," existing in an abstract space-time continuum very different from the moment to moment present. He sees the two participants as identified both in terms of a hierarchical position in the social system, and in terms of a past history and future aspirations. This process deals with *conservation of the self*. The *self* can be differentiated from the immediately present surroundings, in a manner which in principle is similar to that in which a given *volume* of liquid can finally be understood to be the "same" no matter what its immediately present dimensions happen to be.

The notion of the "conservation of the self" in the use of the term conservation according to Piaget, has an interesting corollary in some of the problems observable in actors. The actor has the problem of putting himself temporarily in the role of the character he is portraying. To do this requires that he perform actions foreign to himself as a member of his family, for instance. The beginning actor finds it a problem to put himself into an embarrassing situation without himself being embarrassed; he must come to be able to dissociate himself from his own situation in order to put himself thoroughly into the role. If therefore, the actor has too structured a demand on himself as to his own public behavior, he will find it difficult to be convincing to the audience. On the other hand, there is the reciprocal difficulty that certain persons only feel content when playing somebody else, (e.g., the "as-if" character described by Helene Deutsch). Such a person's own sense of identity may be so incomplete that he relieves his chronic anxiety by taking the part of somebody else.

RESOLUTION

In applying this general line of argument to the process of psychotherapy, there are two points at which crucial developments take place. First, there is the initial decision as to whether to undertake psychotherapy or not. Here the ability of the patient to enter into an as-if system in which he is to play the role of "himself," speaking lines fed to him by his "unconscious," is an essential element in the initial stages. But at the other end of the procedure, the opposite trend is essential, that is, that the patient must eventually come to the decision that the procedure has gone on long enough, that he has learned enough to get along without the preceptor, and that the time has come for him to decide for himself what roles he will and will not play. When the patient can immerse himself in the psychotherapeutic situation for an intensive experience, then dissociate himself from it at a point of diminishing returns, he is likely to have a useful and helpful experience. If he cannot join in the common enterprise, he is a poor or "unsuitable" patient; on the other hand, if he cannot eventually come to the decision that he has had it, he is likely to be a candidate for an "interminable analysis," chronically subject to dislocation abandoned by the therapist.

REFERENCES

1. SZASZ, T. S.: The Myth of Mental Illness. N. Y., Harper and Bros., 1961.
2. FREUD, S.: Postscript to a Discussion on Lay Analysis (1927). Coll. Papers Vol. V. London, Hogarth Press, 1956, pp. 205-214.
3. SHANDS, H. C.: Thinking and Psychotherapy. Cambridge, Harvard Univ. Press, 1960.
4. PIAGET, J.: The Psychology of Intelligence. N. Y., Harcourt, 1950.
5. JAMES, W.: Varieties of Religious Experience; A Study in Human Nature. N. Y., Longmanns Green, 1941.
6. DURKHEIM, E.: Suicide; A Study in Sociology. Glencoe Free Press, 1951.
7. FRANK, J. D.: Persuasion and Healing; A Comparative Study of Psychotherapy. Baltimore, Johns Hopkins Press, 1961.
8. ERIKSON, E. H.: Childhood and Society. N. Y., W. W. Norton and Co., 1950.
9. WITKIN, H. A., DYKE, R., FATERSON, H., GOODENOUGH, D., AND KARP, S.: Psychological Differentiation; Studies in Development. N. Y., John Wiley & Sons, 1962.
10. SHAKOW, D.: Segmental set. Arch. Gen. Psychiat., 6: 1-7, 1962.

Research in Psychotherapy

by ALBERT E. SCHEFLEN, M.D.*

A RICH FOUNDATION of theory for psychotherapy has been laid down
in the last seventy years and more recently the practice of
psychotherapy has been extended to the treatment of depression, psychoses, groups and families. However, systematic research has lagged far
behind theory and clinical application. We have an extensive literature
on therapeutic techniques and intrapsychic phenomenology; but other
dimensions of psychotherapy have hardly been explored. We do not even
have an agreed-upon definition of psychotherapy. Some say psychotherapy is what the therapist does; some say it is a series of personality
changes in the patient; others see psychotherapy as an interaction. We
have not systematically examined the position of psychotherapy in relation to larger social systems nor have we compared it with other social
institutions. Many of our terms are ill defined, for example, movement,
support, resistance. We do not know how the various events in psychotherapy are organized. It remains a matter of debate whether there is
one basic method of psychotherapy with variations in application or
whether there are multiple basic methods.

Some believe that these problems will be settled by more research.
This cliche is hard to refute, but how useful research will be will depend
upon what questions are asked and how adequate the methods are of
arriving at an answer. Currently, there are two general approaches to
research in psychotherapy. These are: (1) participant-observation, followed by the recall of incidents and the forming of abstractions and
generalizations, viz., the clinical method, and (2) the isolation of pre-
selected variables and their statistical treatment, viz., the so-called
"American experimental method."

The clinical approach has several limitations. The clinician, trained in

*This research has been sponsored by the Eastern Pennsylvania Psychiatric
Institute and aided by a grant from the Benjamin Rosenthal Foundation awarded
to the Institute for the Study of Psychotherapy at the Temple University Medical Center.

the method, has learned certain hypotheses and constructs which he takes for granted. In fact, these theories have tended to become reified and dogmatized. His approach to them is limited by certain a *priori* convictions and his viewpoint is of necessity focused upon "practical" issues, such as technique or improvement. In addition, his emotional involvement and the limitations of memory, make it difficult for him to record the incredible complexity of human interaction while he is busily engaged in managing a session.

The use of film recording and third-party observation do not necessarily obviate these limitations. If observers are trained psychotherapists they also have *a priori* convictions; if they are not, ignorance and negative biases may be added to the project. Film recording aids in remembering data but is of no additional value if the data are not utilized systematically.

Much of current formal research in psychotherapy has consisted merely of fragmenting highly organized events and counting the artifically dissected elements. What are counted are usually *a priori* constructs which are treated as if they were anatomic structures. Despite the fact that the American experimental approach has such high status that naive researchers consider it *the* method of science, the method is quite inadequate to deal with intact systems that have a high degree of interaction or interdependency.

However serious these objections to current methods are, they are not the only limitations of current research in psychotherapy. George Gaylord Simpson[1] has stated that the study of any phenomenon requires the answer to *four* questions about it: (1) what is it?, (2) how is it made up?, (3) what is it for?, and (4) how did it come about? By and large, formal research in psychotherapy has been preoccupied with components and mechanisms, i.e., Simpson's Question 2.

Study of the nature of psychotherapy requires a much broader approach or a wider series of research questions than has customarily been asked. We* have modified Simpson's list and recommend that the following four questions constitute the scope of research in psychotherapy:

(1) What field is being examined?
(2) How are the behaviors organized level by level?
(3) What is the "meaning" of a unit?
(4) What changes occur in psychotherapy as it is examined through time?

The purpose of this chapter is to discuss the question "What is

---

*This "we" is not editorial. Dr. Ray L. Birdwhistell and the author have jointly developed these ideas; thus, the pronoun "we" is used when reference is made to concepts of this joint research.

psychotherapy?" in terms of these four subquestions. The reader can see that this series of questions cannot be answered merely by the isolation of variables, although such a procedure plays an essential role in answering Question 2. Clinical observation is also essential but it must be systematized, enlarged in scope, and disciplined. In other words, current methods are not incorrect but they *are* incomplete.

The four questions will be explained by a device—an analogy to the game of baseball. We shall try not to carry the analogy far enough to get into the usual difficulties of such explanation. Baseball is chosen for two reasons: most of us know the structure of baseball; and discussion of the game in this context is not so ladened with affect as to interfere with cognition of the points.

Psychiatric theory is indebted to the distinction made by the Menninger Group[2] between outcome research and process research. In this report we will be concerned with research into psychotherapy structure and processes. The greatest space will be devoted to Question 1, because our basic ideas, prerequisite to understanding the other questions, are explained in this section.

QUESTION 1

WHAT FIELD IS BEING EXAMINED?

A field is a configuration of events. We do not know in advance if it constitutes a naturalistic unit or entity. The delineation of the field appropriate for a given research requires consideration of four concepts: *configuration, level, frame of reference,* and *completeness.*

Configuration

The field should represent a naturalistic, rather than an arbitrary, unit. It may be difficult to know in advance what unit is naturalistic, as boundaries of a unit may become clear only when the research is well advanced, and any popular or *a priori* notion of the naturalistic unit may prove to be mythological on examination. For example, our research indicates that in one psychotherapy session (which is customarily considered to be one unit) there is often a pattern of interaction about twenty minutes in duration, which is then repeated before the session is terminated. In other words, there are often two, not one, major naturalistic units per session.

Researchers commonly isolate certain configurations that are clearly arbitrary and not naturalistic. Some of these that are currently popular are: (1) events occurring in five minutes of a psychotherapy session;[3-4]

(2) one modality of communication, i.e., speech-ignoring, body movement, touch, and other modalities; and (3) one type of statement taken out of context, i.e., the interpretation. When it is not known what configurations belong to a unified whole or system, it is preferable to examine an excessively large field and work out the units by experimentation rather than to bisect a field and try to make sense of incomplete fragments. The rule is that the inclusiveness of a unit must be determined by its nature not by the convenience of the researcher or by using traditional *a priori* constructs.

Examine this theoretical point about a field in relation to baseball. We know that there is a unit called a half-inning in baseball that consists of three outs. If we were to believe erroneously that two outs or four outs made up a unit we would not be able to explain retirement of a side or make any sense out of the changeover from offense to defense. The unit, three outs, is the natural unit at this level for baseball. The origin of popular isolates (arbitrary fields) is partly a matter of tradition. In psychotherapy, certain early constructs have been clinically useful and have become popular and doctrinal. These are not necessarily useful as naturalistic units for research.

For any given field there is likely to be an actual configuration and a mythical configuration. These may not be the same. Experience indicates that members of a social institution, like a hospital procedure or psychotherapy, view the nature of their institution quite differently than an outsider would. In a mental hospital certain procedures that reduce the costs or otherwise serve the convenience of the hospital are interpreted as being in the service of the patient.[5] For example, the use of a patient to carry messages or rake leaves is called industrial therapy. These belief systems are not simply useless rationalizations but come to be believed in by the members and then assume important functions such as maintaining staff morale or aiding patient adaptation.

The disparity between what observers report and what therapists and patients believe about psychotherapy has been discussed elsewhere.[6] The researcher, then, may be confronted with multiple configurations depending upon who defines the field. Because of the adherence of members of an institution to belief systems and because of the important social function, unconscious pressure will be exerted to define the field so as to select those data which sustains the mythology.*

---

*This "pressure" is also felt at other points in the process of research, e.g.: (1) the kinds of design for which money is granted; (2) selectivity of behaviors, revealed and concealed; or (3) public acceptance of the results.

Level

The idea of level is often used in psychiatry, but it is not always recognized that phenomena fall into clearcut hierarchies of levels. Construction of these hierarchies follows clearcut rules. In this usage levels are not equivalent to "layer" as in concepts of levels of consciousness. Any phenomenon consists of constituents, each of which, in turn, consist of constituents, and so forth as we proceed "downward" in a hierarchy. We can also think of an "upward" progression in which constituents are organized into more complex units, which, in turn, are organized into still more complex units, and so on. Any phenomenon, then, is simultaneously a unit in itself at one level and a component of a larger unit (at the level above).

For example, two, of the many possible hierarchies of baseball units, might be as follows:

Baseball
League
Team
Infield
Second baseman

Such a hierarchy for psychotherapy is conceivable:

Unit	Example
Social systems for dealing with deviancy	
Psychotherapy as an institution	Psychotherapy
A school of psychotherapy	Psychoanalysis
A course of psychotherapy	A psychoanalysis
A phase of psychotherapy	Development of transference
A strategy	Impersonality
A tactic	Withholding answers

Such levels are called levels of methodology or *abstraction*. Complexity increases as we ascend upward, so the more complex units are said to be at a "higher" level.[7] Each higher level consists of an abstraction which covers the combinations of the units at the level below.

Some hierarchies do not represent abstractions but have come into being through evolution. Such levels are called levels of *organization*.[1,8,9] The hierarchy is schematized as follows:

Social levels
Organismic level

Organic
Cellular
Molecular
Atomic

A choice of level is a necessary decision in selecting a field for investigation. It is legitimate science to choose any level for research, but we must not confuse parts with wholes, i.e., mix levels. Our goal must be to ascertain and state the levels at which we are working, and to select the lens or measure appropriate to this level of events. The failure to do this mistake has seriously confused research in psychotherapy. At present, psychotherapy is likely to mean any of the following: (1) a relation or interaction of participants; (2) what the therapist does (techniques); or (3) the changes of intrapsychic processes within the patient. These different fields of study are not at the same level. Techniques, for example, are a component of therapists' behaviors, which are a component of a psychotherapy.

Any of these levels are valuable to investigate, but a principle cannot be violated. We must not ignore organization and assume that the level above is merely a *collection* of components from below. This tendency, called reductionism,[10] is widespread in research. One example of reductionism in research in psychotherapy is an operational definition stating that psychotherapy is that which psychotherapists do. Actually, psychotherapy is an organization of behavior* of therapists and patients.

Let us examine reductionism in the baseball analogy. There are 27 x 2 outs in a regulation baseball game. Yet one game does not consist only of 27 x 2 outs. It consists of a particular *organization* of 27 x 2 outs. Every three outs the team at bat is changed. It does not take 27 outs to retire a side, because the baserunners are eliminated after every three outs. Analogously, we do not assume that a course of psychotherapy consists of some total of interpretations, tactics, or insights.

We cannot learn the nature of a total unit at any level by studying some other level. Since complexity increases "upward", the study of parts does not enable us to comprehend wholes. We cannot know about the liver as a whole by studying the hepatic cell, or about the double play from a study of the second baseman alone or about the course of psychotherapy from analysis of a session. By the same token, the study of water (an organization of hydrogen and oxygen) does not tell us about the hydrogen atom. The study of symbiosis does not tell us about one person in an interaction.

---

*The word behavior in this paper is used in the general sense that is used in science, i.e., the observable activities of any system. It does not mean solely complex motor acts.

Frame of Reference

The natural configuration of a unit will be the same regardless of what we select to study, but we can define the same field in various ways, i.e., according to various frames of reference. In psychotherapy research, the observable data constitute human behavior. We can proceed from observations of behavior in four ways. Two of these have already been described, namely: (1) to study the relations of the behavior to other behaviors and determine the unit to which they belong (at a given level),[7] and (2) analyze the components of the behavior at the level below. We can also reconstruct the sequence of behaviors that forms a pattern through time. Finally, as is characteristic in psychiatry and psychology we can make inferences about the intrapsychic processes associated with the behavior.

These possibilities can be seen in 3 dimensions as diagrammed:

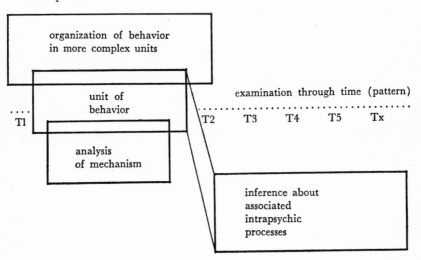

For example, we can take an out in baseball and study its relations to other outs and to getting on base in a larger unit, the half-inning. We can analyze the out as consisting of strikes, ground balls, flies, etc. We can study the sequences of outs in innings and games. Finally, we can, by interview or other means, make inferences about a player's morale, thoughts, motivations and so on, or value judgments about his skill, personality, cooperativeness and the like. Any or all of these are legitimate approaches but they must not be confused or mixed. For example, the intrapsychic processes of any one ballplayer are irrelevant to the *structure* of baseball or to the social function of baseball. The game is similar no matter who plays shortstop.

Intrapsychic phenomenology and variation in techniques belong to a level below questions of rules, ethics, and structure of psychotherapy. Intrapsychic concepts belong to one or another frames of reference within this individual level, e.g., mental economics, psychodynamics, self-concept and identity, affects and so on.

Completeness

All behaviors that occur in the field chosen must be recorded and taken into account. We cannot preselect our observations within a field if we are to have complete data, so that we can organize it meaningfully.

Consider an example in our hypothetical research in baseball. We are studying the activity of the pitcher in baseball. We are told that a good pitcher uses his head and has a good fast ball and a good curve. So we decide *a priori* to record only actions that involve the pitcher's head and his throwing arm. Our data sheet includes scratching of the head, squinting, talking to the catcher, grimacing and throwing. Try organizing this list. Some items refer to being a pitcher and some to being a human being, and some items essential to pitching are excluded.

Absurd, you may say—but this arbitrary selection is not different in kind from nearly universal practices which have traditionally been used in studies of psychotherapy, e.g., using only transcripts of what was said. Most psychotherapy research has been based upon the psychotherapist's description of what he says during the session. This method unwittingly omits body motion, paralanguage and any other behavior of which the therapist is not conscious. Much of what the psychotherapist has learned in training has been implicit, probably by identification. Too, the therapist has a belief system, as described earlier, which may obscure his total behavior. And, most important, much of human interaction has yet to be conceptualized and given language.

The selection of observations according to beliefs about what is important or what is conscious can lead to misapprehension of a field. One well-known clinical example is the belief that we do not communicate with a patient when we do not speak or when we are out of his line of sight. Actually, analysis of motion picture films shows that literally thousands of cues are exchanged in a session through paralanguage, body noise, and movement which we know to be communicational in our culture and which can be shown to affect the patient's behavior. By recording only lexical data from a session, this illusion can be maintained "experimentally."

But, it may be contended, it is perfectly legitimate science to isolate variables. Of course it is. But this isolation then gives us units at the level below and shatters the gestalt of the level we started with (see Question 2). Let us propose several rules of thumb about making observations in a field. Record *all* the data. Do not decide in advance what is relevant (unless you wish to work only with some component of the level below).[12,13] Look upon the unit, not in isolation, but in the context of the hierarchical levels of the gestalt.

QUESTION 2

How Are the Behaviors Organized Level by Level?

Listing the Behavior

Suppose we record every observable behavior in a second baseman. We will have a long and quite disorganized list of such items as: catches ball, runs to right, lowers glove, scratches nose, takes off cap, leaves field, thumps glove, makes sign of the cross, and advertises razor blades. We can develop a similar list for a psychotherapist. We may record these items: bends forward, speaks, asks questions, answers telephone, scratches head, writes notes, and so on.

How can these behaviors be organized? Which behaviors are necessary to playing second base? Which are idiosyncratic for one player? Which are traditional to ball playing even if not necessary by rule? Which relate to the fact that he is a poor fielder or an Irish Catholic? In a psychotherapist which behaviors are necessary for therapy? Which are nontherapeutic or antitherapeutic? Which belong to his culture, his tactics, his doctrine or to some unique personality characteristic?

Determining Contexts of Behaviors

There is a systematic and reliable way in Context Analysis[12] to determine the position of each item, if one understands the principle of levels. Each item is examined in each context in which it occurs. If such actions as bending over, lowering glove, catching ball and throwing to first base all necessarily belong together in the context, "one out," and do not appear (in this configuration) in any other context, then these items belong to an organization at the next higher level which we already know to be called "fields ground ball." Similarly, this organization, combined with catches fly ball, covering second base, tagging runner and so forth, are organized into a more complex unit called "playing second base." The organization, playing second base, when combined with similar ones carried out by three other players, constitutes an organization called "the infield."

"Scratching nose," however, belongs to another context. We can observe it off the field or on the field. We can observe it in all ball-players and in non-ballplayers. What it means we do not know, but it is not a *necessary* part of the organization, "ballplaying," unless of course, it is some part of special signal. The sign of the cross, we might discover, is found in religious contexts and occurs only in second basemen who are Catholic. By this procedure we can determine the context and the organization to which each behavior belongs. In this way we can organize the elements level by level.

This is precisely what we have been doing in our film analysis of psychotherapy in the communicational frame of reference. The task is exacting and tedious. It took eighteen months to complete the first session analyzed, but our efficiency increases and once the units are known they are readily identifiable and do not have to be retested for each session or psychotherapy.

We know a great deal about the lowest levels of communication in psychotherapy because they have been worked out for English speech by the structural linguists[14,15] and for body motion in Americans by Birdwhistell.[12,16] These lower levels are patterned for all members of a culture, but little appears at these levels that is characteristic for psycho-therapy. We know much less about units more complex than syntactic sentences and gestures. At the next level, which combines several syntactic sentences, kinesic complexes, and postural units,[13] certain elements characteristic for psychotherapy begin to appear; tactics, resistances and other clinical concepts can be interpreted as appearing. Strupp's[17] categories of therapists' lexical behaviors seem to be at this level. At this level, too, are found striking immobility (the dampening or absence of movements that are culturally characteristic) on the part of therapists. Presumably, these actions are inhibited.

At higher levels there is in a session a characteristic progression of postures on the parts of therapists which do not appear in any other situations we have observed. In these more complex organizations we expect we will find techniques like encouraging rapport or insight. But we have not yet determined what the naturalistic units for communica-tional systems are at these higher levels.

Defining a Unit

The principle of organizing elements when we do not know to what units they belong is as follows: that configuration (and only that configuration) that is a necessary occurrence to maintaining the structure at the level above constitutes one naturalistic unit. For example, all of those behaviors and only those which inevitably lead to a batter's retiring constitute the unit "one out." (There can, of course, be sub-units related to it: ground out, strike out, fly out, etc.) By this method we are working toward the experimental demonstration of such supposed units as "achieving an insight" or "establishing rapport."

We must constantly remind ourselves that a unit at the higher level is an *organization* of a specific type, not just a set, or group, or collection of behaviors. If the specificity and completeness are lacking, the unit does not have the communicational or social significance that defines it. It is not perceived as a gestalt, not reacted to, not recognized. It does not, therefore, "function" in the system. For example, the occurrence of a strike in baseball is indicated by a specific gesture on the part of the plate umpire. In order to convey the meaning "Strike!" all the essential muscular components of the gesture must be performed or there is ambiguity, which can result in major disruption, as any baseball fan or umpire can tell you—a "rhubarb." Analogously, in psychotherapy, the failure of a therapist to complete a definition of the rules of doctor-patient relationship may lead to ambiguities which can foster consider-able acting-out.

QUESTION 3

WHAT IS THE "MEANING" OF A UNIT?

When we organized the behaviors level by level, our preliminary delineation of a field was replaced by an experimentally defined field, or unit. We can now deal with a very difficult and usually nebulous concept, meaning. The meaning of any unit is its uniqueness, i.e., how it differs from any other unit (at the same level) *and* its reference,[18] i.e., its function in, or its effect upon, the larger units to which it belongs. For example, the meaning of second baseman behavior is that it is not first baseman behavior, and that it functions in a pivotal way in an infield. Interpretation, assuming that it is effective, may some day be specifically defined in terms of (a) its difference from forms like com-pliment, insult and confrontation, and (b) the change it produces in communicational patterns in which the patient is subsequently involved.

Suppose our unit is as inclusive as baseball or psychotherapy as a whole. What are the "meanings" of such units? Baseball is not football and not basketball, but it appears in a unique set of contexts, which belong to the class, sports. Psychotherapy apparently contrasts with academic teaching, military indoctrination, parent-child rearing, and penal correction. These tentative social units appear to belong to an organization that we might tentatively call—using the term very broadly —institutions for correcting and preventing deviancy. The meaning of psychotherapy, then, lies in its difference from other institutions and its function in the social system.

Question 4

What Changes Occur in Psychotherapy?

Just as units can be observed as organized in cross-sections of structure, so they can be seen as events in sequence through time. A relation of events is a phase, a collection of phases a larger stage, and so on. Psychotherapy appears to consist of an organization of occurrences which appear stage by stage.

Just as a baseball game is not a succession of 27 x 2 outs, but occurs inning by inning (in stages), so clinical experience indicates that a course of psychotherapy consists of stages. A course may not be the completion of so many sessions, but a progression of different relationships. An organization of insights or trials or expressions of support might make up one stage, which may require completion before a new set of behaviors can be meaningfully introduced. The model for such an idea would look like a staircase with each rise representing a parameter.

A systematic study of change requires the careful plotting of pattern step by step. Patterns of behavior in psychotherapy prove to be highly stereotyped and repetitive.[19] This regularity makes it easy to recognize change in an accurately plotted pattern, provided the pattern has been followed long enough to know its natural cycling. In practice, this is difficult since one oscillation or phase can last for months or even years. This, in practice, is the difficulty of studying change. A patient who has mood swings from depression to mania may remain in one phase for months, and the beginnings of euphoria may be mistaken for new maturation. By careful recording of pattern, however, it is possible accurately to identify parameters and shifts. In our film material, this has been done quite lucidly. It will be through this method that strategies of psychotherapy and the evaluation of their efficacy can ultimately be investigated with rigor.

Change must be examined level by level, however, for the different orders of change occur in the psychotherapy relationship than those which are seen in the individual behavior of the participants. Thus, we may have to plot events synchronically for psychotherapy: for one school of psychotherapy, for representative courses, for given sessions in the relationship, for each participant, and so on.

There is a history of the institution of psychotherapy about which we know little. We assume some evolution from primitive shaman-patient to doctor-patient to psychotherapist-patient relations. There has been evolution in psychoanalysis, and so on. Any single course, or therapist, or patient also has a history. So, in smaller units of time, does an interpretation, or a rejection, or even a scowl.

Our results indicate that psychotherapeutic tactics are programmed; i.e., they are introduced in an orderly step-by-step progression in accordance with set intervals of time or given changes in patient behavior. The beginnings of a generic definition of psychotherapy can be made: psychotherapy is a *programmed institutionalized interaction:*

As a whole, it is a social level phenomenon. Individual behaviors are components at lower levels. Psychotherapy itself is an interaction, an organization of relationships with established form and steps. A given therapist or patient merely enter into an ongoing social structure. They do not create or invent it.

REFERENCES

1. SIMPSON, G. G.: The status of the study of organisms. In: Am. Scientist, March, 1962.
2. MENNINGER, K.: Theory of Psychoanalytic Technique. New York, Basic Books, 1958.
3. PITTENGER, R. E.; HOCKETT, C. F., AND DANEHY, J. J.: The First Five Minutes. Ithaca, N.Y., Paul Martineau, 1960.
4. GOTTSCHALK, L. A. (Ed): Comparative Psycholinguistic Analysis of Two Psychotherapeutic Interviews. New York, Intern. Univ. Press, 1961.
5. SCHEFLEN, A. E.: A Psychotherapy of Schizophrenia: A Study of Direct Analysis. Springfield, Ill., Charles C Thomas, 1960.
6. FEIBLEMAN, J. K.: Theory of integrative levels. Brit. J. Phil. Sc., 5:59, 1954.
7. BERTALANFFY, L. V.: Problems of Life. New York, Harper Bros., 1960.
8. ——: An outline of general systems theory. Brit. J. Phil. Sc., 1:134, 1950.
9. ENGLISH, H. B. AND ENGLISH, A. C.: A Comprehensive Dictionary of Psychological and Psychoanalytic Terms. New York, Longmans, Green and Co., 1958, p. 529.
10. GOFFMAN, E.: Asylums. New York, Doubleday, 1961.
11. MAHLER, M.: On child psychosis and schizophrenia. In: Psychoanalytic Study of the Child, vol. VII, New York, Intern. Univ. Press, 1952, p. 286.
12. BATESON, G., BIRDWHISTELL, R. L., BROSIN, H., FROMM-REICHMAN, F., HOCKETT, C., AND McQUOWN, N. A. In McQuown (Ed.): Natural History of an Interview (in press).
13. SCHEFLEN, A. E., ENGLISH, O. S., HAMPE, W. W., AND AUERBACH, A.: An Analysis of a Psychotherapy: Whitaker and Malone (to be published).
14. GLEASON, H. A.: An Introduction to Descriptive Linguistics. New York, Holt, Rinehart, and Wiston, 1955.

15. HOCKETT, C. F.: A Course in Modern Linguistics. New York, MacMillan, 1958.
16. BIRDWHISTELL, R. L.: Introduction to Kinesics. Louisville, Ky., Univ. of Louisville Press, 1952.
17. STRUPP, H. H.: A multi-dimensional system for analyzing psychotherapeutic techniques. Psychiatry, 20:293, 1957.
18. BIRDWHISTELL, R. L.: An approach to communication. In: Family Process, Vol. 1, 2, Sept. 1962.
19. SCHEFLEN, A. E.: Communication and regulation in psychotherapy. Psychiatry (in press).

PART II

TECHNIQUES OF PSYCHOTHERAPY

Free-Operant Conditioning and Psychotherapy[1]

by OGDEN R. LINDSLEY, PH.D.[2,3]

I N OPERANT CONDITIONING the frequency of a response is altered by locating and arranging suitable consequences (reinforcement). This conditioning of responses by altering their consequences is contrasted with Pavlovian conditioning, in which responses are conditioned by arranging their antecedents.[4] If an organism being conditioned is at all

[1]The research was supported by grants MH-977 and MY-2778 from the National Institute of Mental Health, Public Health Service.

[2]The assistance of Jack R. Ewalt, M.D., and Elvin V. Semrad, M.D., of the Mass. Mental Health Center in interpreting the results of the psychotherapeutic evaluation is gratefully acknowledged. The patient contact program of the student nurse therapists was directed by Teresa J. Mouid, R.N., M.S., Boston College School of Nursing, and included classes given by Fr. William P. Sullivan, Metropolitan State Hospital. Therapy described in detail in this paper was conducted by Thomas Housenecht, M.D., Mass. Mental Health Center, and Marion Donahue, R.N.

[3]The cooperation of the staff and patients of Metropolitan State Hospital, Waltham, Mass., (William F. McLaughlin, M.D., Superintendent) is gratefully acknowledged. Appreciation is extended to Sol Sherman, M.D., Chief Psychiatrist, who arranged that somatic therapies would not confound our psychotherapeutic evaluations.

[4]If both controlling antecedents and controlling consequences were located for the same response, then the response could be both classically and operantly conditioned. Therefore, we see that the type of conditioning is a controlling procedure, rather than an iron-clad characteristic of the response. Theoreticians would be happier if nature's categories and man's methods did not overlap, but in most cases they do overlap. The natural scientist realistically accepts these overlaps and often uses them to his advantage for independent measurement.

times free to emit the response and to receive the arranged consequence, and if more than one response can occur within a given experimental session, then we use the term *free-operant conditioning*. The adjective *free* separates this form of conditioning from controlled-operant conditioning, in which only one response can be emitted per trial.

Free-operant conditioning provides *a method of experimentally analyzing behavior in the laboratory*. By isolating an individual within an appropriate enclosure, all variables which affect the behavior under study are experimentally rather than statistically controlled. The behavioral response and any environmental manipulations whose effects on the response are being studied are automatically and continuously recorded. This environmental control and automatic continuous recording qualify the method as a laboratory natural science, comparable to chemistry, physics, and biology.

The topography of the response is usually kept as simple as possible (e.g., pressing a small lever) in order to minimize peripheral effector variables and permit more exact study of general behavioral processes. The functional meaning of the response is primarily determined by the nature of its experimental consequence, or reinforcement. Usually only a small portion of the responses is reinforced (intermittent schedules of reinforcement) in order to generate a high frequency of responding without satiation and to study discriminations demanded by particular patterns of reinforcement (Ferster and Skinner, 1957). Rate of response emission is of primary interest and is continuously recorded as the slope of a cumulative response record. Since the method is sensitive to subtle changes in an individual's rate of responding, it is especially useful for longitudinal studies of single organisms.

Rapid development and wide application of the method of free-operant conditioning has opened up to scientific control and laboratory investigation the type of behavior which was once considered "voluntary." The discovery that such behavior is subject to control by its consequences makes it unnecessary to explain the behavior in terms of hypothetical antecedents. Although antecedents may eventually be found and objectively measured, it seems more profitable at this time directly to manipulate and analyze behavior in terms of its consequences.

Free-operant methods are especially appropriate to the problems of psychotherapy, because both fields (1) emphasize behavioral modification and control, (2) deal with single individuals, (3) use frequency of response over a period of time as a datum, (4) concentrate on the consequences of behavior, and (5) are interested in the functional and dynamic relationships between individuals and their social and non-social environments.

A sensitive and appropriate method, free-operant principles and techniques may provide psychotherapy with: (1) a fresh theoretical background, (2) refinements of current therapeutic practices, (3) new therapeutic methods, (4) independent evaluations of therapeutic effects, and (5) direct experimental analyses of therapeutic processes. Several recent exploratory experiments support these suggested areas of application. The particular studies which will be mentioned merely indicate the kind of research that has been done. They should not be considered a summary of research to date.

A Fresh Theoretical Background

Free-operant conditioning principles can provide a fresh, exciting, and highly relevant theoretical background for the practice of office, group, and ward psychotherapy. Time-worn habitual practices can be re-evaluated and revised as information is reshuffled according to the new descriptive nomenclature. For such an application it is not necessary to purchase complicated controlling and reinforcing apparatus. Although information derived from carefully controlled experiments has higher scientific credulity than information derived from the application of principles, new descriptive and theoretical approaches can lead to important advances.

Ayllon and Michael (1959), for example, had marked success in training ward nurses to make the behavior of their psychotic patients more socially acceptable. Entering the nurses' office, talking psychotically, and sitting or lying on the floor were disturbing responses which were successfully extinguished by the nurses' use of free-operant principles. By dropping food on patients' clothing while feeding them, the nurses were able to generate self-feeding in patients who previously had to be spoon-fed. This mild punishment for spoon-feeding, accompanied by the positive reinforcement of self-feeding and the nurses' talking to the patients while they fed themselves, successfully conditioned the patients to feed themselves.

Refinement of Current Therapeutic Practices

Rado (1962) has recently stressed the need for determining the truly important aspects of current psychoanalytic practices. Free-operant experimental methods appear to be useful for this purpose. Slack (1960), for example, conducted an experiment to determine the importance of the therapist's presence during therapeutic sessions. Neurotic patients spoke into a microphone while alone in a small chamber. Patients never saw the therapist but were told that he would listen to tape recordings of their talk. The patients were reinforced for talking by being given points on a counter placed in front of them during the sessions. Regardless of speech content, high rates of talking were reinforced with high scores. At the end of each session scores were converted to money. Therapeutic results suggested strongly that patients developed insight and worked out their problems as rapidly as they would have in non-directive office counseling.

New Therapeutic Methods

Free-operant conditioning techniques promise to provide therapists with methods of directly manipulating the behavior of patients in controlled laboratory settings. These methods involve placing the patient alone in a controlled experimental environment with a suitable operandum which automatically records the behavior being manipulated. Suitable reinforcing events are automatically presented to the patient as a consequence for appropriate responding. Conditioning sessions are usually held each week-day for at least one hour.

Strengthening Normal Responses

If pulling a small plunger competes with a major symptom of a chronic psychotic, intermittently presented reinforcement (candy or cigarettes) for plunger-pulling increases the rate of plunger-pulling to within the normal range in 25 hours of conditioning (Lindsley, 1956, 1960). The rate of symptom display decreases and does not return even during subsequent extinction (non-reinforcement) of plunger-pulling. Symptom display outside of the experimental environment is also reduced.

Attempts at direct reinforcement of psychotic symptoms themselves have not been successful. This observation suggests that a *psychotic symptom* can be objectively and functionally defined as a frequently occurring response not currently under the control of its immediate environmental consequences.

As a patient is slowly conditioned, it is possible to increase the therapeutic value of experimental environments by successively approximating more complex situations. Gradual addition of interpersonal factors should maximize therapeutic potential (Lindsley, 1954). King, Armitage, and Tilton (1960), for example, have recently shown that 30-minute sessions of operant-interpersonal therapy given three times a week have a greater therapeutic effect than verbal and recreational control therapies. Initially, with the therapist present, patients made simple operant responses for candy, cigarettes, and presentations of colored slides as reinforcers. Increasingly complex manual and verbal tasks were incorporated in accordance with the patients' therapeutic progress. At maximum complexity, the method required verbal communication and cooperation between two patients together in an experimental room.

Brady and Lind (1961) reinforced a patient, who had been hysterically blind for over two years, with points on a counter for correct responses to the presence of a light. The points were exchanged for canteen coupons after each session. Gradually the patient began to respond only when the light was on. This reconditioned sight transferred to extra-experimental situations, with the patient regaining his sight.

Decreasing Rate of Symptoms

Flanagan, Goldiamond, and Azrin (1958) successfully reduced the rate of stuttering in stutterers by making a 1-second blast of loud noise contingent upon the stuttering. They were also able to increase rate of stuttering by making termination of the noise contingent upon stuttering. Barrett (1962) was able to reduce the rate of multiple tics in a neurological patient by allowing the patient to hear pleasant music of his own choice while he did not tic and making brief periods of silence contingent upon ticing.

EVALUATION OF THERAPEUTIC EFFECTS

There is a great need for an objective laboratory technique to evaluate independently the effects of various therapeutic treatments. Individual differences in type and severity of mental illness and in degree and direction of therapeutic response are so great that techniques which demand grouping data from different patients are unsuitable. Furthermore, many patients show high day-to-day and hour-to-hour variability in degree of behavioral deviation. The practical impossibility of controlling important variables such as personal interaction on the wards and home visits makes evaluation of therapy even more difficult.

Free-operant methods may provide psychiatry with an objective evaluative device. With further modification and higher clinical relevance, these methods promise to provide sensitive differential measurement of the effects of single therapeutic sessions.

Experiments conducted in our laboratory have shown that even the simplest free-operant design (pulling a single plunger for intermittent candy reinforcement) is sensitive to the effects of psycho-active drugs, insulin and electro-shock coma, and psychotherapy on the rate of response of individual psychotic patients (Lindsley, 1960). Figure 1 shows the effect of psychotherapy sessions on the rate of response of an inactive chronic schizophrenic. This patient had previously participated in 659 experimental sessions, during which he usually made less than 10 responses per hour, except for eight spontaneous improvement phases lasting two to four weeks. During these improved periods, the rate of response rose as high as 1,500 responses per hour. Including the experimental sessions shown in Figure 1, this experimental baseline covers six calendar years with a few brief experimental interruptions.

Therapy sessions, conducted by a student nurse three times a week, began at the first arrow. At the second arrow the patient stopped swearing at the nurse during therapy. At the third arrow the nurse, who had become quite involved with the patient, became very emotional and directive. She told the patient that he would not get well unless he stopped listening to his voices and paid attention to her. As the nurse began to cry, the patient also began to cry, for the first time in six years. In the experimental session immediately following this therapy session, the rate of response climbed to 350 responses per hour. In the second session after this, the rate increased to 750 responses per hour, and in the third session to 2,450 responses per hour. Responding was maintained at this high rate, which is well within the "normal" range, even on the two days each week that the nurse did not see the patient. During this time, the patient did not hallucinate on the wards or hospital grounds.

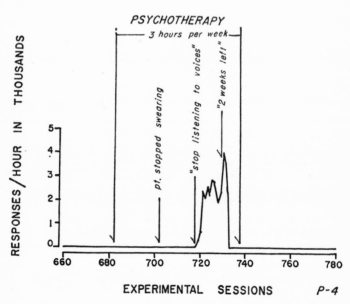

Fig. 1. Effect of psychotherapy sessions on free-operant response rate of a chronic schizophrenic.

At the fourth arrow, the nurse informed the patient that her affiliation with the hospital would be over in two weeks. Immediately after this notice of termination, the patient's rate of response jumped to almost 4,000 responses per hour. This responsing peak appears to be an objective measure of the "flight into health" often described by experienced therapists. Within two experimental sessions, however, the rate fell to zero as the patient again "withdrew into his psychosis." On the 734th session the nurse took the patient to Boston for a day's outing, with no therapeutic effect. The nurse saw the patient for the last time at the fifth arrow.

Attempts to reproduce this psychotherapeutic effect using student-nurse therapists have succeeded with only one of four patients. Since three months of student-nurse therapy is not notably effective and since chronic psychosis is so resistant to therapy, the method was modified to increase its sensitivity to therapeutic relationships. After seeing their patients three times a week for 10 weeks, student-nurses went into the experimental rooms with their patients during an experimental session. There were two experimental conditions, one in which the nurse told her patient she would keep him company and simply sat with him for 15 minutes, and another in which the nurse requested her patient to get her some candy or gum. In addition, there were two 15-minute control periods with the patient alone in the experimental room. Table 1 shows the number of responses emitted by patients during each of these four 15-minute periods. Note that all four patients showed significantly increased rates of responding when answering the requests of their nurse-therapists.

TABLE 1.—*Effect of Therapist's Presence on Free-Operant Responding of Chronic Schizophrenics for Candy and Cigarette Reinforcement*

| Patient No. | No. of Responses in Successive 15-Min. Periods of One Experimental Session | | | |
	Patient Alone	Therapist's Company	Patient Alone	Therapist's Requests
P-4	0	4	0	14
P-5	1	0	0	15
P-6	0	0	0	11
P-60	0	0	0	714

Since student nurses are a relatively homogeneous group, nurses who had no previous contact with the patients were used as control subjects. Table 2 contains the number of responses emitted by patients in the company of these strange student nurses and the number of responses emitted in answer to the strangers' requests. It appears that when they served merely as company, neither significantly affected the patients' rates of responsing, but that when they requested reinforcers, therapists produced much higher rates of responding than strangers. This difference suggests that a slight therapeutic relationship can be developed even under these limited conditions and that its effect can be measured with free-operant methods.

TABLE 2.—*Effect of Stranger's Presence on Free-Operant Responding of Chronic Schizophrenics for Candy and Cigarette Reinforcement*

	No. of Responses in Successive 15-Min. Periods of One Experimental Session			
Patient No.	Patient Alone	Stranger's Company	Patient Alone	Stranger's Requests
P-4	0	10	0	8
P-5	0	0	0	4
P-6	0	0	0	0
P-60	0	0	0	0

DIRECT EXPERIMENTAL ANALYSIS OF THERAPEUTIC PROCESS

Perhaps the most exciting application of free-operant methods to psychotherapy would be the direct measurement of the viewing and listening responses of patient and therapist during psychotherapy. Direct measurement of leadership in cooperation and competition has been previously accomplished and demonstrates the utility of the free-operant for analysis of social behavior (Cohen, 1962; Lindsley, 1961).

With a patient in one small room and a therapist in another, the degree and direction of visual and auditory communication could be controlled by using closed-circuit television. The patient would have two switches in front of him. A rapid rate of pressing one switch would bring the therapist into view on a closed-circuit television screen in front of the patient. A rapid rate of pressing the other would increase the intensity of the therapist's voice, heard over a speaker in the patient's room. The immediate reinforcing effects of the therapist's movements and speech would be indicated by variations in the patient's rates of pressing the viewing and listening switches. These two rates of responding would be separately but simultaneously recorded in another room on cumulative response recorders.

Fluctuations in rates of responding would indicate subtle changes in communication and the degree of transference within therapeutic sessions.

Correlation of rate variations with the verbal content of communication between patient and therapist would reveal and test many of the dynamics supposedly involved in the therapeutic process.

In a more complex experimental design, the therapist could have two switches parallel with the patient's switches. If a patient failed to operate either switch, permitting the therapist to revert to visual and auditory oblivion, the therapist could lend support by pressing his own switches to present himself visually and auditorily to his patient.[5] Since all responses by both patients and therapist would be simultaneously recorded, the interplay of these operations could be manipulated or experimentally analyzed.

Other refinements and variations of the method may permit analysis of even more subtle effects. For example, the importance of the content of the therapist's speech could be tested by breaking the connection between the therapist's microphone and the patient's speaker. The therapist could have two switches, one to light a sign in the patient's room saying "yes" and another to light a sign saying "wonderful." The therapist could use these signs to reinforce specific behavior in his patient. The effects of such contentless reinforcement could be compared with therapeutic effects of full speech. The effect of catharsis could be determined by having the patient respond to produce movies or tape recordings of his arguments with his spouse or of arguments between couples with similar problems.

CONCLUSION

Exploratory experiments have shown that free-operant principles and methods have wide application in social and clinical behavioral research. The method shows promise in the analysis of psychotherapy behavior and process.

At this time, further refinements and applications appear to be limited only by the originality of the investigator and the behavioral accuracy with which the clinical problems are interpreted. When clinical relevance is wedded to methodological refinement, the magic of the word may be strengthened by the power of the number.

---

[5] "Support" appears to be used in another, quite different way by therapists. Not only does it mean fairly direct positive reinforcement of socially appropriate responses by the patient, but also it means letting the patient emote without consequent punishment, in ways that are socially disapproved. In other words, some therapists use the word "support" to describe the provision of a non-punishing audience.

REFERENCES

AYLLON, T., AND MICHAEL, J.: The psychiatric nurse as a behavioral engineer. J. Exper. Anal. Behav., 2:323-334, 1959.

BARRETT, B. H.: Reduction in rate of multiple tics by free operant conditioning methods. J. Nerv. Ment. Dis., 135:187-195, 1962.

BRADY, J. P., AND LIND, D. L.: Experimental analysis of hysterical blindness. Arch. Gen. Psychiat., 4:331-339, 1961.

COHEN, D. J.: Justin and his peers: An experimental analysis of a child's social world. Child Develpm., 33:697-717, 1962.

FERSTER, C. B., AND SKINNER, B. F.: Schedules of Reinforcement, New York, Appleton-Century-Crofts, 1957.

FLANAGAN, B., GOLDIAMOND, I., AND AZRIN, N.: Operant stuttering: The control of stuttering behavior through response-contingent consequences. J. Exper. Anal. Behav., 1:173-177, 1958.

KING, G. F., ARMITAGE, S. G., AND TILTON, J. R.: A therapeutic approach to schizophrenics of extreme pathology: An operant-interpersonal approach. J. Abnorm. Soc. Psychol., 61: 276-286, 1960.

LINDSLEY, O. R.: Discussant for B. F. Skinner, A new method for the experimental analysis of the behavior of psychotic patients. J. Nerv. Ment. Dis., 120: 403-406, 1954.

——: Operant conditioning methods applied to research in chronic schizophrenia. Psychiat. Res. Rep., 5: 118-139, 1956.

——: Characteristics of the behavior of chronic psychotics as revealed by free-operant conditioning methods. Dis. Nerv. Sys., monogr. suppl., 21:66-78, 1960.

——: Experimental analysis of cooperation and competition. Paper read at Eastern Psychol. Assn., Philadelphia, April 1961.

RADO, S.: Towards the construction of an organized foundation for clinical psychiatry. In P. H. Hoch & J. Zubin (Eds.) The Future of Psychiatry. New York, Grune & Stratton, 1962, pp. 116-126.

SLACK, C. W.: The automatic interview machine: A system for reinforcing verbal behavior in the absence of an interviewer. Mimeographed Rep., Harvard Center for Research in Personality, 1960.

The Confrontation Technique

by H. H. GARNER, M.D.

REQUESTS FOR INTERVENTION

ACTIVE INTERVENTION is requested by patients for all manner of problems. Patients who feel a need to control the therapist and look upon his interventions for them as evidence of their ability to regulate the relationship will constantly try to manipulate the therapist into activity on their behalf. Certainly a very large number of any therapist's patients seek to have the therapist instruct, command, forbid, inform, show methods, give advice, etc., e.g., "What should I do?"

Basic activities in psychotherapy have been categorized by Bibring,[1] Wolberg,[2] and others in attempts to delineate the elements present in the communication process of psychotherapy. The therapist's verbal and explicit expressions usually are found to fall within the following descriptions of verbal interventions.

(1) Asking questions is an activity which is almost always permissible. Questions, when used within reason, are usually acceptable and create many effects in the therapeutic situation. For instance, they can give the feeling that the therapist is participating in the relationship. They can be seen as intended to improve evaluation of the patient's difficulty (diagnosis) or encourage the process of uncovering to further the work of psychotherapy, e.g., "Why?" "For instance?"

(2) Reassurance—To placate and pacify. Statements may be directed at elevation of the patient's sense of importance and significance. Individuals unable to mobilize from their own self-appraisal a feeling of worth, significance, adequacy, lovability, goodness, and desirability may seek an outside source for replenishing such feelings. Statements or questions may be so designed as to elevate the patient's feeling of self-esteem.

Some therapists may respond by almost always, if not always, reassuring the patient. Others may create a prerequisite to the patient's expectations by declaring that if he does what is required of him, he will get well. The implication is, "Tell me everything, and after three months or longer you will be well." In psychoanalytic therapy such requests ordinarily do not elicit a response and the patient may be treated with silence. The silence here supposedly implies, "Proceed with whatever is uppermost in your mind."

Activity by the therapist to deal with his needs and the patient's for some kind of response can be quite effective without responding to the patient's desire for reassuring statements. The patient may be asked questions which call for further exploration. "Apparently you have some doubts about your health, although you have had repeated examinations, etc. I wonder why you still have such doubts?"

(3) Advice—The concept of the therapist as an educator who directs the patient to engage in activities intended to foster correction of attitudes, behavior and the diversion of interest from self to external life situations was altered by the psychoanalytic concept of no advice giving. Freud[3] warned against the analyst who finds himself in the position of having freed the patient from inhibitions then being tempted to point out new aims. The danger of the physician being responsive to his own wishes rather than the capacities of the patient and the absence of ability to sublimate in many neurotics were noted as reasons.

(4) Suggestion is a particular reaction to a perception which may be exogenous in origin, e.g., the spoken word, or endogenous, secondary to sensations arising from viscera. This reaction is characterized by acceptance of the implication of the perception with assent and without any reflection on its significance. Such a state occurs as a result of feelings being aroused by the perceptions which do not permit of reflection or because of a state of fatigue which prevents good reflective action. In the case of suggestions arising as a result of visceral stimuli, ideas occur in association with the stimuli to which emotional responses are attached.

The significance of suggestion in hypnosis has been related to the basic hysterical defense tendencies of individuals. Hypnosis has been defined as a state of increased suggestibility by Forel[4] and Bernheim.[5] Freud[6] described hypnosis as analogous to falling in love, and Ferenczi[7] stressed the regressive nature of the hypnotic experience in terms of its being an experience in which the patient accepts a child-parent relationship to the therapist. It must not be forgotten that psychotherapeutic relationships have been described in exactly the same terms.

Freud,[8] in the case history of an infantile neurosis indicated that certain past experiences could help explain the patient's difficulty. The completion or reconstruction of these experiences could be accomplished with the help of the therapist. Freud felt that the interpretations which were helpful in bringing about a genetic reconstruction of the past had no significant suggestive importance since they either brought about immediate confirming associations or were rejected by the patient.

Many analysts have pointed to the element of suggestion in the psycho-analytic process. As Fliess[9] indicated, "The analyst is immobile as was the hypnotist while the patient lies on the couch as did the subject, and the analyst acquires, by sitting behind the patient, the hypnotist's invisi-bility after the subject has closed his eyes." It is obvious that the situation intended to produce free association may prove to have suggestive influences as strong as those of the hypnotic situation. The significance of suggestive influences in any interpretation is indicated by Grinker.[10] He says that we have demonstrated in our experiments that the patient-subject interprets almost everything that the psychiatrist says as having therapeutic meaning. There is little possibility that the patient will refute the hypothesis (interpretation) of the therapist.

The adoption of the therapist's values as evidence of suggestive influences in psychotherapy is shown in studies by Rosenthal.[11] The patients who improved were those who adopted the moral values of the therapist. Glad,[12] in studies by himself and others supervised by him, found that persons in a psychotherapy group behave in patterns con-sistent with the particular psychotherapy theory as expressed in the leader's methods.

The fact that words may be expected to have magic effects is allied to the use of suggestion or the fact that patients respond to therapeutic efforts by creating changes in thoughts and behavior as if they were responding to suggestion. Evidence of the acceptance of language as having magical qualities is seen in special prayers, incantations, ritualistic use of words to ward off unfavorable influences, and in adolescent words of special and secret significance. Words, and word patterns have been considered to be very important elements in the therapeutic efforts of many institutions and systems, such as Christian Science, Coue therapy, and the Will therapy of Low. It must be recognized that therapeutic effects supposedly due to insight and working through of intrapsychic conflicts may be a mere verbalization of material accepted by the patient during therapy. The reverbalization of such magic words are accepted by some therapists as a cure and may explain why some patients with seemingly good insight show no real change in their attitudes or behavior.

An interesting aspect of suggestion in psychoanalytic therapy that has been mentioned by some therapists is an unintended negative suggestion in classical psychoanalytic therapy. The emphasis on abnormality, and complexes, and dwelling on the unconscious, i.e., on the reprehensible qualities, and failure to appreciate and respond to the patient's positive qualities produces this sort of negative suggestion.

(5) Clarifying statements may be directed at educating and informing when the patient's lack of information, inadequate knowledge, or false concepts can be altered by additional or corrective information. Such activity has the effect of producing security through a mastery (knowing), while at the same time it tends to create the sense of protection that the patient may need by making him feel that any inadequacies and errors will be tested and help given in correcting them. On the other hand, clarifying statements may be responded to with hostility, the patient implying that the therapist is being critical and directing without reason.

(6) Interpretation, the basic activity in psychoanalytic therapy, was directed at making that which was unconscious conscious. The interpretation was intended to make the patient aware of the repressing forces; the goal was, as Freud[13] saw it, "a return of the repressed." The controversy over what to interpret has often narrowed to whether the interpretation should be of content, transference or resistance. The tendency to make interpretations of resistance or transference exceeds the tendency toward content interpretations. The interpretations may be so ordered as to attempt to follow a kind of peeling process as recommended by Reich[14] or, in some therapy, one may see what is explained as an intuitive response exemplified by Reik.[15]

The tendency to make interpretations prematurely was described by Freud[16] who emphasized the need to wait until repressed material comes to the surface. The therapist frequently makes broadly applicable interpretations with little or no relevance to the problem which is the basis of the patient's struggle at that time; the patient may use blanket interpretations as a means of resisting real understanding. Feldman,[17] in describing examples of such blanket interpretations, re-emphasizes this problem. Making interpretations tentative—"I wonder if"—has been suggested by many therapists. Important for the understanding of the response of a patient to the interpretations made in therapy, is the fact that what we perceive is dependent upon the need to understand that which one wishes to understand. Cantril[18] writes: "What we perceive is, as already emphasized, in a large part our own creation and depends upon the assumptions we bring to the particular occasion. We seem to give meaning and order to sensory impingements in terms of our own needs and purposes, and this process of selection is actively creative."

(7) To Persuade, Command, or Forbid. In psychotherapy of a less intense nature, the periods between visits may be associated with considerable anxiety. To offset the weakening of the relationship between doctor and patient and foster the early development of a transference relationship, it may become necessary to make statements which include evidence of the therapist's personal and intense interest in the patient, control of impulses which the patient feels are beyond his personal capacity for control, and the possibility that his desire for dependent gratification may be fulfilled and protection afforded him. In intensive psychotherapy, the patient may infer the presence of many of the supportive aids which in psychotherapy of a briefer nature are supplied through supportive and controlling statements. It should be quite obvious that the dependency and transference phenomena produced by such activity will require working through, if more than supportive effects are expected from treatment. Cameron[19] uses persuasion in converting passivity into self-assertion; specific interventions are used to convert passivity into normal self-assertion in patients whose constant response to hostility in others is passivity. After a key figure is identified toward whom the passive attitude is most prominent and the manifestations of the attitude are known, the patient is urged to be self-assertive.

The therapist has generally been described as being careful of expressing disapproval. However, where it is evident that the patient is exposing himself to real danger or irreparable harm, the therapist may attempt to use persuasion to discourage him.

(8) Exclamations: "Really," "well," "perhaps," "it could be so," "naturally," are statements used in nearly all psychotherapeutic procedures. Several interesting kinds of activity are mentioned by Dollard and Miller.[20] By noticing certain things and ignoring others, the patient's responses are strengthened. The therapist's attention is a strong reward. "Uhuh" may be used in some sentences and not in others. "Mmmm hmm" may be used similarly. Repeating something which is contradictory to something previously said in a questioning manner, "But you can be more independent now?" can encourage the patient away from dependency.

(9) Cliches are used as part of a basic character tendency or may be used in the treatment situation as a resistance against expressing conscious or unconscious content. Trite phrases which have lost their precise meaning are often accepted and used by the patient. "Such a phrase by becoming stereotyped loses the meaning it once had and becomes employed as resistance." (Stein[21]) The therapist who uses such expressions as "you are resisting" readily produces feelings of lack of acceptability and

a need for compliance or disobedience which may be expressed in many ways, depending on the characteristic pattern of reacting and the transference situation at the time. Cliches used by the therapist create the tendency to substitute ready-made phrases for meaningful expressions.

(10) Passivity is activity. Although favoring almost complete non-intervention in psychotherapy, Menninger[22] feels that the process of treatment is expedited by pointing to the existence or possible existence of connections, the implications of certain verbalizations, and reminding the patient of forgotten experiences. He would point out discrepancies, self-contradiction, a misrepresentation or unrecognized obvious omissions.

One recognizes the explicit verbal activities of the therapist readily; the significance of *non-verbal communications* as potent elements seen by the patient as active interventions whether intended or not by the therapist is less evident (Ruesch,[23] Birdwhitsell[24]). The significance of passivity in the therapy situation of the psychoanalytic model technique has been explored by the author.[25] Permissiveness as a psychotherapeutic concept is likewise related to elements in the psychotherapeutic process which have been generally seen as non-interventions.

Freeman[26] and Finesinger[27] have described the concept of permissiveness as seen by the patient as containing elements of active intervention. Finesinger described two basic attitudes toward permissiveness. To some psychiatrists permissiveness is not a desirable value. As a result of this, we are told, our patients always remain dependent and immature; our treatment never grapples with the patient's defenses. We never intervene to point them out and avoid locking horns with the basic and fundamental problems of the patient. To other psychiatrists, permissiveness is a highly desirable value, and, to them, reflects man's struggle throughout the last thousand years in establishing the primacy of the individual, the development and utilization of personality resources along personal and individualistic lines. The idea of external control is not a therapeutic possibility, but actually repugnant.

Intervention: The what, why, and how of an intervention is best considered by how what the therapist does or does not do is seen by the patient. He may see it as an intervention intended to influence him, a neutral position, or a situation where the therapist is being influenced by him. The significance of interventions, active or passive, verbal or non-verbal, intended or unintended, can also be seen as follows.

a. The intervention repeats the situation of an earlier life experience in which the parent, parent surrogate, or older person is communicating to the child. It therefore suffers from the parataxic distortion (Sullivan[28]) of the transference situation. Rado's[29] description of the hierarchic levels at which the psychotherapeutic process takes place is revelant.

Each intervention, whether intended or accidental, must be understood in relation to the nature of the doctor-patient relationship at the time. This relationship is such that most interventions are seen in the context of therapist as parent and patient as child. Individuals doing so-called uncovering psychotherapy feel that the problem of the transference neurosis is readily dealt with through interpretations intended to disclose the distortions of the patient, bring about insight into the nature of the parataxic distortions with the therapist, and relate the present transference neurosis to a repetition compulsion in that present distortions tend to be repeated frequently in the course of therapy.

b. The intervention represents a relatively neutral exchange between equals, an adult to adult relationship. In psychotherapy, the "hello!" "goodbye!" and some interchange of communication seen by the patient as "just conversation" are included in this category. It may reflect a mature acceptance of the role of student to educator.

c. The intervention may represent an instructive educational effort directed at increasing the breadth, depth and ease with which one person in a two party interchange is enabled to learn and acquire new information. The intervention may be seen as correcting information no longer valid. Where no emotional resistance to the intervention exists, there is relatively little hindrance to the correction. Where motivational factors and effective resistance to correct previously acquired learning exists, the correction will not take place or will take place with considerable resistance to change.

Most interventions in psychotherapy are verbal and, as such, have the generalized abstract significance to the patient of any symbol. "Words, like all other symbols, also have 'meanings' only with reference to their specific connotations for each individual and even these meanings may vary widely not only with the context of the phrase, sentence, paragraph and oration but also with the current circumstances and emotional state of the writer, speaker, reader or hearer." (Masserman[30])

Crucial to all interventions for patient insight, uncovering, giving up of resistance, maturation, etc., is the degree to which the patient sees intervention and reacts to it with uncritical compliance. The significance factor to which improvement can be attributed in patients whether following suggestion, persuasion, seemingly neutral discussion, authoritarian directives, questions or non-verbal communication is the uncritical compliance of the patient. Insofar as parentifying the therapist and compliant attitudes are predominant, the therapeutic interventions closely simulate those seen in hypnosis. When the patient can deal with interventions with critical appraisal he approaches a state of increased maturity and realistic evaluation of his interpersonal relations and his environment. The more such critical appraisal occurs during therapy, the more the patient may be seen as responding to therapy in a manner different from responses made as a result of neurotic patterns, or as a result of the transference neurosis.

The Confrontation Technique: The successful utilization of a confrontation technique in psychiatric treatment was previously described.[31-37] This technique has a problem-solving rather than a permissive or coercive approach. The technique has been utilized in hundreds of patients with diverse psychiatric, medical and surgical problems. The technique of the confrontation treatment is as follows.

Several methods of wording statements are used, followed by the question, "What do you think of what I told you?" For instance, one method is to use an authoritative statement directing the patient to control certain drives, impulses or desires which were creating conflict and anxiety. The statement is then followed by the question, "What do you think about what I told you?" The use of a confrontation by the therapist has value in that it creates a situation wherein the patient feels if his ability to control the undesirable impulse or to function independently is impaired, such control will emanate from sources outside of himself. In headlong flight from reality, controls, and object relations, the patient finds himself confronted by the therapist in such a way that his line of retreat is cut off. If he wishes to evade reality now, he must think about why. But thinking about reasons for evading is secondary process activity. It requires differentiating among reasons, evaluating them and choosing how to behave. The patient's crumbling controls are re-enforced. His anxiety is reduced. He is invited to explore what he is doing with the help and support of someone who has done his part in bridging the communication barrier.

The confrontation technique can be applied with a variety of psychotherapeutic approaches. Its development has been within the framework of uncovering psychotherapy in which interpretations and questions are intended to overcome transference resistance, bring about varying degrees of reconstruction of the past, an understanding of the pathological defenses and an awareness of the personality structure in concepts expressed by terms such as: drives, needs, desires, anxiety, controls, social conventions, superego, conscience, adaptive functions and reality testing. An awareness of the influence of past on present interpersonal relations and their importance for transference phenomena is included. The basic psychotherapy framework in which the technique has evolved might be described as psychoanalytically oriented psychotherapy. When insight is not involved because of the technique used, or the goals for the treatment of the patient are limited, transference interpretations, or dealing with the relationship of past and present, may be totally avoided, the goal being to bring about change in symptoms, rather than to focus on the mental or emotional structure.

Controlling a patient through methods which re-establish the authoritarian parent-child relationship is generally frowned upon, or may be considered, at best a form of supportive psychotherapy. However, it reassures the patient that his own controls will be strengthened further by an external control, and thus helps relieve acute panic states and anxiety. Authoritarian directives intensify transference phenomena and the tendency to repeat a behavior pattern previously executed without question as to its significance. However, the patient is invited to work out a mutually satisfactory solution to conflicts rather than being simply instructed or left to wander alone by the question, "What do you think of what I told you?" The question creates a desire in the patient to test the significance of the controls, and to evaluate these further on a realistic basis. In other words, it fosters reality testing in contradistinction to fostering transference neurosis. The use of the confrontation may also strengthen the patient's favorable feelings of hope for recovery and restoration to health. Since the patient has lost a great deal of faith in his ability to recover, the promise of health through authority increases his capacity to deal with his anxieties to the degree where he can be more realistically aware of the conflicts creating his anxiety. The patient, freed from anxiety, can construct more wholesome and more realistic adaptations. The struggle of impulses seeking expression against internalized controls becomes partially transferred to a conflict between impulses and an external parental figure and leads to an awareness of the attitudes toward such impulses in the general sociocultural milieu of the patient. French[38] suggested that as a guide to therapy, attention should be constantly focused upon the "integrative task," the problem the ego is trying to solve at each particular moment. The use of this technique, which I have called "confrontation" tends to highlight the integrative task for the patient. The statement with which the patient is confronted will vary in the light of his clinical picture and the nature of the relationship at the initial use of the confrontation. The area of conflict selected will vary from case to case. It is determined by the therapist's acuity in ascertaining the area of immediate conflict, whether it be sexual, sibling rivalry, or some other area of conflict. The patient may be confronted with: (1) a prohibitive statement, "You must never, under any circumstances, masturbate!" (2) an expressive or permissive statement, "It would be better if your husband dies!" or (3) an adaptive statement, involving a mature value orientation, "I want you to continue to work at your job." By and large, all of the confrontation statements may be classified in one of these three categories. When one is formulated, it is used continuously, an important advantage.

The essence of all modern psychotherapeutic endeavor is the interpersonal exchange between the patient and the psychiatrist. This means that the medium in which the psychotherapist operates has a complex pattern which includes all the variables and intangibles inherent in each of the two persons and their interactions. Although transference and counter-transference, empathy, and intuition with their various experiential components constitute specific elements in the doctor-patient relationship, they have defied scientific description and evaluation. I agree that our aim is to replace intuition with understanding, and to convert the intuitive truths with which all psychotherapy works into scientific truths, so that they may become public property. Our hypotheses should be able to be used, tested, questioned, probed, and experimented with by anyone interested in science.

REFERENCES

1. BIBRING, E.: Psychoanalysis and dynamic psychotherapies. J. Am. Psychoanalytic A., 2:745-69, 1954.
2. WOLBERG, L. R.: The Technique of Psychotherapy. New York, Grune & Stratton, 1945.
3. FREUD, S.: Recommendations for Physicians on the Psychoanalytic Method of Treatment. Collected Papers, Vol. 2. London, Hogarth Press, 1946.
4. FOREL, A.: Hypnotism: or Suggestion and Psychotherapy. (Trans. H. W. Armit) New York, Rebman, 1907.
5. BERNHEIM, H.: Suggestive Therapeutics. (Trans. C. A. Herter) New York, Putnam, 1900.
6. FREUD, S.: The Dynamics of Transference. Collected Papers, Vol. 2. London, Hogarth Press, 1946.
7. FERENCZI, S.: Suggestion in Psychoanalysis. Further Contributions to the Theory and Technique of Psychoanalysis, Vol. 2. New York, Basic Books, 1952.
8. FREUD, S.: From the History of an Infantile Neurosis. Collected Papers, Vol. 3. London, Hogarth Press, 1946.
9. FLIESS, R.: The hypnotic evasion. Psychoanalyt. Quart., 22:497, 1953.
10. GRINKER, R. R.: A Philosophical Appraisal of Psychoanalysis. Science and Psychoanalysis, Vol. 1: Ed. Jules Masserman. New York, Grune & Stratton, 1958.
11. ROSENTHAL, D.: Changes in some moral values following psychotherapy. J. Consult. Psychol., 19: 431-4, 1955.
12. GLAD, D.: Operational Values in Psychotherapy. New York, Oxford University Press, 1955.
13. FREUD, S.: A General Introduction to Psychoanalysis. (Trans. Joan Rivere) Garden City, Garden City Pub. Co., 1943.
14. REICH, W.: Character Analysis. New York, Orgonne Inst. Press, 1949.
15. REIK, T.: Listening with the Third Ear. New York, Farrar, Straus and Young, 1949.

16. FREUD, S.: "Observations on 'Wild' Psychoanalysis." Collected Papers, Vol. 2. London, Hogarth Press, 1946.
17. FELDMAN, S.: Blanket interpretations. Psychoanalyt. Quart., 28:205-15, 1959.
18. CANTRIL, H.: Perceptions and interpersonal relations. Am. J. Psychiat., 114: 119-26, 1957.
19. CAMERON, E.: The conversion of passivity into normal self-assertion. Am. J. Psychiat., 108:98-102, 1951.
20. DOLLARD, J., AND MILLER, N. E.: Personality and Psychotherapy. New York, McGraw-Hill Book Co., 1950.
21. STEIN, M.: The cliche. J. Am. Psychoanalyt. A., 6:263-77, 1958.
22. MENNINGER, K. A.: Theory of Psychoanalytic Technique. New York, Basic Books, 1958.
23. RUESCH, J., AND KESS, W.: Non-Verbal Communication. Berkeley, University of California Press, 1956.
24. BIRDWHISTELL, R. L.: Contributions of Linguistic Kinetic Studies to the Understanding of Schizophrenia—An Integrated Approach. Ed. A. Auerbach. New York, Ronald Press, 1959.
25. GARNER, H. H.: Passivity and activity in psychotherapy. Arch. Gen. Psychiat., 5:411-417, 1961.
26. FREEMAN, R.: Contaminants of permissiveness in hospital care. Am. J. Psychiat., 110:52-4, 1954.
27. FINESINGER, J. E., AND KELLAM, S. G.: Permissiveness—its definition, usefulness and application in psychotherapy. Am. J. Psychiat., 115:992-6, 1959.
28. SULLIVAN, H. S.: Conceptions of Modern Psychiatry. Washington, D.C., William Alanson White Psychiatric Found., 1947.
29. RADO, S.: Recent Advances in Psychiatric Treatment. Ed. S. Bernard Wortis. A. Res. Nerv. Ment. Dis. Proc., Baltimore, Williams & Wilkins Co., 1953.
30. MASSERMAN, J.: Principles of Dynamic Psychiatry. Philadelphia, W. B. Saunders Co., 1961.
31. GARNER, H. H.: A confrontation technique used in psychotherapy. Am. J. Psychotherapy, 8:18-34, 1959.
32. ——: A nascent somatic delusion treated psychotherapeutically by a confrontation technique. J. Clin. & Exper. Psychopath. & Quart. Rev. Psychiat. & Neurol., 20:135-43, 1959.
33. ——: A Confrontation Technique Used in Psychotherapy, Progress in Psychotherapy. Ed. Jules Masserman and J. L. Moreno. New York, Grune & Stratton, 1960.
34. ——: A confrontation technique used in psychotherapy. Comp. Psychiat., 1:201-11, 1960.
35. ——, AND JEANS, R. F.: Confrontation technique in psychotherapy—some existential implications. J. Exist. Psychiat. To be published.
36. ——, AND WALDMAN, I.: The Confrontation Technique as Used in the Treatment of Adolescent Schizophrenia, Read at Central Neuropsychiatric Society Meeting. Chicago, October, 1961.
37. ——, AND JEANS, R. F.: Treatment of Nascent Schizophrenia by a Confrontation Technique. To be published Proc. World Psychiatry Congress, Toronto, June, 1961.
38. FRENCH, T.: The Integration of Behavior, Vol. 1. Chicago, University of Chicago Press, 1952.

Present Trends in Psychoanalytic Therapy

by SANDOR LORAND, M.D.

URING THE PAST 30 years psychoanalytic rationale about therapy and the technical handling of patients has changed considerably. In 1945 I wrote, "before the 1920's analysis was more of an intellectual process and the emotional content of the transference situation was not analyzed. With preconceived ideas in mind, based on theoretical knowledge, the unconscious was investigated with a view to uncovering what the analyst presupposed to be there. The principles of technique were applied, not as the need arose, or according to the personality and flexibility of the therapist, but in accordance with a basic rule to interpret the unconscious. The technique was at times a hit and miss proposition with little or no elasticity in the application of technical rules."[39]

Freud originally defined psychoanalysis as mainly applicable to "the transference-neuroses, phobias, hysterias, obsessional neuroses, and besides these such abnormalities of character as have been developed instead of these diseases. Everything other than these, such as narcissistic and psychotic conditions is more or less unsuitable."[19] Since then, however, various reformulations and revisions have influenced the therapeutic interest, trends and clinical evaluation in analyses. Our outlook and evaluation of therapy were the direct results of a revised interest in ego psychology. Analysts with wide therapeutic experiences in somewhat different approaches tried out and added innovations, modifications to our therapeutic armamentarium in treating the borderline neuroses, cases with ego weaknesses, perversions, etc. New elaborations of the entire method were added based on clinical findings and experiences and we all make use directly or indirectly of these new technical approaches. But nearly all publications in the field maintained that the basic principles of the technique of psychoanalytic therapy, as initiated by Freud, remain valid today. Having been derived from his clinical experiences, they remain the fundamental guide in analytic therapy, although later elaborated and modified. Much attention is now given to preoedipal stages and the entire problem of early object relationships, with emphasis on their relationship to the therapy of borderline neuroses, perversions, etc. These investigations made it possible to evaluate for therapeutic purposes patients who were considered not amenable for analysis.

Ego psychology also helped us gain deeper insights into the pathology of character neurosis, perversions, moral masochisms and schizophrenic regressions, and added to our better evaluation and therapeutic management of these cases. As Anna Freud wrote, . . . "the investigation of the id and its mode of operation was always only a means to an end and the end was invariably the same correction of abnormalities and the restoration of the ego with its integrity."[16] This followed Freud's earlier statement: "The quantitative factor of instinctual strength in the past opposed the efforts of the patient's ego to defend itself, and now that analysis has been called in to help, that same factor sets a limit to the efficacy of this new attempt. If the instincts are excessively strong the ego fails in its task . . . we shall achieve our therapeutic purpose only when we can give a greater measure of analytic help to the patient's ego."[17] This does not have to be taken as the ego having priority over everything else in analytic therapy, but it emphasizes the reaction of the ego to unconscious processes. All resistances, whether of the ego, superego, or id, are in the center of our therapeutic approach and have to be dealt with equally and constantly.

In the therapeutic relationships we try to strengthen the ego, but the more we can explore the earliest stages of ego development, the more fundamental factors we understand from early object relationship, the better we will be able to help the patient re-experience early frustrations and his patterns of reaction, which are then repeated in the transference relationship.

To establish a transference with patients who, as a result of early disturbances in object relationship acquired in severe neuroses with ego weakness, defects and deep regression, the analyst has to approach therapy with a special attitude. Freud referred to this when he wrote, "The ego has been weakened by the internal conflict; we must come to its aid. The position is like a civil war which can only be decided by the help of an ally from without. The analytical physician and the weakened ego of the patient, basing themselves upon the real external world, are to combine against the enemies, the instinctual demands of the id, and the moral demands of the super-ego. We form a pact with each other. The patient's sick ego promises us the most complete candor, promises, that is, to put at our disposal all of the material which his self-perception provides; we, on the other hand, assure him of the strictest discretion and put at his service our experience in interpreting material that has been influenced by the unconscious. Our knowledge shall compensate for his ignorance and shall give his ego once more mastery over the lost provinces of his mental life. This pact constitutes the analytic situation."[18]

But coming to the aid of the ego implies a number of difficulties. The patient whose object relationship in early childhood were bad, may try to maintain this bad relationship with the analyst. To prepare the groundwork for analytic therapy, the transference has first to be developed by making interpretations to the patient acceptable and well enough tolerated so as not to increase his defences.

How to reduce regression, when to stop it, when to encourage it and to what degree, is a permanent problem during the therapy. In order to undo the harm done to his ego development by his early environment, we must surmount constantly negative therapeutic reactions in the early phases of therapy. In later periods of analysis the patient's transference demands may become so violent that they demand constant attention.

The variety of opinions expressed about the theoretical as well as technical aspects of regression, give it an important place in current psychoanalytic therapy. One has to be more active in order to further the relationship with the patient and sometimes a preanalytical period is necessary to strengthen the patient's ego and help create a transference relationship.

The therapeutic management of such patients necessitates modifications and deviations of the classical psychoanalytic approach. Sometimes devices which would be called not strictly psychoanalytic are used. In furthering therapeutic success we have to change our attitudes to suit the patients' behavior. They are prone to acting out frequently in the analytical situation, which again imposes special difficulties and tolerance on the analyst. In this connection Glover stated: "Even in so-called classical analysis of the psychoneurosis, the approach of different analysts varies not only in numerous points of detail but also in many important points of policy[22] [p. 165. techniques of greater activity were adopted] due, respectively, to unsatisfactory results and to widespread feeling among analysts that analytic therapy must be speeded up."[22] (p. 166.) Glover then reminds us that long before the issue of active treatment became controversial, the technique of psychoanalysis came to include new measures of "active type." One was in the nature of a prohibition, i.e., that analysis should be carried out in a state of abstinence; the other was the positive injunction that certain cases suffering from phobias should at certain times begin to face rather than avoid situations which induce anxiety.

We accept the fact that we cannot analyze all patients the same way, and within the basic framework of established methods we have to alter our therapeutic technique. It is nearly impossible for an entire analysis to be completed without the analyst at some time interfering with the patient's acting out in his social relationship and perhaps business affairs, and also in his pleasure-seeking tendencies. The therapist must manipulate the transference, dose interpretation and help the patient in an extra-analytical way. All this activity is utilized to deal with the patient's resistance and to promote analysis.[47] Again to quote Glover: "It should therefore be our object to reinforce those parts of the ego which are less affected by guilt processes and through which the patient's capacity for positive contact can be increased. The same policy should be followed when encouraging the patient to make decisions regarding his life and work which owing to a feeling of inertia he is unable to make himself."[22] (p. 241.)

Therapy, then, begins with giving some support directly to the patient to help him tolerate and cope with his daily conflicts and current difficulties. We do not attempt reconstruction or interpretation—instead we guide the patient in his everyday contacts. We then may make some inroad and modify the rigidity and resistance of the patient. Thus a transference relationship will slowly be established.

Deviation from regular procedures may be based on the personality and temperament of the analyst and yet achieve a degree of success. But deviation from classical technique should not be based on the analyst's personality and temperament alone if it is to have success in the long run. Obviously it may be connected with and have implications for the analyst's countertransference, but when it is too obviously so, results are invariably bad. What is going on in a given case must be understood apart from personal, subjective feelings on the matter. Active measures always derive out of the analyst's objectivity and understanding, and indicate empathy with his patient. Tactful application of active measures and manipulations of them will put more demands on the analyst's tolerance, elasticity and objectivity. Manipulations arising out of the analyst's countertransference imperfections, will have their effect on the therapy and its results. The post-Freudian expansion of ego psychoanalysis enriched and widened our technique of psychoanalytic therapy and placed strong emphasis not only on technical methods but also on deeper clinical investigations of technical problems in psychoanalysis.

REFERENCES

1. ALEXANDER, F.: Development of the Ego Psychology. Psychoanalysis Today, ed. Sandor Lorand. New York, International Universities Press, 1950.
2. ——: Fundamental of Psychoanalysis. London, Allen and Unwin; New York, W. W. Norton & Co., Inc., 1949.

3. ARLOW, J.: Sublimation: panel report at midwinter meeting 1954. J. Am. Psychoanal. A., 3:515, 1955.

4. BALINT, M.: The final goal of psychoanalytic therapy. Int. J. Psychoanal., 18:206, 1936.

5. ——, FAIRBAIRN, FOULKES, AND SUTHERLAND: Criticism of Fairbairn's generalisation about object relations. Brit. J. Phil. Sc., 7:——, 1957.

6. BRIERLEY, M.: Trends in Psychoanalysis. London, Hogarth Press, 1951.

7. EISSLER, E. R.: Searchlights on Delinquency. New York, Inter. Univer. Press, 1949.

8. FAIRBAIRN, W.: Endopsychic structure considered in terms of object-relationships. Psycho. Quart., 5:541, 1946.

9. ——: Obect-relationships and dynamic structure. Int. J. Psychoanal., 17:30, 1946.

10. FENICHEL, O.: Identification (1926). The Collected Papers of Otto Fenichel, First Series. New York, W, W. Norton & Co., Inc., 1953.

11. FERENCZI, S.: The Further Development of the Active Therapy in Psychoanalysis (1921). Further Contributions to Psychoanalysis. London, Hogarth Press, 1950.

12. ——: Contra-Indications to the 'Active' Psychoanalytical Technique (1926). Further Contributions to Psychoanalysis. London, Hogarth Press, 1950.

13. ——: The Elasticity of Psycho-Analytical Technique (1928). Further Contributions to Psychoanalysis. London, Hogarth Press, 1950.

14. ——: The Future Development of the Active Therapy in Psychoanalysis (1921). Further Contributions to Psychoanalysis. London, Hogarth Press, 1950.

15. —FREUD, A.: Ego and the Mechanisms of Defense. London, Hogarth Press, 1936, p. 4.

16. FREUD, S.: Analysis Terminable and Interminable. Collected Papers V, pp. 331-332.

17. ——: An Outline of Psychoanalysis. Trans. James Strachey. New York, W. W. Norton & Colk, Inc., 1949, pp. 62-63.

18. ——: New Introductory Lectures on Psychoanalysis. New York, W. W. Norton & Co., Inc., 1933, p. 212.

19. GITELSON, M.: On ego distortion. Int. J. Psychoanal. 39:245, 1958.

20. GREENACRE, P.: Problems of infantile neurosis: A discussion. Psycho. Study Child, 9:16-71, 1954.

21. ——: Trauma, Growth and Personality. New York, W. W. Norton and Co., Inc., 1952.

22. GLOVER, E.: The Technique of Psychoanalysis. New York, Inter. Univer. Press, 1955.

23. GUNTRIP, H.: Recent developments in psychoanalytical theory. Brit. J. M. Psychology, 29:82, 1956.

24. ——: Ego weakness and the hard core of the problem of psychotherapy. Brit. J. M. Psychology, 33:163, 1960.

25. HARTMANN, H.: The mutual influences in the development of ego and id. Psychoanal. Study Child, 7:9, 1952.

26. ——, AND HEINZ, AND KRIS: The genetic approach in psychoanalysis. Psychoanal. Study Child, 1:11, 1945.

27. ——, KRIS, AND LOEWENSTEIN: Comments on the formation of psychic structure. Psychoanal. Study Child, 2:11, 1946.

28. HOFFER, W.: Mouth, hand, and ego-integration. Psychoanal. Study Child, 3-4:49, 1949.
29. KATAN, M.: Contribution to the panel on ego distortion (as-if and pseudo as-if). Int. J. Psychoanal, 39:265, 1958.
30. KHAN, M. R.: Dream psychology and the evolution of the psychoanalytic situation. Int. J. Psychoanal., 63:21, 1962.
31. ———: Regression and integration in the analytic setting. Int. J. Psychoanal., 61:130, 1960.
32. KUBIE, L. S.: Problems and Techniques of Psychoanalysis: Validation and Progress. Psychoanalysis as a Science, ed. E. Pumpian-Mindlin. Stanford, Calif., Stanford University Press, 1952.
33. LORAND, S.: Comments on the Correlation of Theory and Technique (1948). Clinical Studies in Psychoanalysis. New York, Inter. Univer. Press, 1950.
34. ———: On regression: technical and theoretical problems. Tokyo J. Psychoanal., 19:2, 1961.
35. ———: (Ed.): Psychoanalysis Today. London, Allen and Unwin; New York, Inter. Univer. Press, 1950.
36. ———: Psychoanalytic therapy of religious devotees. Int. J. Psychoanal., 63: P. 1, 1962.
37. ———: Technique of Psychoanalytic Therapy. New York, Inter. Univer. Press, 1946.
38. PETO, A.: Infant and mother: observations on object relations in early infancy, (1936). Int. J. Psychoanal., 30:260, 1949.
39. SPITZ, R. A.: Relevancy of direct infant observation. Psychoanal. Study Child, 5:66, 1950.
40. STONE, L.: The Psychoanalytic Situation. New York, Int. Univer. Press, 1961.
41. ———: The widening scope of indications for psychoanalysis. J. Am. Psychoanal. A., 2:567, 1954.
42. SZASZ, T. S.: On the theory of psychoanalytic treatment. Int. J. Psychoanal., 38: A., Parts 3-4, p. 166, 1957.
43. WINNICOTT, D. W.: Collected Papers: Through Paediatrics to Psychoanalysis. London, Tavistock Publications; New York, Basic Books, Inc., 1958.
44. ———: The Child and the Family. London, Tavistock Publications; New York, Basic Books, Inc., 1957.

Existential Theory and Therapy

by ROLLO MAY, PH.D.

AND

ADRIAN VAN KAAM, PH.D.

WILLIAM JAMES once said that every new theory goes through three stages. First, it "is attacked as absurd; then it is admitted to be true, but obvious and insignificant; finally it is seen to be so important that its adversaries claim that they themselves discovered it."[1]

Existential psychotherapy certainly went through plenty of the first stage, lasting until about two years ago. It also has survived the second stage. The most recent period seemed marked by the third stage; everyone claimed his school invented it. There were voices which said that existential psychology is Adlerian, others that it was all in Jung, others that it was encompassed in Freud, still others that it was identical with Zen Buddism and anti-intellectual trends on one hand; or with a super-intellectual philosophy composed of untranslatable German terms on the other. It was said to be therapy which everyone does when he is doing good therapy, and also to be—especially in its classical phenomenological wing—a philosophical analysis which has nothing to do with the practice of therapy as such. These spokesmen seemed blithely unaware of their patent contradictions: if existential psychotherapy is one of these things, it cannot be the others.

But more and more the attitude of psychiatrists and psychologists in America seems to have become a serious and questioning interest in the existential approach; and it is therefore finding its constructive way into our thinking. Increasingly the books coming off the press as outlines or surveys of psychology and psychiatry have their chapter on this approach. The difficulty, of course, experienced by the authors of most of these books lies in the fact that this psychology does not fit our usual categories. In America we try to test our psychologies behavioristically, but the existential viewpoint denies that this is possible: its concept of "being-in the

---

[1] W. JAMES,: Pragmatism: A New Name for Some Old Ways of Thinking. New York, Longmans, Green, and Co., 1949, p. 198.

world" implies that no item of behavior can be understood apart from its subjective meaning to the person involved, just as there is no subjective meaning which does not have its objective pole. Also in books on psychotherapy we tend to categorize therapies in terms of techniques: but although existential psychology has made and will make significant and in some ways radical contributions to many therapists' manner of treatment, it is not essentially a technique, and therapists of many different technical schools may rightly be called existential.

A number of psychiatrists and psychologists who have been important for the development of psychotherapy in this country have held viewpoints to a greater of lesser degree existential long before that term was heard in America. William James, Adolph Meyer, Harry Stack Sullivan, Gordon Allport, Carl Rogers, Henry Murray, Abraham Maslow are examples. But what has been lacking (with the possible exception of William James) has been a consistent underlying structure which would give unity to the work of these psychiatrists and psychologists who are concerned with man in his immediate existence. This underlying structure must necessarily be both on the philosophical and psychological levels. We propose here that the existential approach, re-cast and re-born into our American language and thought forms, can and will give this underlying structure.

By good fortune several of the classical works in existential psychiatry and psychology have just been translated and are in process of being published in English. One of these is Erwin Straus' The Primary World,[1] a basic treatment of sense experience in psychiatry and psychology. Another is a collection of Straus' papers, including such works as the widely quoted "Upright Posture."[2] Medard Boss' Psychoanalysis and Daseinsanalysis will also be available in 1963.[3] Prof. Herbert Spiegelberg's two-volume work on phenomenology makes that field at last accessible to us in English.[4] A number of other basic works are appearing, and thus the serious student will be able to study original works and come to his own judgments.

Principles Underlying Theory

Since any adequate psychotherapy rests upon a theory of personality, we shall present here several principles indicating how a comprehensive theory can be and is being developed in the existential approach.

---

[1] To be published in 1963 by Free Press, Glencoe, Illinois.
[2] To be published by Basic Books, New York.
[3] To be published by Basic Books, New York.
[4] The Phenomenological Movement, A Historical Introduction, Martinus Nijhoff, The Hague, Holland, 1960.

A comprehensive theory of psychotherapy presupposes the integration not only of findings in various schools of psychology and psychiatry but also of their interrelationships with one another and with human nature as such. Such an over-all integration is feasible only on the basis of a synthesizing idea or theoretical construct concerning man's nature which is comprehensive enough to connect all those findings without distorting their original contribution. First, *phenomenological descriptions* are necessary in order to uncover the original phenomena on which the interpretations of the various schools are based. Second, in order to find what binds those phenomena with one another and with the nature of man, we need the method of *existential* phenomenology, which tries to describe man's nature as such, that is, its essential characteristics.

The construct of "existence" is one of those comprehensive concepts and thus refers to the fact that it is man's essence to find himself bodily together with others in the world. This concept unites the subjective, physiological, objective and social aspects of the reality of man. The student of psychology has to split up this reality of man into many aspects in order to study them in isolation. As a result we are confronted with a variety of psychologies, such as social, behavioristic, physiological, introspectional, psychoanalytic and so on. In contrast, the existential approach seeks to *reintegrate* the phenomena which are discovered when man has been studied from those various, isolated viewpoints. But this reintegration presupposes a return to the original experience of man in his unity before he was split up into a variety of profiles by the various methodologies. It is for this reason that the construct of man's existence is used in psychology and psychotherapy as an integrational construct. In this context we define an integrational construct as: *a concept that refers to observed phenomena and that can be used for the integration of the greatest number and variety of phenomena and relationships observed by the different schools of psychology and psychiatry.*

Although "existence" or "existential" is the fundamental construct used in this comprehensive theory of personality, many more constructs are needed to develop a full theory. We shall here call them subordinated constructs, such as "mode of existence," "existential world," "existential transference," "the centered self," "ontological security and insecurity," and so on. They have the function of connecting the phenomena uncovered by the various schools of psychotherapy with the fundamental construct of existence.

The existential psychotherapist profits from the work of various existential philosophers without aligning himself with any particular school or system of philosophy. He borrows some of their existential concepts which prove useful for his integrating task. The status of the concepts, however, in a scientific psychological theory differs essentially from their previous position in philosophy. First, the existential psychologist neither affirms nor denies their ontological validity. For this would imply a philosophical statement which the psychologist and psychiatrist with only empirical methods at his disposal cannot make. Second, he changes them into hypothetical constructs from which he derives postulates which can be put to the empirical test. Third, he allows the original meaning of these constructs to change while being attuned to the phenomena uncovered in the various areas of psychology and psychiatry.*

THE EXISTENTIAL APPROACH TO THERAPY

We may now consider the application of the existential constructs to the practice of psychotherapy in one area, namely, *will* and *decision*. The capacity for self-conscious will and decision (we shall define these terms later) is taken as one of the essential, distinguishing characteristics of the being called man.†

The existential approach in psychology and psychotherapy holds that we cannot leave will and decision to chance. We cannot work on the assumption that ultimately the patient "somehow happens" to make a decision, or slides into a decision by ennui, default, or mutual fatigue with the therapist, or acts from sensing that the therapist (now the benevolent parent) will approve of him if he does take such and such steps. The existential approach puts decision and will back into the center of the picture—"The very stone which the builders rejected has become the head of the corner." Not in the sense of "free will against determinism"; this issue is dead and buried. Nor in the sense of denying what Freud describes as unconscious experience; these deterministic "unconscious" factors certainly operate, and the existentialists, who make much of "finiteness" and man's limitations, obviously know this. We hold, however, that in the revealing and exploring of these deterministic

---

*An example in theoretical physics of the change of the meaning of such a construct during the dialogue between philosophical concepts and observed data is the hypothetical construct "atom" that was first formulated by Democritus.

†It is well known that the existential thinkers such as Kierkegaard, Nietzsche, Sartre, Paul Ricoeur and Tillich have dealt centrally with the problem of will and decision. "Man becomes truly human only in moments of decision," stated Tillich in his demonstration that "will" is one of the essential characteristics of man as man. Probably the most accessible and readable book in this whole area is *The Courage to Be* by Paul Tillich (Yale: 1952). The endeavor has also been made to formulate psychologically the problem of will and decision; see Rollo May, "Existential Bases of Psychotherapy," *American Journal of Orthopsychiatry,* October, 1960, Vol. 30, No. 4.

forces in his life, the patient is orienting himself in some particular way to the data and thus is engaged in some choice, no matter how seemingly insignificant; is experiencing some freedom, no matter how subtle.

But the existential attitude in psychotherapy does not at all "push" the patient into decisions. Indeed, we are convinced that it is only by this clarification of the patient's own powers of will and decision that the therapist can avoid inadvertently and subtly pushing the patient in one direction or another. The existentialist point is that self-consciousness itself—the person's potential awareness that the vast, complex, protean flow of experience is *his* experience—brings in inseparably the element of decision at every moment. This conative element is present to some degree in experiences as simple and non-world shaking as any new idea one finds oneself entertaining, or any new memory that pops up in a seemingly random chain of free association. It is these and similar considerations which have led the existential psychotherapists to be concerned with the problems of will and decision as central to the process of therapy.

But when we turn to the endeavor to understand will and decision themselves, we find our task is not at all easy. Our problem hinges upon the terms "will" and "wish" and the interrelation between the two. The word "will," associated as it is with "will power," is at best dubious, and perhaps no longer helpful or even available. But the reality it has historically described must be retained. 'Will power" expressed the arrogant effort of Victorian man to manipulate nature and to rule nature with an iron hand (*vide* industrialism and capitalism) and to manipulate himself, rule his own life in the same way as an object (shown particularly in Protestantism but present in other modern ethical and religious systems as well). Thus "will" was set over against "wish" and used as a faculty by which "wish" could be denied. We have observed in patients that the emphasis on "will power" is often a reaction formation to their own repressed passive desires, a way of fighting off their wishes to be taken care of; and the likelihood is that this mechanism had much to do with the form "will power" took in Victorianism. Victorian man sought, as Schachtel has put it, to deny that he ever had been a child, to repress his irrational tendencies and so-called infantile wishes as unacceptable to his concept of himself as a grown-up and responsible man. Will power was then a way of avoiding awareness of bodily and of sexual urges or hostile impulses that did not fit the picture of the controlled, well-managed self. The process of using will to deny wish results in a greater and greater emotional void, a progressive emptying of inner contents which must ultimately impoverish intellectual experience as well.

In attacking these morbid psychological processes, Freud produced his far-reaching emphasis on the *wish*. In view of the fact that in our post-Victorian day we still tend to impoverish the word by making it a concession to our immaturity or "needs," let us hasten to say that the term "wish" may be seen as related to processes much more extensive than the residue of childhood. Its correlates can be found in all phenomena in nature down to the most minute pattern of atomic re-, action; for example, in the context of what Whitehead and Tillich describe as negative-positive movements in all nature. Tropism is one form in its etymological sense of the innate tendency in biological organisms to "turn toward." However, if we stop with "wish" as this more or less blind and involuntary movement of one particle toward another or one organism toward another, we are inexorably pushed to Freud's pessimistic conclusion of the "death instinct," the inevitable tendency of organisms to move back toward the inorganic. Therefore, in human beings "wish" can never be seen without relation to "will."

Our problem now becomes the inter-relation of "wish" and "will." We shall offer some suggestions which, although not intended to make a neat definition, show us some of the aspects of the problem that must be taken into consideration. "Wish" gives the warmth, the content, the child's play, the freshness and richness to "will." "Will" gives the self-direction, the freedom, the maturity to "wish." If you have only will and no wish, you have the dried up Victorian, post-Puritan man. If you have only wish and no will, you have the driven, unfree infantile human being who as an adult may become the robot man.

We propose the term "decision" to stand for the human act which brings both will and wish together. Decision in this sense does not deny or exclude wish but incorporates it and transcends it. Decision in an individual takes into the picture the experiencing of all wishes, but it forms these into a way of acting which is consciously chosen.

THERAPEUTIC DIMENSIONS

The process of therapy with individual patients involves bringing together these three dimensions of wish, will and decision. As the patient moves from one dimension to the next in his integration, the previous level is incorporated and remains present in the next.

In practical therapy, the first dimension, wish, occurs on the level of *awareness*, the dimension which the human organism shares with all nature. The experiencing of infantile wishes, bodily needs and desires, sexuality and hunger and all the infinite and inexhaustible gamut of wishes which occur in any individual, seems to be a central part of practically all therapy. Experiencing these wishes may involve dramatic and sometimes traumatic anxiety and upheaval as the repressions which led to the blocking off of the awareness in the first place are brought out into the open. On the significance and necessity of unmasking repression—the dynamic aspects of which are beyond the scope of our present discussion—various kinds of therapy differ radically; but we cannot conceive of any form of *psycho*therapy which does not accord the process of awareness itself a central place. The experiencing of these wishes may come out in the simplest forms in the desire to fondle or be fondled, the wishes associated originally with nursing and closeness to mother and family members in early experience, the touch of the hand of a friend or loved one in adult experience, the simple pleasure of wind and water against one's skin; and it goes all the way up to the sophisticated experiences which may come, for example, in a dazzling instant when one is standing near a clump of blooming forsythia and is suddenly struck by how much more brilliantly blue the sky looks when seen beyond the sea of yellow flowers. The immediate awareness of the world continues throughout life, hopefully at an accelerating degree, and is infinitely more varied and rich than one would gather from most psychological discussion.

From the existential viewpoint, this growing awareness of one's body, wishes and desires—processes which are obviously related to the experiencing of identity—normally also brings heightened appreciation of one's self as *a* being and a heightened reverence for Being itself. Here the eastern philosophies like Zen Buddhism have much to teach us.

The second level in the relating of *wish* to *will* in therapy is the transmitting of awareness into self-consciousness. This level is correlated with the distinctive form of awareness in human beings, consciousness. (The term *consciousness,* coming etymologically from *con* plus *sciere,* "knowing with," is used here as synonymous with self-consciousness.)*
On this level the patient experiences I-am-the-one-who-has-these-wishes. This is the level of accepting one's self as having a world. If I experience the fact that my wishes are not simply blind pushes toward someone or something, that I am the one who stands in this world where touch, nourishment, sexual pleasure and relatedness may be possible between me and other persons, I can begin to see how I may do something about these wishes. This gives me the possibility of *in-sight,* of "inward sight," of seeing the world and other people in relation to myself. Thus the previous alternatives of repressing wishes because one cannot stand

---

*The relationships of awareness to self-consciousness have been developed elsewhere, (May, op. cit.). Strictly speaking, "self-consciousness" is redundant: consciousness already implies relation to the self.

the lack of their gratification on one hand, or being compulsively pushed to the blind gratification of the wishes and desires on the other, are replaced by the experience of the fact that I myself am involved in these relationships of pleasure, love, beauty, trust and I hopefully then have the possibility of changing my own behavior to make these more possible.

On this level *will* enters the picture, not as a denial of wish but as an incorporation of wish on the higher level of consciousness. To refer to our example above: the experiencing of the blue of the sky behind forsythia blossoms on the simple level of awareness and wish may bring delight and the desire to continue or renew the experience; but the realization that I am the person who lives in a world in which flowers are yellow and the sky so brilliant, and that I can even increase my pleasure by sharing this experience with a friend, has profound implications for life, love, death, and the other ultimate problems of human existence. As Tennyson remarked when he looked at the flower in the crannied wall, ". . . I could understand what God and man are."

The third level in the process of therapy is that of *decision* and *responsibility*. We use these two terms together to indicate that decision is not simply synonymous with will. Responsibility involves being responsive, *responding*. As consciousness is the distinctively human form of awareness, so decision and responsibility are the distinctive forms of consciousness in the human being who is moving toward self-realization, integration, maturity. Again, this dimension is not achieved by denying wishes and self-assertive will, but incorporates and keeps present the previous two levels. *Decision* in our sense forms the two previous levels into a pattern of acting and living which is not only empowered and enriched by wishes and asserted by will but is responsive to and responsible for the significant other persons who are important to one's self in the realizing of the long-term goals. This sounds like an ethical statement, and *is* in the sense that ethics have their psychological base in these capacities of the human being to transcend the concrete situation of immediate self-oriented desire and to live in the dimensions of past and future and in terms of the welfare of the persons and groups upon which one's own fulfillment intimately depends. The point, however, cannot be dismissed as "just" ethical. If it is not self-evident it could be demonstrated along the lines of Sullivan's interpersonal theory of psychiatry, Buber's philosophy and other viewpoints, that *wish, will* and *decision* occur within a nexus of relationships upon which the individual himself depends not only for his fulfillment but for his very existence.

PART III

PSYCHOPHYSIOLOGIC
FACILITATIONS

Pharmacotherapy in Children's Behavior Disorders

by Barbara Fish, M.D.

Since 1940, amphetamines, anticonvulsants and antihistamines have been used to treat children with behavior disorders. The introduction of chlorpromazine and reserpine enlarged the scope of pharmacotherapy, but it also heightened the controversy about the role of drugs. Glib claims of "improvement" were countered by dire warnings about the effect of drugs on learning and the psychotherapeutic relationship.[1] Controlled studies are needed to establish specific indications and contraindications, using criteria that can be compared in different centers. Pending such definitive studies, one must draw upon the accumulated clinical experience of the past twenty years to establish a practical modus operandi.

What Drugs Can and Cannot Do

Drugs are most effective in reducing psychomotor excitement. Optimally the reduction of impulsivity and irritability is accompanied by lessened anxiety and improved attention-span. To a lesser extent drugs can increase spontaneous activity and affective responsiveness in states of apathy and inertia.

The response of complex behavior patterns to physiological treatment is far less predictable. Hallucinations, perceptual distortions and thought disorders subside in some children with the lessening of psychomotor excitement; other children retain residual defects. Whether drugs can improve intellectual functioning has still to be determined. Children with severe mental retardation, associated with organic brain disease or schizophrenia show the least response to drugs. The more severe, unchanging deficits in function appear to have the same prognostic significance in children as do long duration and chronicity of symptoms in adults.[2]

Drugs may modify a child's responsiveness to current and past experiences but chemicals alone cannot undo previously learned behavior, alter character patterns or neurotic attitudes. Thus aggressive behavior may respond to drugs only if it is associated with gross psychomotor disturbance. Less disturbed children frequently resent the physiological changes produced by drugs and the threat to their autonomy which such manipulations represent.

If drugs cannot alter established patterns in the most severe psychoses or the mildest conduct disorders, they can modify appropriate target symptoms in moderately severe schizophrenia and chronic brain syndromes, or in severe behavior disorders. In addition some neurotic children with persistent anxiety, inhibitions and phobias become more spontaneous and increase their adaptive functioning if given drugs. The younger the child, the more is psychiatric disturbance of any type expressed in hyperexcitability, hyperactivity, and disorganized behavior which can respond to medication. Symptomatic pharmacotherapy may enable severely disturbed children to participate in group activities and special classes; it helps others to become amenable to psychotherapy and education which would otherwise be impossible; it can accelerate the therapy of less disturbed children.[3,4]

When to Introduce Drugs into Treatment

Good medicine dictates that one must first evaluate the child's psychopathology and the relation of his symptoms to his family and environment before introducing any foreign agent into this complex situation. The child's ability to change in the new setting of ambulatory or institutional psychiatric treatment should be observed for two to four weeks before starting a trial of drug therapy. If an acute crisis demands immediate medication, drugs can be withheld later, to evaluate the child's own capacity for reintegration.

If symptoms disappear completely, in the child's usual environment, with full resumption of social and academic activities, using social manipulation and psychotherapy alone, obviously no additional treatment is indicated. However, if considerable anxiety or a limitation in function persists after four weeks, one should not withhold drugs which could accelerate recovery, even if the child is responding slowly to other measures. Medical judgment must weigh the slight chance of harm from drugs against the limitation in the child's function and the strain imposed on his family if drugs are withheld. A potentially useful treatment may be withheld in a controlled experiment comparing different treatments; it should not be postponed merely to satisfy the therapist's desire for psychotherapeutic omnipotence.

DRUGS AND PSYCHOTHERAPY

Pharmacotherapy need not interfere with the subtler interpersonal operations of psychotherapy if the physician has a constructive and common sense attitude toward drugs and is alert to the transference problems which may arise. The therapeutic meaning of biologic measures, verbal interpretations or environmental restrictions depends upon the conscious and unconscious attitudes of all the participants. Drugs would destroy therapy if the doctor used them as a quick expedient to avoid responsibility for the child's complex problems in living, or if he saw drugs as the ultimate weapon of authority to enforce compliance on a problem child, or if he felt drugs were a measure of desperation to be used only after all other measures failed.

If drug therapy is put into its proper perspective by the physician, the auxiliary use of drugs does not permit parents to minimize the child's problems. Parents should be told that at best drugs produce only quantitative changes and the child will not be cured or "made over." Discussions of all the other measures needed to help the child emphasize this point. Even very young children can understand that medicine just "helps the way your stomach feels when you're scared," or "angry," or "jumpy" and that once they feel better it is easier to do something about these other problems.

The use of drugs will not alarm parents about the seriousness of the child's disturbance, if the doctor does not wait for a desperate or hopeless situation to force his hand, but uses drugs for specific indications of varying severity. The physician must relieve parents' anxieties by explaining the effects of drugs and by being available between appointments to discuss any questionable side effects. Children are usually reassured by the information that their "funny feelings" are not unique, and by finding out that these feelings can be helped by medication. Seriously disturbed children who need maintenance drug therapy need to understand that this is to help their "over-sensitivity" at the times in their life when this is necessary.

The child does not experience medication as a weapon of authority when his own distress is made the mutual concern of himself and the therapist, and he is given the responsibility to report which medicine makes him feel better, or sleepy or jumpy. The management of medication between child and doctor can become part of a new and constructive experience for a child who is not used to being listened to or taken seriously by an adult.

When parents are helped to understand the child's symptoms in terms of anxiety or disturbances in development, the emphasis of treatment is shifted away from blaming the child for being "bad," or the parent for being inadequate. Specific goals should be set for increasing the child's function so that medication becomes a positive tool and not a way to make the child "behave." Additional precautions must be taken to prevent the actual giving of medication from becoming an issue between mother and child. First, medicine is given regularly at specific times; the mother is not to offer it to the child just when he becomes upset, or if he happens to annoy her. Second, the mother does not adjust the dose herself for what might be subjective reasons. Finally, if a child objects to drugs, the mother should not force the issue. The child's feelings about pills, as about any other aspect of treatment, are a matter for him to discuss with his doctor.

Children typically tend to deny physical and psychological difficulties, and are all too ready to terminate medication as soon as their distress is lessened. Rarely, an older neurotic child may use medication in the interest of his hypochondriasis or secondary gain. If the physician himself is sceptical about the effects of medication and is alert to these transference complications, they can be readily resolved.

The regulation of medication creates transference complications, but these can be handled just like the similar problems encountered in the absence of drugs. Medication itself can be readily accepted by parent and child as simply another way in which the doctor tries to help the child. In the interest of good medical and psychotherapeutic management, the psychological and pharmacological aspects of treatment should not be split between two therapists.

INDICATIONS FOR SPECIFIC DRUGS

In general the more severe the disorder the more potent is the drug required to produce a response. The standard diagnostic categories serve as a gross guide to severity. Within a diagnostic group, severity increases with greater intellectual, perceptual, and neurological impairment, and with greater affective and motoric disturbance.[2] Hyperactive and hypoactive children may react differently to drugs and there are also individual differences in response to the sedative and stimulating properties of medications.

The clinician should become familiar with a few representative minor and major tranquilizers and stimulants which span the spectrum of potency and differential effects. Additional drugs may be used if sensitivity to previous drugs makes substitution necessary.

The following discussion is limited to children's behavioral and central nervous system responses. The clinician should be familiar with the possible systemic, allergic and other toxic effects, and should observe all the precautions which are taken with adults.[5,6] Any of these drugs may also produce undesirable exaggerations of their therapeutic effects on the nervous system, if the dose is too high for the particular child. However, excessive sedation or irritability readily subside if the dose is reduced.

MINOR TRANQUILIZERS

These drugs are primarily useful in mild to moderately severe neurotic and "primary" behavior disorders, comparable to their use in adult patients. Unlike adults and adolescents, prepuberty children do not tend to become addicted to medication. Children with moderately severe organic and schizophrenic reactions are frequently helped by certain of the mild medications, as if their patterns were more malleable than adults', or the immature nervous system reacted differently to drugs.[2,3]

Diphenylmethane Derivatives

Diphenhydramine (Benadryl) has been used for over ten years to treat disturbed children.[3,7,8] It is most effective in behavior disorders associated with hyperactivity, but it also reduces anxiety in very young children who are not hyperactive and may be helpful in moderately severe organic or schizophrenic disorders. Unlike the other drugs, diphenhydramine drops in effectiveness at puberty. In young children it reduces anxiety without producing drowsiness or lethargy; after ten years of age children respond like adults: the drug frequently produces fatigue or drowsiness and is most useful as a bedtime sedative.[3] Hydroxyzine (Atarax) and Azacyclonol (Frenquel) appear to be weaker and more variable in their action than diphenhydramine. Captodiamine (Suvren) is similar chemically to diphenhydramine, and has been reported to be effective in organic brain disorders.[9]

Substituted Diols

Meprobamate (Equanil, Miltown) is effective in neurotic and behavior disorders including those associated with mild organic brain disease.[8] I found it less effective for hyperactivity than diphenhydramine in the same subjects, but unlike diphenhydramine it continues to be effective in neurotic children into adolescence.

Miscellaneous

Promethazine (Phenergan) is structurally related to the phenothiazines but acts as a mild tranquilizer. It has been reported to be effective in severely disturbed children,[7] but I found it less effective than diphen-hydramine in the same subjects. *Chlordiazepoxide* (*Librium*) is apparent-ly comparable in potency to the most effective minor tranquilizers, but preliminary work suggests that it may also have excitatory effects which require further exploration.[10]

ANTICONVULSANTS

Early studies reported encouraging results in the use of hydantoin compounds in the treatment of children whose behavior disorders were associated with non-specific EEG abnormalities.[11,12] Later reports failed to confirm these findings,[8,13] and my own experience agrees with this latter impression.

HYPNOTICS

These drugs have not been demonstrated to be effective in psychiatric disorders of prepuberty children. Barbiturates may actually increase anxiety and disorganization in severely disturbed children. When night-time sedation is needed, chloral hydrate or the more effective mild tranquilizers usually suffice.

MAJOR TRANQUILIZERS

Phenothiazines

Extensive experience has demonstrated that these compounds are highly effective in severely disturbed children with "primary" behavior disorders, schizophrenia, or organic brain disease. Used with the proper precautions,[6] these drugs are safe enough to warrant use in disorders which resist milder therapies.

Dimethylamine Series

These drugs are relatively less potent than the piperazine series. They show a predominance of sedative over stimulating effects, are very effective against psychomotor excitement, but small doses may depress less agitated children. Extra-pyramidal reactions are rare in disturbed children and can be terminated promptly by reducing the dose.

Chlorpromazine (*Thorazine*) serves as the standard of comparison for the others. *Promazine* (*Sparine*) is about half as potent as chlorproma-zine and intermediate in action between the major and minor tran-quilizers. *Triflupromazine* (*Vesprin*) is two to three times as potent as chlorpromazine.

Piperidine Series

Thioridazine (*Mellaril*) has not yet been shown to have any advantage

over chlorpromazine for children that outweighs the possible complication
of toxic retinitis. It has a low incidence of extra-pyramidal symptoms in
adults, but this is not a problem in children. *Mepazine* (*Pacatal*) has a
relatively high incidence of severe toxicity in adults.[6]

Piperazine Series

These drugs are useful especially in hypoactive schizophrenic or
severely neurotic children and children who tend to be depressed by the
administration of chlorpromazine. Severely apathetic schizophrenic children with IQ's under 70 may require relatively large doses by body
weight. However, most children tend to be more sensitive than adults to
the stimulating effects of these drugs and may show irritability, agitation
and then dyskinesia with small doses. The adult dose adjusted strictly for
body weight, may be two to five times too high for a child.[3] This may
well account for the high incidence of dystonic effects reported.

Trifluoperazine (*Stelazine*) may be 20 to 100 times as potent as
chlorpromazine in the same child. Its stimulating effects are especially
indicated to increase alertness and motor drive in severely apathetic,
withdrawn, schizophrenic children. If these children are very young the
drug may even increase motor skills, social responsiveness, and language.
Fluphenazine (*Permitil, Prolixin*) has effects similar to trifluoperazine
but is more potent. *Prochlorperazine* (*Compazine*), *Perphenazine* (*Tri-
lafon*), *and Thiopropazate* (*Dartal*) are about five to ten times as potent
as chlorpromazine in the same child. Their sedative and stimulating
properties are intermediate between the dimethylamine group and
trifluoperazine.

Rauwolfia Alkaloids

These drugs have a less reliable action than the phenothiazines and
are now generally reserved for severe schizophrenics who have not
responded to phenothiazines.

MINOR STIMULANTS

Amphetamines have been used for over twenty years to treat children
with behavior disorders. They stimulate overly inhibited neurotic children
and are especially useful in prepuberty children with school phobias and
those who are disturbed by sexual preoccupations and fantasies. Many
workers report that doses up to 40 mg. per day also quieted hyperactive
children including those with organic brain disorders.[14,15] Others have
not confirmed this effect using a maximum, however, of 20 mg. per
day.[3,7,8] In my own experience, children complained of uncomfortable

side effects if given more than 20 mg. *Methylphenidate* (*Ritalin*) and *Pipradol* (*Meratran*) have not yet been demonstrated to have any advantages in children over the amphetamines.

MAJOR STIMULANTS AND ANTIDEPRESSANTS

Since psychotic retarded depressions are rare before midadolescence, these drugs are being tested primarily in apathetic schizophrenic children, but effectiveness and safety have not yet been established.

TABLE 1.—*Suggested Dosages for Children's Psychiatric Disorders**

Name of Drug	Dose Range (mg./Kg./day)	Average Dose (mg./Kg./day)
Amphetamine	0.15- 0.80	0.2
Diphenhydramine (Benadryl)	2.0 -10.0	4.0
Meprobamate (Equanil, Miltown)	4.0 -30.0	15.0
Chlorpromazine (Thorazine)	1.0 - 8.0	2.0
Trifluoperazine (Stelazine)		
a) hypoactive schizophrenic children	.1 - 1.0	0.5
b) all others	.02- 0.2	0.1

An Approach to Regulating Medication

Pharmacotherapy should start with the mildest drug which might be effective for a particular child. The dose is gradually increased until symptoms disappear or the first signs of excess dose appear (mild headache, fatigue, irritability, etc.), to make certain that the useful dose range has been fully explored. The child's response may indicate that a more sedative or more stimulating agent is required. If drug-susceptible symptoms persist with the highest tolerated dose of a mild drug, more potent drugs should be explored in the same way. The optimal dose is the level which reduces symptoms and increases function without causing discomfort. In disturbed children with severe impairment of function, one must carefully weigh the positive and negative effects of increasing dosage.

In mild disorders where symptoms disappear with mild medication, drugs need only be continued for a brief period, to give the child and his family sufficient time to establish a new level of adaptation in the

---

*Physicians who plan to use these drugs should consult the recommendation on dosage provided by the manufacturers. The dosages presented above are used by the author in in-patient and out-patient psychiatric treatment with children but they are intended only as a general guide, to indicate the relationship of children's doses to adults'. *See text also.*

absence of symptoms. In severely disturbed children who do not get complete relief of symptoms even with potent medication, pharmacotherapy must be maintained just as it is in chronic adult patients, readjusting the medication as indicated. There have been no reports to date that maintenance medication of the phenothiazines continued for five to six years leads to any disturbance of growth or endocrine development in adolescence.

Until much more is known about the mechanism of action of these drugs, and the physiological and psychological factors that make up individual differences in responsiveness, pharmacotherapy will continue to be on an empirical basis. But even so, it provides an invaluable adjunct to the total psychiatric treatment of the disturbed child.

REFERENCES

1. FISHER, S., (Ed.): Child Research in Psychopharmacology. Springfield, Illinois, Charles C Thomas, 1959.
2. FISH, B.: Evaluation of psychiatric therapies in children. Delivered at the American Psychopathologic Assn. Meeting, February 1962.
3. ——: Drug therapy in child psychiatry: pharmacological aspects. Comprehensive Psychiatry, 1:212-227, 1960.
4. ——: Drug therapy in child psychiatry: psychological aspects. Comprehensive Psychiatry, 1:55-61, 1960.
5. NYHAN, W. L.: Toxicity of drugs in the neonatal period. J. Pediat., 59:1-20, 1961.
6. SCHIELE, B. C., AND BENSON, W. M.: Tranquilizing and Antidepressive Drugs. Springfield, Illinois, Charles C Thomas, 1962.
7. BENDER, L., AND NICHTERN, S.: Chemotherapy in child psychiatry. New York State J. Med., 56:2791-2796, 1956.
8. FREEDMAN, A. M.: Drug therapy in behavior disorders. Pediatric Clinics of North America. Baltimore, W. B. Saunders Company, 1958.
9. LOW, N. L., AND MYERS, G. G.: Suvren in brain-injured children. J. Pediat., 3:259-263, 1958.
10. KRAFT, I. A.: Personal communications, September 1962.
11. LINDSLEY, D. B., AND HENRY, C. E.: Effect of drugs on behavior and electro-encephalograms of children with behavior disorders. Psychosomatic Med., 4:140-149, 1942.
12. WALKER, C. F., AND KIRKPATRICK, B. B.: Dilantin treatment of behavior problem children with abnormal E.E.G.'s. Am. J. Psychiat., 103:484-492, 1947.
13. PASAMANICK, B.: Anticonvulsant drug therapy of behavior problem children with abnormal encephalograms. Arch. Neurol. & Psychiat., 65:752, 1951.
14. BRADLEY, C.: Benzedrine and dexedrine in the treatment of children's behavior disorders. Pediatrics, 5:24-37, 1950.
15. LAUFER, M. W., DENHOFF, E., AND SOLOMONS, G.: Hyperkinetic impulse disorder in children's behavior problems. Psychosomatic Med., 19:38-49, 1957.

Pharmacologic Facilitation of Psychoanalytic Therapy

by C. C. DAHLBERG, M.D.

PSYCHOANALYSTS, from the beginning of the science, have engaged in the search for techniques which would help lay bare the roots of neurosis. It was Freud's radical view that treatment aimed at remembering was superior to treatment aimed at forgetting. His original tool was hypnosis.

This report deals with certain drugs (LSD, and briefly mescaline, Psilocybin, Sernyl, and Ditran) which are being investigated for their value in helping uncover memories and emotions, and evoke fantasies without interfering with subsequent memory of the drug-induced event. Drugs formerly used for this purpose such as barbiturates, ethyl alcohol and CO_2 have all seriously interfered with memory and therefore left the patient in roughly the same condition as before taking the drug, insofar as his conscious-unconscious axis was concerned.

In analysis, the free associative process is designed among other things to facilitate the flow of unconscious material into consciousness. Unfortunately many persons who would most profit from this process, such as obsessional neurotics and detached schizoid personalities, are least susceptible to it. They tend to be repetitious, unemotional and intellectual.

A number of drugs are being experimented with for their value in breaking through these defensive systems. Lysergic Acid Diethylamide, better known as LSD 25 or LSD, is the substance in this group which has been used the most and the one with which I have worked. The main body of this report will be confined to the use of LSD; brief mention of other substances will follow.

LSD, a relative of the ergot alkaloids, was synthesized in 1943. Psychotherapeutic studies go back to 1950.[1] Oral doses of 300 mcg. can produce schizophrenic-like states with hallucinations, thinking disorders and mood changes. Doses of 50-100 mcg. are subhallucinatory and cause milder effects.

Therapy with hospitalized alcoholics and obsessionals has been successful using the larger dosage in a single treatment.[2-9] Powerful abreaction occurs and the function of the therapist is supportive and sometimes exhortative.

My work has been with repeated doses of under 100 mcg. on psychoanalytic patients functioning in the community. All that is necessary for analysis with LSD is the drug itself, a room for the patient to wait in while the effects are coming on, an ampule of Thorazine, a syringe, a competent attendant and time.[10-23]

Suitable patients are offered the drug and a few days allowed to elapse for discussion about its use. On the first LSD session, slightly less than 1 mcg./Kg. is given orally on an empty stomach. Within 30-60 minutes sympathomimetic effects appear which are on the order of mild nausea, muscular irritability, light flashes, chills and flushing. These soon pass. The main psychic effects are at their peak in about two hours, and last 4 to 6 hours. A long (2-4 hour) analytic session then takes place following which the patient is sent home with an attendant who remains on call 8-12 hours. The only restrictions are on alcohol and driving.

Patients like LSD. They find the experience stimulating and exciting as well as terrifying at times. I have never had the experience get out of hand but if it should, 25-50 mg. of Thorazine intramuscularly will quickly bring matters under control. A hospital should be available if needed. Time and dosage can be adjusted in later sessions.

What happens under the drug which can have therapeutic value? Clinically, I have noted:

1. The expression of emotion is quite open.
2. Patient's expression of feeling toward the therapist is open and there tends to be an increase in dependency feelings.
3. Fantasies are rich.
4. Forgotten episodes are remembered with the appropriate emotion.
5. Associations are rich and free.
6. There is a curious exaggeration of the patients fundamental way of relating so that the patient, with intense emotion, acts this out with the analyst and/or in fantasy while simultaneously or alternately observing himself and commenting to the analyst and himself on his actions and feelings.
7. Embarrassment is at a minimum and matters which have previously been held back are spoken of more freely.
8. The problems come to the foreground and defensive measures may be discarded.
9. On some occasions, certain simple reassurances, interpretations, well placed expressions of confidence, etc. are very convincing.
10. Post LSD recall is usually remarkable. This is because the experiences are so sharp and clear that they are unforgettable and consciousness is not clouded. The patient is very impressed with what has come out of him.

This last point is what makes the drug superior to all others which have been used similarly. The ego or self system is not bypassed. Memory is good and the gained information has a chance to be integrated into the personality. Clearly then, if this integration is to take place, it has the best chance in a therapeutic setting and it is in this way that I am using the drug. It is not a substitute for psychoanalysis or psychotherapy but a facilitating agent.

LSD can be used in any psychoneurotic whose defensive system does not allow him to open up sufficiently with ordinary analytic techniques. Psychosis as well as pre-psychotic or borderline conditions rule out the drug. Epilepsy and any organic brain condition are contraindications and one would not want to use it in a pregnant woman. A seriously depressed person should have LSD only in a hospital because of the danger of suicide.[24]

I insist upon at least 6 months of analysis and psychological studies to confirm the absence of a hidden psychotic process before starting with LSD. I start out giving the drug every three weeks. In analysis three times a week, this allows 8 sessions in which to work through the LSD material before the next time. Such a rigid schedule is useful at first to minimize dependence upon the drug and to counteract possible resistance. Since LSD mobilizes conflicts, resistance[25] may increase. If the patient has to make a fresh decision about each session he may well decide against it, just when he could find it most valuable. For this reason, a reasonably rigid schedule of treatments is necessary.

As time goes on, variations in the timing of the LSD session and the length of time given to it are useful. The following have been tried successfully:

1. A three month vacation from LSD to catch up with the insights.

2. Two sessions 3 days apart to mobilize a certain defensive system and work it through in the first session; then take advantage of that in the second session before the defenses are reconstructed.

3. Absence of the doctor during the entire session but having an attendant in the next room. This was useful in a patient who had never been given privacy during his childhood and needed the chance to experience this special event alone and report on it later.

The following case illustrates the special abreactive and transference qualities that can occur with LSD.

The patient is a 30 year old dependent, lonely, negativistic, withdrawn, depressed professional man. Three persons had acted as "mother" in his life; the second was Mrs. A., a housekeeper, who had the greatest success. She was superseded by Louise, a rejecting, demanding step-mother. All the mothers were dead when analysis started. He had had four years of analysis with four different analysts, the greater part with two. His regular analytic session was generally dull and lifeless.

The following session started two hours after taking 75 mcg. of LSD.

After a slow beginning, he reported the following dream. "I was in a tunnel. I asked directions of someone. He was using the memory code system to give them to me and I explained that I understood the code. Only a few people do." He continued: "It's as if I were communicating with two different means. I think Mrs. A. and I had this special code of our own. Your being here scares the life out of me. We communicated in one way when Louise was there and one way when she wasn't."

I asked him if my threat was that I would break the code and he said that the real threat came when he forgot the code.

"I'm afraid of establishing the code with you. I denied that I told you about the system. It's true that I just gave you the general idea. It's interesting that I spent a long time recently explaining the system to this girl I liked. I trans_ lated the word 'normal' for her and explained it. Curious. With my cousin, Pete, the last thing he said was in the code. We play with it."

I remarked that people who love each other have a code, a special language, shared associations.

He laughed and remembered asking Mrs. A. when he was about 5 if he knew everything. She had replied that if he did he wouldn't ask that question. "It's the sort of thing I was always asking. You still scare the life out of me but I feel better just remembering a few things like that."

I said I thought it had to do with his letting me in and I continued that the most heartening thing that had happened in his analysis is the change in the people he lets himself know. He told me not to build it up too much. "It's a real feeling I can't let you in on. It was the feeling that she was on my side. It wasn't until later that I realized that. I took it for granted. I didn't care about her false teeth which had made her inferior at one time. That only meant she was old and might die and go away some day."

"This tremendous feeling a baby has of wanting to live—you know, participate, grow." I said, "The opposite of what you've described all the early part of the session."

"Right," he replied through his sobs, "Tremendous. This was the feeling of self hatred. That nobody could do this for me. I know vaguely that she did one time. I went over to the enemy and didn't live—I was in an artificial, dead, dream world. I hate Dad for taking me into that. He didn't know what it was all about. I'm sure the beatings and lectures I got were to break up the special code. But before Louise came he didn't mind. He even approved. Maybe Mrs. A.'s daughter minded a little my calling her mother 'Mommy'." I asked if "Mommy" was the code word. "Yes, I think so. I'm very scared. It is . . ." and he cried bitterly. "This is when she got the message that I had to close her out, when she said I hadn't called her 'Mommy' for a long time. I didn't really want to. I just refused to think of it for a long time. It was a terrible thing."

It can be noted in this case that LSD helped release memories and emotions in the dream analysis. More importantly, elements of the transference dependency and hostility were made clear, and the patient went on to work out many of his problems very well.

The most convincing psychological theory of how LSD works is that it is like sensory deprivation[26,27,39] in that the ordering effect of external reality is diminished and the internal reality is therefore increased in relative importance. Thus, condensations are decreased and the defensive limitations on associations is dissolved. Transference distortions may then be related back to their original interpersonal sources with release of accumulated affect and be replaced by a normal perception of the analyst as a helping person. This can only take place if the analyst is actually present and helping. Since psychic conflicts are so readily mobilized under the influence of the drug, it is important that the resulting anxiety be minimized by the presence of a friendly, reality orienting person. This is why an attendant must always be with the patient after he leaves the analyst's office.

A few other points need be mentioned. LSD is physiologically safe in the doses used. It is not addicting and placebo effects have been adequately tested and ruled out. Tolerance develops in 3 successive days of use.

The extension of the time[28] of the analytic session has been singled out as possibly accounting for some of the effects. However, early analysts who worked with variations in time and frequency did not find that prolonging the session gave them results comparable to these, so this does not seem to be a serious criticism.

One final point should be mentioned. There is considerable opposition to the use of this drug on outpatients,[29-37] the contention being that it can produce prolonged psychotic reactions or violent acting out. My own experience, as well as the experiences of others[10-13,15,19,38] who have used it on outpatients, convinces me that LSD is safe in the hands of an experienced psychoanalyst who employs the technique I have described.

To recapitulate, the analyst must know his patient well, use doses under 100 mcg., provide adequate supervision of the patient, and be prepared to handle an upsurging of repressed material and affect.

PSILOCYBIN

The newest of the three most important drugs in this group, Psilocybin, is a derivative of the Mexican hallucinogenic mushroom Psilocybe mexicana and can now be synthesized. It is chemically related to LSD, having an indole nucleus and is a tryptamine derivative related to reserpine.

Physiological and psychological effects are remarkably similar to LSD.[40-43] The two main differences are in dosage and duration of effect. Oral dosage of Psilocybin is about 100 times that of LSD and lasts half as long (about 4 hours). This would seem to offer advantages in outpatient psychotherapy, being less disruptive to the doctor's schedule and the patient's life.

No important psychoanalytic reports have as yet been published on this drug, but it would seem to have potentialities as great as LSD. Malitz[44] noted some "blocking, associational impairment and flight of ideas" possibly due to dosage or personality variations, so we must await further elucidation.

MESCALINE

The oldest of the three most important drugs in this group, mescaline, has been chewed from the peyotle cactus for centuries. The pure alkaloid was isolated in 1894. Chemically it is unlike LSD, since it is related to epinephrine.[45]

The psychological effects are nearly identical to those of LSD, but again a dose about 100 times as great is necessary. Sympathomimetic effects are more severe than with LSD which is a disadvantage in analytic treatment. Nausea and vomiting are common and may be persistent. A few workers have used this drug to facilitate psychotherapy for over a decade.[18,46]

PHENCYCLIDINE (SERNYL)*

An intravenous anesthetic compound which created difficult nursing problems in some patients because of bizarre behavior, echolalia and logorrhea, Sernyl has been considered an "interoceptive sensory blocking agent.[47] Investigation has been principally into its psychotomimetic capacities; the cardinal features of which are changes in body image, disorganization of thought, estrangement, negativism, drowsiness and apathy.[48] In small doses (3.5-4.5 mg. intravenously) it has been used to facilitate psychotherapy, principally as an abreactive agent.[49,50] There is no evidence that specific psychotherapeutic or psychoanalytic procedures were used on the five psychoneurotic patients in this study. One patient, however, did seem to acquire some insight into his problems and became available for psychotherapy following 16 Sernyl sessions. Another patient received both LSD and Sernyl. Comparison of the effects of the two drugs revealed much livelier fantasy experiences with LSD. After the drugs had worn off, memory of the events and symptoms were increased with LSD and diminished with Sernyl. This points up the necessity for adequate psychotherapeutic handling of the conflictual material when LSD is used.

On the basis of published data, Sernyl does not seem to be particularly useful in facilitating therapy based on insight but may be useful for other procedures.

---

*Park-Davis; C I 395.

DITRAN*

This is one of a number of anticholinergic drugs[51] which produces a psychotic-like state resembling a toxic delerium. In intramuscular doses of 15 mg., Ditran has been used with some success to treat patients with severe depressions; however, the patient tends to withdraw from human relationships and is relatively uncommunicative.[52,56]

REFERENCES

1. BUSCH, A. K., AND JOHNSON, W. C.: LSD 25 as an aid in psychotherapy. Dis. Nerv. System, 11:241, 1950.
2. COOPER, H. A.: Hallucinogenic drugs. Lancet, 1:1078, 1955.
3. CUTNER, M.: Analytic work with LSD 25. Psychiat. Quart., 33:715-757, 1959.
4. DAY, J.: The role and reaction of the psychiatrist in LSD therapy. J. Nerv. & Ment. Dis., 125:444, 1957.
5. DITMAN, K. S., WHITTLESEY, J. R. B., AND HAYMAN, M.: Subjective claims following the LSD experience. Unpublished observations.
6. LEWIS, D. J., AND SLOANE, R. B.: Therapy with LSD. J. Clin. & Exper. Psychopath., 19:19, 1958.
7. MARTIN, A. J.: LSD treatment of chronic psychoneurotic patients under day hospital conditions. Internat. J. Soc. Psychiat., 3:188,1957.
8. SMITH, C. M.: A new adjunct to the treatment of alcoholism: the hallucinogenetic drugs. Quart. J. Studies on Alcohol, 19:406, 1958.
9. HOFFER, A.: Introductory Remarks, The Use of LSD in Psychotherapy. Josiah Macy, Jr. Foundation, p. 18, 1959.
10. ABRAMSON, H. A., JARVIK, M. E., LEVINE, A., AND WAGNER, M.: LSD I, physiological and perceptual responses. J. Psychol., 39:3, 1955.
11. ——: LSD 25 III. As an adjunct to psychotherapy with elimination of fear of homosexuality. J. Psychol., 39:127, 1955.
12. ——: LSD 25 XXII. Effect on transference. J. Psychol., 42:51, 1956.
13. ——: LSD 25 XIX. As an adjunct to brief psychotherapy with special reference to ego enhancement. J. Psychol., 41:199, 1956.
14. ——, ROLO, A., AND STACKE, J.: LSD antagonists: chlorpromazine. J. Neuropsychiat., 1:309, 1959-60.
15. CHANDLER, A. L., AND HARTMAN, M. A.: LSD 25 as a facilitating agent in psychotherapy. Arch. Gen. Psychiat., 2:286, 1960.
16. COHEN, S., AND EISNER, B. G.: Use of LSD in a psychotherapeutic setting. Arch. Neurol. Psychiat., 81:615, 1959.
17. EISNER, B. G., AND COHEN, S.: Psychotherapy with LSD. J. Nerv. & Ment. Dis., 127:528, 1958.
18. FRIEDERKING, W.: Intoxicant drugs (mescaline and LSD) in psychotherapy. J. Nerv. & Ment. Dis., 121:262, 1955.
19. HAYES, J. S.: Clinical investigations with LSD 25. Research Dept. Bulletin, No. 1 of the Phila. Mental Health Clinic (undated) mimeo.
20. LANGNER, F. W.: Six years experience with LSD therapy. Unpublished paper delivered at the meeting of the National Association of Private Psychiatric Hospitals, January 23, 1961.

*J.B.329, Lakeside Laboratories.

21. SANDISON, R. A.: Psychological aspects of the LSD treatment of the neuroses. J. Ment. Sc., 100:508, 1954.

22. ——, AND WHITELAW, J. D. A.: Further studies in the therapeutic value of LSD in mental illness. J. Ment. Sc., 103:332, 1957.

23. WHITELAW, J. D. A.: A case of fetishism treated with LSD. J. Nerv. & Ment. Dis., 129:573, 1959.

24. COHEN, S.: LSD: side effects and complications. J. Nerv. & Ment. Dis., 130:30, 1960.

25. SAVAGE, C.: The resolution and subsequent remobilization of resistance by LSD in psychotherapy. J. Nerv. & Ment. Dis., 125:434, 1957.

26. Harvard Medical School Symposium, Sensory Deprivation. Harvard University Press, Cambridge, Mass., 1961.

27. DAHLBERG, C. C.: LSD as an aid to psychoanalytic treatment. Ed. In: J. H. Masserman, Science and Psychoanalysis, Vol. 7. New York, Grune & Stratton, 1963.

28. FINK, M.: Discussion of reference 27.

29. CATTELL, J. P.: Influence of mescaline on psychodynamic material. J. Nerv. & Ment. Dis., 119:233, 1954.

30. ——: Use of drugs in psychodynamic investigations. In: Experimental Psychopathology. New York, Grune & Stratton, 1957, pp. 218-233.

31. HOCH, P. H., CATTELL, J. P., AND PENNES, H. H.: Effects of Mescaline and LSD 25. Am. J. Psychiat., 108:579, 1952.

32. ——, ——, AND ——: Effects of drugs: Theoretical considerations from a psychological viewpoint. Am. J. Psychiat., 108:585, 1952.

33. ——: Remarks on LSD and Mescaline. J. Nerv. & Ment., Dis., 125:442, 1957.

34. ——: Pharmacologically induced psychoses. In: American Handbook of Psychiatry, S. Arieti, ed. New York, Basic Books, 1959.

35. ——: Methods and analysis of drug induced abnormal mental states in man. Comprehensive Psychiat., 1:265, 1960.

36. MORSELLI, G. E.: Contribution a la psychopathologie de l'intoxication par la Mescaline. Le probleme d'une schizophrenie experimentale. J. Psychol. Norm. Path., 33:368, 1936.

37. STEVENSON, I., AND RICHARDS, T. W.: Prolonged reactions to Mescaline: a report of two cases. Psychopharmacologia, 1:241, 1960.

38. Editorial: Hallucinogenic drugs. Lancet, 1:445, 1961.

39. POLLARD, J. C., BAKKER, C., UHR, L., AND FEUERFILE, D. F.: Controlled sensory input: a note on the technic of drug evaluation with a preliminary report on a comparative study of Sernyl, Psilocybin, and LSD 25. Comprehensive Psychiat., 1:377, 1960.

40. ISBELL, H.: Comparison of the reactions induced by Psilocybin and LSD 25 in man. Psychopharmacologia, 1:29, 1959.

41. ABRAMSON, H. A.: LSD 25: The questionnaire technique with notes on its use. J. Psychol., 49:57, 1960.

42. HOLLISTER, L. E.: Clinical, biochemical and psychologic effects of psilocybin. Arch. Int. Pharmacodyn, 130:42, 1961.

43. ——, PRUSMACK, J. J., PAULSEN, J. A., AND ROSENQUIST, N.: Comparison of three psychotropic drugs (Psilocybin, J.B. 329 and IT 290) in volunteer subjects. J. Nerv. & Ment. Dis., 130:428, 1960.

44. MALITZ, S., ESECOVER, H., WILKENS, B., AND HOCH, P. H.: Some ob-

servations on Psilocybin, a new hallucinogen, in volunteer subjects. Comprehensive Psychiat., 1:8, 1960.

45. DRILL, V.: Pharmacology in Medicine, 2nd Ed. New York, McGraw-Hill, 1958, p. 249.

46. CHOLDEN, L., Ed.: Lysergic Acid Diethylamide and Mescaline in Experimental Psychiatry. New York, Grune & Stratton, 1956.

47. LUBY, E. D., COHEN, B. O., ROSENBAUM, G., GOTTLIEB, J. S., AND KELLY, R.: Study of a new schizophrenomimetic drug-Sernyl. Arch. Neurol. & Psychiat., 81:363, 1959.

48. MORGENSTERN, F. S., BEECH, H. R., AND DAVIES, B. M.: An investigation of drug induced sensory disturbances. Psychopharmacologia, 3:193, 1962.

49. DAVIES, B. M.: A preliminary report on the use of Sernyl in psychiatric illness. J. Ment. Sc., 106:1073, 1960.

50. ——, AND BEECH, H. R.: The effect of 1-Arylcyclohexylamine (Sernyl) on twelve normal volunteers. J. Ment. Sci., 106:912, 1960.

51. BIEL, J. H., NUHFER, P. A., HOYA, W. K., LEISER, H. A., AND ABOOD, L. G.: Cholinergic blockade as an approach to the development of new psychotropic drugs. New York Acad. Sciences, 96:251, 1962.

52. MEDUNA, L. J., AND ABOOD, L. G.: Studies of a new drug (Ditran) in depressive states. J. Neuropsychiat., 1:1, 1959.

53. BERCEL, N. A.: Clinical experience with a new type of antidepressant drug: Ditran. J. Neuropsychiat., 2:271, 1961.

54. GERSHON, S., AND OLARIU, J.: J.B.329—A new psychotomimetic. Its antagonism by Tetrahydroaminacrin and its comparison with LSD, Mescaline and Sernyl. J. Neuropsychiat., 1:283, 1960.

55. LEBOVITZ, B. Z., VISOTSKY, H. M., AND OSTFELD, A. M.: LSD and J.B.318: A comparison of two hallucinogens. Arch Gen. Psychiat., 7:39, 1962.

56. JANSSEN, W. C.: Asst. Dir. of Clinical Research, Lakeside Laboratories, Inc., Milwaukee, Letter dated January 17, 1962.

Progressive Leucotomy

by H. J. Crow, M.A., M.B., Ch.B., R. Cooper, Ph.D. and
D. G. Phillips, F.R.C.S.

I N PATIENTS whose disabling psychological symptoms seem to be caused
or maintained by an otherwise ineradicable anxiety-tension state or
obsessional syndrome, some form of frontal leucotomy is a treatment to
be seriously considered.

Since many such patients are young adults, of good intelligence and
personality, and sometimes have heavy responsibilities, surgeons have
been striving in the past decade and more to relieve the symptoms without producing the emotional blunting and intellectual and social deterior-
ations which only too often followed the earlier forms of frontal
leucotomy. The trend has been towards smaller lesions in more carefully
selected regions of the frontal lobes. These developments have greatly
reduced the frequency and severity of unwanted side-effects, and many
psychiatrists have been glad to turn again to a form of treatment that,
for a time, fell into disfavour.

Despite the advances achieved in delicacy of psycho-surgery, undesirable side effects still do occur, and the search continues for greater
refinement and better control in the surgical procedures. There are,
however, fundamental difficulties facing the surgeon in his quest for
improved techniques. These arise partly from individual variations in
neuranatomy but mainly from the serious lack of knowledge concerning
the anatomical and physiological basis of most psychiatric symptoms; it
is difficult to predict with consistency the effect of a certain size and
site of lesion in any particular patient. An operation in which the site
and size of a brain lesion is determined without any knowledge of the
patient's reaction to it can take only a crude cognisance of the variability
and idiosyncrasy of man's anatomy, thinking, feeling and behaving.

Temporary, trial leucotomy has been attempted by injection of pro-
caine in, or by cooling of the frontal tissues, but these techniques are
seriously limited in their scope and delicacy. White, Sweet, and Hackett[1]
devised a method of leaving one or two coagulating electrodes in each of

the frontal lobes for some time, to allow the lesion to be enlarged at a later date if the clinical state indicated the need. The electrodes could be partly withdrawn and more coagulation performed, thus permitting treatment of different sites along the line of the electrode.

Since 1958 we have been using a method of leucotomy in which a large number of very small electrodes are implanted in the frontal lobes and left in place for periods up to 7 months. Electro-coagulation of tissue is performed, in progressive steps, by passing direct current through selected electrodes. This technique has several advantages over other methods.

(1) By recording the EEG during electrical stimulation it is possible to test whether the electrodes are in white or grey matter and thus avoid the formation of scars in the orbito-frontal grey matter which is known to be especially epileptogenic.

(2) The region of frontal white matter, the destruction of which is most likely to help the patient, can often be selected by a "polarizing" technique (see below). This is, in effect, a trial and reversible error leucotomy of a very small region of white matter, the site of which is clearly defined radiologically.

(3) The sites for destruction having been selected from the results of the "polarizing" tests and by inspection of roentgenograms, the size and number of lesions can be graded to match the patient's symptomatic and personality needs. Since the size and number of lesions are gradually increased over a period of weeks and months, undesirable side effects can be avoided or minimised.

(4) Since the plug assembly of the electrodes, which is strapped to the scalp, is quite small, and completely hidden under normal headgear, the patient can go outside the hospital, and even home, and to work, during the course of treatment. In this way, the benefits of treatment can be tested under the real environmental stresses of the world to which he must return.

(5) Since the actual treatment is undertaken some time after the surgical intervention and is planned and conducted by the psychiatrist, the doctor-patient relations are continuous and personal; this encourages combination of psychotherapeutic and physical treatment in tranquil and familiar surroundings.

The method has been described in detail elsewhere[2] and details not discussed here will be found in that paper. Briefly, the technique involves the stereotactic implantation through two burr-holes of ten sheaves of insulated wire, providing twenty-four to thirty-four gold electrodes (4 mm. long, 150 μ diameter) in each frontal lobe (fig. 1 and 2). A few days after implantation, electrical stimulation and recording at each electrode enables identification of the electrodes which are lying in or

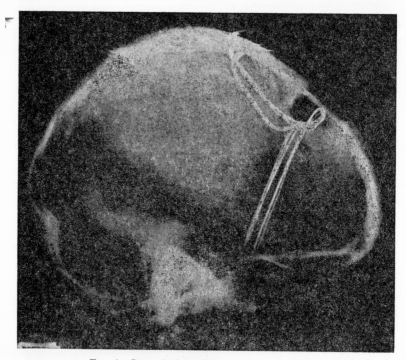

Fig. 1. Lateral view of the electrode sheaves.

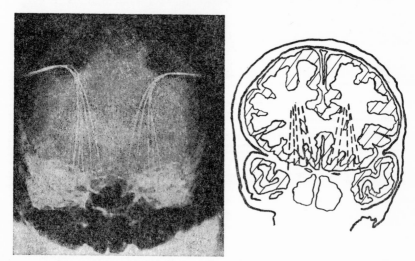

Fig. 2. Left, antero-posterior view of the electrode sheaves. Right, diagram showing the disposition of the individual electrodes in the brain tissue. The cross hatched portion represents the grey matter. (The section is taken from Cranio-Cerebral Topometry in Man by Delmas and Pertuiset, published by Masson & Cie, Paris, and Blackwell Scientific Publications, Oxford).

near to grey matter. These electrodes are never used for coagulation. When the patient is well recovered from the effects of the insertion (which may itself produce some slight symptomatic relief), testing and treatment is commenced. All these procedures are performed with the patient fully conscious and alert, cooperating to his maximum ability in the estimation of the clinical effects of the electrical manipulations of his brain state. Whilst any tests or treatments are being performed the clinician sits at the bedside talking to the patient, exploring the psychiatric problems, asking for subjective impressions from the patient, and noting any objective changes in his state.

The electrolytic lesions are made by passing direct current between selected electrodes and a cathode on the arm. The current can be preset to any value up to 20 mA, and the time of rise and fall, to and from this value, is variable from 1 to 60 seconds. In this way undesirable stimulating effects are reduced.

With the patient fully conscious and lying comfortably on a bed, low currents (1 mA for 15 sec.) are passed in turn through each of the electrodes lying in frontal white matter. (A more rapid procedure is to connect two or three electrodes together and double or treble the current). We have found that it is possible to relieve symptoms when certain electrodes are "polarised" in this way, and that this relief may persist for periods varying from 15 minutes to 24 hours. This temporary relief may be due to very small amounts of permanent damage, with other fibres later taking over the function of those destroyed; or it may be due to temporary electrotonic change in fibres which subsequently recover. After symptoms have returned polarization of the same electrode at the same time or slightly higher current value (for the same length of time) will again produce temporary relief. Thus is achieved a reversible focal functional leucotomy.

In cases where "polarization" does not produce any obvious relief to the patient, we select regions for coagulation where previous experience of others and ourselves leads us to expect benefit.

Coagulation of the selected brain regions is achieved by passing progressively larger quantities of electricity through the electrodes. The steps are usually 2 mA for 15 sec., 5 mA for 15 sec., 10 mA for 60 sec., and mounting usually to 20 mA for 180 sec. Occasionally in selected regions we have passed 20 mA for 6 minutes through the electrode. In a session lasting about an hour, up to six electrodes can be treated in this way.

Experiments on fresh cadaver brain have shown that 10 mA passed for 3 minutes through a gold electrode, 4 mm. long and 150 μ diameter, produces a macroscopic lesion 5 by 3 mm.

CLINICAL RESULTS

During the four years since this procedure was introduced we have completed treatment in 14 patients. The follow-up periods range from 2 months to 3½ years. The smallness of this series is an indication of the conservative criteria for the selection of patients and the deliberation with which the progressive technique has been developed.

Our criteria for selecting patients for this treatment probably do not differ very much from those used in recent years in most psychiatric clinics where frontal leucotomy is practised. The essential requirement is that the patient should have been seriously disabled for a long time, and has not had a prolonged remission with non-surgical treatments.

All the patients in this series have been afflicted by strong anxiety-tension feelings, either chronically or repeatedly over a prolonged period. In all but one case the anxiety-tension could be said to be basic to the illness (primary fear state). In the cases selected for treatment other symptoms (such as unreality feelings, specific phobias, including fear of organic disease, so-called depressions, difficulty in concentrating, hallucinatory experiences, and mild drug addictions) were considered to be secondary to the basic propensity to fear. Unlike some psychological theorists, we do not distinguish, in quality, between anxiety and fear. We believe that they represent different intensities of the same specific physiological activity in the brain.

We have not considered for leucotomy patients suffering from the classical thought disorder of schizophrenia as described by Bleuler.[3] We also excluded those whom we considered were unlikely to be able to co-operate in the treatment either because of defective intelligence or because of the severity of the loss of self-control induced by the illness.

The effectiveness of the trial leucotomy by "polarization" has varied greatly from patient to patient. However, in 9 of our 14 patients, we obtained some clinical changes, guiding us to particular regions for destruction by electro-coagulation.

The results of treatment in the 14 cases are summarised in table 1. The comments in the final columns give an indication of the relief from symptoms and an impression of the coarse adjustments that the patients have made in their lives. But what of the fine adjustments which this treatment has been trying to achieve?

In 11 of the cases, social behaviour, tact, and thoughtfulness for others have not fallen below the individual's preoperative standard. In 6 of these patients, these qualities seem to have improved since they were released from their illness.

Intelligence is known to be little affected by the modern fractional leucotomies and our small group also shows this absence of gross effect. In fact a few cases have shown improvement in their I.Q. test scores after treatment, thus supporting what is commonly believed, that anxiety of pathological degree can reduce intellectual efficiency and judgment in an important way.

There are three unsatisfactory results. One (IR) is relapsing in his phobic symptoms, although he is the only patient to show affective blunting. He probably received more treatment than his basic personality structure warranted. The second unsatisfactory result is in a lady (Mrs. D. P.) who is well relieved of her symptoms, with maintenance of her intellect, but who has lost domestic initiative and attentiveness, although her social behaviour is superficially normal. The recent birth of a child has improved the domestic situation, the baby presumably acting as an ever-present psychic stimulant. This is a case in whom too many lesions were made, although this did not become apparent until many weeks after the completion of treatment. In the third case (Miss M. N.) the result is partly unsatisfactory. We deliberately reduced her general attentiveness, since this seemed to be the only way to relieve a very distressing symptom. A long lasting anxiety state had been relieved by a moderate amount of treatment, but another symptom was untouched. To any sudden sound, of even moderate degree, such as a hand clap, her whole body jerked in a massive startle response. She was relieved of this by reduction of her "attentiveness" by further treatment. Her present happiness and satisfactory domestic and social state have been bought at a cost of loss of ability in her previous work. Her basic intelligence is probably little, if at all impaired since the first post-leucotomy I.Q. score had not fallen, although a later one showed considerable apparent loss of intelligence, thought to be due to inattentiveness.

DISCUSSION

Figure 3 is a diagram of a coronal section of brain, about 0.5 cm. anterior to the anterior clinoids, where the electrodes lie. The figure

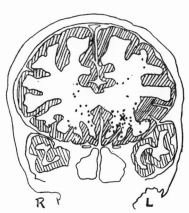

Fig. 3. Composite diagram showing electrode positions at which polarisation has produced temporary relief of symptoms.

TABLE 1.

Case	Sex & Age	Duration of Illness	Nature of Illness	No. of Hospital Admissions	Length of Current Hosp. Stay	Previous Treatments	No. of Lesions	Total Coulombs (Amp. secs)	Follow-up	Degree of Symptom Relief %	Present life
Mrs. R.C.	F36	18 years	Primary fear state, presenting with obsessional fears of murdering, & committing suicide, & unreality feelings	3	3½ years	Psycho-therapy, E.C.T.—several courses, Drugs	16	29	3½ years	100	Living at home, doing normal household duties; diligent and sociable.
Mrs. M.N.	F59	10 years	Primary fear state, presenting as agiated, panic states	3	Admitted for Leucotomy	Psycho-therapy, E.C.T.—several courses, Drugs	19	24	2½ years	100	Living a happy full life at home; sociable and kind
F.S.	M46	6 years	Primary fear state, presenting as inability to meet & talk to people	2	Admitted for Leucotomy	Psycho-therapy, Drugs	32	56	2 years	100	Living at home; resigned from original job because of ambition drive; present work, so far, less remunerative
R.B.	M52	7 years	Primary fear state, presenting as panic attacks	3	Admitted for Leucotomy	Psycho-therapy, Drugs	21	31	1½ years	80	Living at home; working with original efficiency; progressive expansion of social activities
Mrs. I.B.	F50	5 years 3 previous attacks	Primary fear state, presenting as panic attacks, trembling, headaches	5	Admitted for Leucotomy	Psycho-therapy, E.C.T., Drugs	26	79	1 year	95	Living at and managing her home; doing part-time work also; her social life has returned to its usual state
Miss M.N.	F44	14 years intermittent	Primary fear state, presenting with multiple anxieties and guilts	2	10 months	Psycho-therapy, Drugs	35	126	1 year	100	Living happily at home; socially she is completely satisfactory, but her working ability (draughtsman) has dropped considerably
H.M.	M39	16 years	Primary fear state, presenting with multiple anxieties, bizarre twitchings, & sodium amytal addiction	6	Admitted for Leucotomy	Psycho-therapy, Drugs	34	110	1 year	100	Living happily at home; attending business course to fit himself for promotion in his original type of work
Miss F.R.	F34	10 years	Primary fear state, presenting with tensions & weeping panics	3	11 months	Psycho-therapy, E.C.T., Drugs	45	155	11 months	80	Working for first time in 7 years; maintaining herself in lodgings, & taking active part in social life

TABLE 1. (continued)

Case	Sex & Age	Duration of Illness	Nature of Illness	No. of Hospital Admissions	Length of Current Hosp. Stay	Previous Treatments	No. of Lesions	Total Coulombs (Amp. secs)	Follow-up	Degree of Symptom Relief %	Present life
Mrs. D.P.	F36	5 years	Primary fear state, with paralysing terror agitations & guilt feelings, and paranoid tendencies; actively suicidal	4	Admitted for Leucotomy	Psycho-therapy, E.C.T., Drugs	37	88	1½ years	90	Maintaining herself at home; inattentive in domestic affairs but socially nearly normal; the birth recently of a baby has improved her interest in & attention to her domestic life
I.R.	M42	7 years	Primary fear state, with several different phobias. Talk of suicide. Reactive alcoholism.	2	Admitted for Leucotomy	Psycho-therapy, Drugs, Aversion therapy	37	113	10 months	75	Returned to work but working poorly; relapsing in some symptoms; sense of responsibility has deteriorated; no return of alcoholism
Mrs. H.W.	F36	12 years	Primary fear state, with tension & inability to meet people, and intermittent drug addictions	6	Admitted for Leucotomy	Psycho-therapy, Drugs, E.C.T.	21	38	3 months	90	Living at home; has made many social advances; has entertained guests, and made new friends
Mrs. J.W.	F36	Lifelong symptoms. Breakdown 4 yrs. ago	Primary obsessional thinking, with reactive anxieties, & withdrawals into compulsive "thinks"	4	1 year	Psycho-therapy, E.C.T., Drugs	19 *	42 *	2 months	75	Although still in hospital for rehabilitation, there are signs of a fundamental change in her thinking habits, of which she and we are aware; has been on home trial leave for one month, during which she did all house work and looked after husband and 5 year old baby; she has never before been able to do this
M.E.	M40	14 years	Primary fear state, with psycho-somatic manifestations	4	Admitted for Leucotomy	Psycho-therapy, E.C.T., Drugs	30	144	3 months	80	Making optimistic and happy adjustments in home, and making realistic plans for future employment
F.D.	M40	10 years	Primary fear state, with psycho-somatic manifestations, and unable to be outside hospital	2	1 year	Psycho-therapy, E.C.T., Drugs	26	90	3 months	90	Now able to be at home, and elsewhere, for periods up to a month, without difficulty; mild head psycho-somatic symptom persists

*Coagulations performed in region of cingulate gyri (see Discussion).

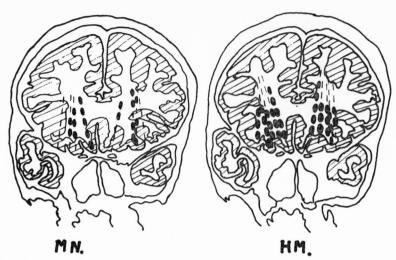

FIG. 4. Comparison of amounts of coagulations in cases H.M. and Mrs. M.N.

represents a composite survey of our 14 patients. Each dot on the diagram marks the position of an electrode, through which the passage of a polarizing current produced a reduction in the anxiety-fear emotion. So well demarcated in this region and so constant the type of response to a current which reduces or abolishes axonal function, that it is suggested that the region is part of a brain "fear system." This name implies greater specificity of action of this brain region than some commentators will allow; but our results do suggest this specificity.

It is in this region of supra-orbital white matter that most of the coagulation has been performed. As was expected there has been a considerable variation in the amount of coagulation required to relieve the illness of the different patients. Figure 4 shows the amount of coagulation performed in two patients, who have both made excellent recoveries. One of the patients required four times more coagulation than the other. This and table 1 demonstrates how widely different patients' needs can vary, and how important it is to attempt to match the lesion to the patient.

We have some interesting examples of how thought processes are modified when the activity of the fear-producing brain region is changed by polarization. One patient (Mrs. R. C.) had a temporary reduction of her chronic fear each time we polarized in the electrode position marked x in figure 3. One day before polarization began, she discussed a complaint of "confusion" which she often had as well as the fear. This was not like an organic type of confusion. It was as if her thoughts were whirling so fast around her head that she could not lay hold of one long enough to complete it satisfactorily. Immediately after polarizing at position x, she relaxed and smiled a little as her fear dissipated. She was straightway asked, "Tell me about your confusion again." She replied "Confusion? I'm not confused." This suggests that excessive activity of the hypothetical fear-producing system can disrupt the normal complex activity of the concept producing regions of the brain.

This patient had other symptoms of abnormality in concept formation. She "saw" a devil in her head, who "told" her to kill her daughter and then herself. These abnormalities also changed and disappeared after the fear was banished by coagulation of the orbital white matter. This sequence suggests that the abnormalities of concept (instead of being the primary causes of fear) were themselves fixed, and made symptoms, by the primary fear state.

Other observations made during testing and treatment suggest that another region of the frontal lobe has a specific function. We have noted that polarization of electrodes in the region of the anterior ends of the cingulate gyri produces a temporary change in performance that could be described as a reduction in the maintenance of attention, with immediate restoration of attention when significant stimulus changes occurred. For example, a patient, after polarization in the para-cingulate region, went off to shave. Once he had arrived in front of the mirror he did nothing except stare at himself in the mirror with a disinterested expression on his face. This continued for minutes, until he was told sharply to get on with his shaving, which he promptly did.

These observations suggest that the anterior part of the cingulate gyrus may play a specific part in the allocation and maintenance of "attention."

On the basis of these observations and ideas we coagulated para-cingulate white matter in two patients. One (Miss M. N.) has already been mentioned. She had a gross startle body-response to quite trivial sudden sounds. This was abolished when four electrodes were used to coagulate the white matter adjacent to the anterior end of each cingulate gyrus.

The second patient (Mrs. J. W.) deserves more notice. She is a married woman (now 36) who had felt since childhood an obsessional need to think out in detail everything she was going to do, and to consider in detail everything that she had done. If she was interrupted in her prolonged cogitations, which she called 'my thinks,' or was otherwise unable to complete them, she became assailed by feelings of guilt and fear. While she was single, she had been able to indulge her obsessional need for 'thinks,' by living a slow and simple life. But when a husband, and a home, and then a child were added to her life, she found the day too short for all the necessary 'thinks.' She broke down in a state of terror, exhaustion, and depression. Electro-convulsive therapy relieved the depression but made no difference to the other symptoms. Three stays in hospital were necessary in the 18 months before the insertion of frontal electrodes.

By the time the electrodes were inserted she had been in hospital for some weeks, and in the simple life there, she had lost all her fear and tension. She was calmly performing her daily 'thinks.' Therefore, apart from her 'thinks' she had no symptoms when treatment was being conducted, and the amount of destruction required could not be tested by clinical emotional response.

Eight lesions (all smaller than those made in more recent cases) were made in each frontal lobe, in the supra-orbital white matter. The wires were then removed, and she was discharged to her home. She was soon back in hospital again, her 'thinks' having been immobilizing her for many hours on end, even when faced all day by her hungry crying baby in the cot. For a further year in hospital she was given all the usual drug and psychotherapies again, without benefit, and she remained unfit to go home.

Our reappraisal of the situation was that anxieties and panics never occurred primarily, but only when she was prevented from completing her 'thinks.' We considered that there was a possibility that her cingulate gyrus, all her life, had been allocating too much "attention" to each conceptual mental event, thus giving her a "compulsion" to carry out her "thinks." Lewin's[4] description of how three obsessional thinkers were improved by anterior cingulectomy lends some support to this thesis.

We therefore introduced a cluster of electrodes into the white matter immediately lateral to the anterior 4 cm. of each cingulate gyrus and coagulated small zones in these regions. She soon began to show changes in her mental habits. She would give answers to simple arithmetical problems (e.g., 100 − 7 etc.) without checking and rechecking each answer in her mind before making her reply. This sort of casual handling of small problems is quite new to her, and she is delighted with this change. She is now progressively dropping out her ritual 'thinks.' She has had a trial month at home (with the electrodes still in place) and she was able to do the shopping, cooking and cleaning, and to look after her 5 year old child and husband, by herself, a thing she had never managed to do before.

She says she is sure that this treatment has made a significant change and improvement in her thinking habits, whereas the first operation did not. She cannot describe what has happened to her thinking; she can only appreciate an increasing freedom from compulsive 'thinks.'

SIDE-EFFECTS

Immediate side-effects of treatment have not been severe and the patients have not been disturbed. Headaches during the passage of the coagulating currents have sometimes been reported. Occasionally peculiar head sensations while the current is passing have been described—'like something moving in my head,' 'a crackling noise,' 'a squeezed feeling' —but usually the patient talks to the doctor as if nothing unusual were happening.

The current, in passing between the cathode on the arm and the anode in the frontal lobe must affect intervening tissues. When the current rises above 3 mA, its passage through tissues including the tongue, gives rise to a metallic taste. Occasionally the patient complains of a transient "flickering" in front of the eyes. This is presumably due to the effect of voltage fluctuations as a small fraction of the current passes through the optic nerves in the optic foramina. No deterioration in vision has resulted.

Sometimes during coagulation a patient has complained of a scalp sensation varying from "prickling" to sharp or burning pains. These are presumably due to the development of tiny holes in the insulation of the electrodes, brought about by continual acute flexure of the electrodes as they leave the scalp. Pethidine has been given to alleviate this pain and we have always been able to press the treatment to its conclusion.

Delayed side-effects of coagulation have included dull headache during the 24 hours after treatment; nausea some hours after treatment occurred in three patients; inattentiveness for some hours up to a few days after treatment has been noticed twice; usually there is a small rise in temperature (0.5 to 1° F.) in the evening after treatment. The patients sometimes sleep for an hour or two later in the day of treatment. Apart from the patients with neusea, all remained ambulant, ate meals in the dining room and mixed with other patients in an ordinary way. Indeed. so gentle and unfrightening is this treatment and so obvious are its effects, that other patients in the wards have been asking for it.

Problems

The most difficult and important practical problem is to know when to stop treatment since the manner and rate of response to intracerebral changes vary very considerably. Three types of reaction to the treatment may be distinguished:

1. Five patients showed improvement, which was maintained, after each treatment session; treatment was continued until a satisfactory clinical state was achieved. These patients have not relapsed seriously.

2. Four patients improved after each treatment, and then quite soon relapsed to some extent. It was a matter of two steps forward, and one step back.

3 Five patients, as treatment progressed over weeks, showed behavioural signs of remission yet they firmly denied feeling any relief of symptoms. Their own appreciation of their improvement came weeks or months later.

In these patterns of response there are two main types of mistake to be guarded against. The first is premature withdrawal of the electrodes. The first patient (Mrs. R. C.) got complete relief of symptoms after coagulating at four electrodes. After a fortnight of continued relief the electrodes were withdrawn but a week later at home she began to relapse, and within ten weeks was as bad as ever. A second insertion of electrodes with adequate treatment has since produced a complete remission. To prevent this sort of error occurring, we now do not remove the electrodes until the patient has maintained himself for at least four weeks after the last treatment in what we consider his optimal clinical state and in his normal social environment.

The second, and more serious mistake is to do too much coagulation in the patients of treatment-reaction type (3). Much weight should be given to their spontaneous day to day conversation and behaviour and general manner. Their refusal or inability to recognise or appreciate the observed improvement should be carefuly evaluated against their personal and cultural backgrounds. Thorough and repeated explanation of the mechanisms which are blinding them to their new potential for normal feeling and thinking will sometimes promote hopeful insight. They should be encouraged and their futures should be practically and optimistically discussed. It is a mistake to strive, by more and more coagulations, to get the patient's complete satisfaction with the treatment. In most of our cases the patients were still dissatisfied with themselves in some respects when we withdrew the electrodes. Subsequently, as the months of near normal feeling and living passed, their satisfaction grew; and eventually most have come to say that they are largely "cured."

Conclusion

Our series is too small, the follow-up in the later cases too short, and our patients too unmatched with those of others, to permit close comparison with the results of other procedures. However, considering that all the patients treated by this method so far had previously failed to obtain relief from the accepted psychiatric, physical and pharmaceutical remedies, the results must be considered promising. With increasing experience and confidence in selection still better results may be expected. Restriction of treatment to those cases with long-standing intractable disturbances must limit the chances of success, and we are now studying methods for earlier recognition of patients likely to benefit specifically from this treatment.

There are four features of the procedure which especially encourage us to persevere. The first is that it is *progressive;* the interference can be developed little by tested little, with ample time to wait and see without risk or disappointment. The second is that it provides for *tailoring* the lesion more neatly to fit the patient's symptoms, personality and social situation. The third is a subtle but important quality of post-therapy *personality.* Most of the patients exhibit a human warmth and friendliness, with a sense of responsibility and consideration that is too rare in post-leucotomy personalities. The fourth is the ease with which the manipulation of brain function can be *combined* over long periods with suitable psycho-therapeutic measures. The surgical operation is merely an incident in the relations between the patient and the therapist, who is able to exploit the obvious progressive changes in constitutional mental state, in order to promote and consolidate fresh and effective attitudes to previously insoluble personal problems.

The greater control thus exercised over the patient naturally imposes upon the psychiatrist a proportionately greater responsibility for accuracy of clinical judgment and therapeutic decision.

REFERENCES

1. WHITE, J. C., SWEET, W. H., AND HACKETT, T. P.: Radiofrequency leucotomy for relief of pain. Arch. Neurol. Psychiat., 2:317-330, 1960.
2. CROW, H. J., COOPER, R., AND PHILLIPS, D. G.: Controlled multifocal frontal leucotomy for psychiatric illness. J. Neurol. Neurosurg. Psychiat., 24:353-360, 1961.
3. BLEULER, E.: Dementia Praecox. (Translation 1950. International Universities Press) 1911.
4. LEWIN, W.: Observations on selective leucotomy. J. Neurol. Neurosurg. Psychiat., 24: 37-44, 1961.

PART IV

SPECIAL APPLICATIONS

The Psychotherapy of Stuttering*

by DOMINICK A. BARBARA, M.D.

T HE DEVELOPMENT of speech therapy has brought with it a greater knowledge of how the speech mechanism works, making for improved skills in the correction of both speech and hearing defects, and an awareness of the deeper, fuller meaning of speech in the complex society of today. If speech therapy is to continue to evolve and serve the needs of the individual, it must become more than a mechanical approach which, at one time, seemed to make the speech therapist merely some type of mechanic making motor adjustments. Today when some aspect of remedial speech work is sought, what is really being asked is help in fields intimately connected with personality and human development.

GENERAL PRINCIPLES OF PSYCHOTHERAPY

Kenneth E. Appel[1] recently defined "psychotherapy as helping the patient handle his feelings, motivations, and behavior more effectively. More formally, it is purposeful experience, providing opportunities for personality growth and improved health through the emotional interaction between patient and therapist, and when appropriate and possible, providing for the mutual exploration of the sources of maladjustment and the possibilities of improvement." Theodor Reik,[2] elaborating on the principle of the liberating effects of psychotherapy, stated: "Unconscious forces announce themselves, reveal their existence and effects; but they are mute or their language is not the one we speak. Their nature and their aims have to be guessed and have to be translated into words . . . What cannot be said or thought in words or word-presentations never happens as far as the conscious mind is concerned. It lies dormant . . .

---

*Summarized from author's edited volume, The Psychotherapy of Stuttering. Charles C Thomas, Publisher; 1962.

The effects of psychoanalysis are, to a great extent, related to bringing to light what is buried in the depths." In more simple, yet direct and comprehensive terms, psychotherapy may be defined as a human situation in which a therapist tends to influence another person—the patient, with words, gestures, thoughts, feelings, etc.; to guide him from a state of neurosis or unproductive living, to one of healthy, constructive or productive self-realization.

Stuttering as a speech impediment is both a personal and social detriment. As a symptom, it can be considered an outward expression of anxiety in conflict, secondary to an unhealthy personality development. The stutterer in his speech difficulty tells us that his lines of communication are broken not only with the world about him, but also in relation to himself. Therefore, it is essential that we approach the stutterer as a whole person, suffering from unhealthy relationships and neurotic difficulties which become expressed overtly when he speaks and especially so at the moment of stuttering. Only after we are able to help him work through his innermost confusion and entanglements, will he find real inner balance and subsequently achieve healthy coordination of his feelings and actions—including that of relaxed and spontaneous speech.

Briefly, the following are some of the essential aims in therapy:

1. To remove those forces which obstruct the patient's motivations for seeking help. People who come into therapy want to be helped because of their stuttering, phobias, headaches, difficulties in speaking or communication, inhibitions in work, etc. However, although these symptoms appear to be sufficient reasons for undergoing treatment and would not require further examination, the essential question to be asked is not "what is being disturbed?," but "who is disturbed?."

2. To help the patient overcome all the needs, drives, or attitudes which obstruct his growth as a whole; so that he can relinquish his illusions about himself and his illusory goals. In so doing, he can develop realistic self-concepts about himself and the world about him, and thus discover his true potentialities, real feelings, wishes, beliefs and ideals. Only when he faces these issues squarely, can he evolve a solid self-confidence, remove his existing conflicts and ultimately have a chance for real integration.

3. Finally, a knowledge of one's self must not remain on the intellectual level, but must become an *emotional experience*.

An understanding of and feeling for what goes on when one person talks and another listens is the foundation stone for modern techniques in the practice of psychotherapy. Disturbances in communication, when properly evaluated, are considered as distortions either in perception (listening) or in transmission (speaking). Therefore, most important as a corrective agent in personality disturbances in the communicative interaction between patient and therapist.

The first section of the therapeutic process takes place primarily on the conscious or verbal level. The patient contacts us, comes to us, verbalizes his psychosomatic ailment, anxieties, dilemmas, etc.; and in the initial meetings attempts to give us a bird's-eye view of himself. We can learn a great deal about these first impressions and instinctive feelings which are communicated either directly or indirectly through verbal, and non-verbal channels. There is meaning for instance in the stutterer's words, in his gestures, facial grimaces, his movements, his tensions, his pauses or silences, his reflections mannerisms, the many other communicating factors. The tone of his voice with its many inflections; the choice of his words; the pattern of his speech; the sense of rhythm and tempo in his gait; are all valuable aids in the total evaluation and understanding of his general make-up. The therapist must be trained to listen and observe holistically, so that he can grasp more astutely what is being communicated to him, not only in the direct, literal and verbal content, but in the many non-verbal expressions of hidden emotions, repressed feelings and symbolic clues, which go on incessantly beneath the more obvious levels of awareness.

After we have gathered pertinent data from our patient, the next step consists in our absorbing the data, deciphering their hidden messages, and then activating our own inner resources for a constructive interaction with him. In this process of communicative exchange, the therapist, while refraining from prejudice, condemnation or adverse criticism, must make conscious efforts to direct the therapeutic process toward producing in his patient a positive forward movement. In so doing, the therapist sets off a process of growth which takes place not only in the patient, but in the therapist as well.

Disturbances of communication, write Ruesch and Bateson,[4] are understood best by a participant-observer attitude, which enables the therapist to decide whether or not a person is suffering from disturbances of communication, and if so, to initiate the necessary processes for their correction.

The ideal psychotherapeutic milieu would adhere to a similar communication system, a spontaneous give-and-take of ideas, feelings and beliefs, and finally, an atmosphere where satisfactory exchange can take place. Though there may be an interchange of messages between two persons with different systems of codification and evaluation, it might so change as to effect meaningful and productive communication. Productivity, in this sense, can stimulate and channel energies in the direction of healthy self-realization, and away from neurotic self-preoccupation.

The dilemma that the therapist is faced with, however, is related to the undimensionality of language. Since observations vary from person to person and situation to situation, by the time the therapist draws any formal conclusions about what he has perceived, more recent sensory impressions have supervened and most of what was originally perceived is lost. The therapist can thus do justice both to his patient and to himself only by listening to the fullest of his capacities, abstracting, and condensing as he goes along (without causing too much distraction or interruption in the communicative system of interrelatedness).

Reusch[5] also believes that disturbances in communication are intimately associated with disturbances in sign behavior, language and symbols and that disturbances in non-verbal language (sign language or gestures, action language and object language) are associated with more severe illness than are disturbances in verbal language.

In language development we can observe a gradual shift from non-verbal to verbal codification. A schizophrenic, for instance, shows evidence that he has never learned to communicate non-verbally and cannot relate to others through movement and action. Manic-depressives show a loss of synchronization between verbal and non-verbal forms of communication. Some psychosomatic patients show a third type of disorder, an ability to use non-verbal but not verbal language. The psychopath uses, for the most part, action rather than words to convey messages to others.

Since the average man must use both verbal and non-verbal forms of language, therapy aims for the achievement of a balanced, complementary use of both forms of language. By helping the patient to use the various forms of codification in an optimal way, the therapist can provide him with the tools for overcoming isolation, increasing his self-respect, and cooperating with others.

The sensitive therapist will adapt his approach, style and technique to the individual patient. If he is to do constructive work with the widely differing syndromes seen in the course of practice, the therapist must, in a sense, be eclectic, drawing upon the many theories and practices available to him.

Working with the Problem of Stuttering

A preliminary survey of *all* symptoms and complaints is of prime importance. The therapist should then ask for information pertaining to the age at onset of stuttering, how and where it started, its connection with any traumatic experiences, and when the patient first began to associate the first objective and subjective feelings of anxiety with his speech defect. It is important to seek data concerning a specific familial history of stuttering, parental attitudes toward his speaking and toward his speech defect, and, most essential of all, the patient's own feelings and attitudes about his stuttering throughout his development, including his present attitudes about his speech impediment, in relation to himself and others. We can now arrive at some beginning working premise of the patient's predominant neurotic solutions, the extent to which he uses his stuttering as a neurotic device, and finally some insight into the degree of alienation present. Since we are treating the personality as a whole, we may question him about his ways of life, his habits, his likes and dislikes, his preference for others, his capacities, abilities, potentialities; and something about his dreams, phantasies, and imagination. As he speaks, we can also arrive at some of his possible reactions to ourselves as therapists; the manner in which he may attempt to avoid direct answers; the use of "bugaboo" words, or means of rituals and distractions, when he feels he may be about to stutter. These and kindred points of observation are some of the unlimited resources we have at hand in the first few initial interviews, which can be of tremendous importance as we proceed with the therapeutic process.

Stutterers for the most part use their verbal productions in such a manner as to set up a screen of resistance between themselves and the therapeutic process. They speak with intellectualizations, imparting a "broken record" quality to their communications. They take a great deal of pride in "wisdom" and "intellect," using their language to impress the therapist, rather than attempting to communicate effectively with him. They think mainly in terms of absolutes and, because of their fear of feelings, they are compelled to seek for logical and clear-cut answers to their problems. In their attempts to keep their conflicts at a distance, they tend to compartmentalize and rationalize a great deal of the time.

Stutterers use word associations whose communicative coloring is usually not free and spontaneous in quality. They may bring to the therapeutic interview an abundance of material, yet have little real feeling connected with it. As do compulsive neurotics who tend to experience their conflicts on the verbal level (doubts, compulsive thoughts) stutterers have strong defensive reactions against spontaneous emotional experiencing. They are interested mainly in talking, and in impressing others that they are willing to talk about everything. These are the individuals who may compulsively insist on reminding the therapist of their intellectual honesty and frankness. Since this interferes with the progress of treatment, it is imperative that the stutterer be educated and made aware of this blocking early in therapy, in order to promote a more "down-to-earth" atmosphere in the therapeutic relationship. The therapist should be on the alert, so as not to be deceived by this intellectual activity, and should attempt to aid the patient in looking "behind the scenes" of his own productions.

The following brief illustration of one of my patient's associations indicates the extent of blockage which interferes with spontaneity and freedom in communication:

"I couldn't paint my feelings, or express them verbally. They bubbled over and over in my mind. The only way I could express them was to write them down . . . I'm like a robot waiting for an electric charge, I feeling nothing . . ."

Dreams are also valid indications of our true inner behavioristic patterns. Stutterers have their own particular dream symbols. The stutterer, for instance, is a chronic blocker and hesitator in both the waking and sleeping states. It is not uncommon to find that in his dreams, many of his activities and other forms of expression—including that of speaking —become symbolically illustrated with all of their inhibitions and blockages. Stutterers, in dreams, see themselves as going in the wrong direction, as having slipped upon an icy pavement; unable to move their feet; having their mouth stuffed; their breathing stopped; their many actions and movements blocked. Their dream sequences are rarely completed because of numerous unexpected interruptions, such as fires, riots, explosions, and other unforeseen eventualities. All of these symbols are indicative of the stutterer's feelings of indecisiveness, procrastination and self-doubts.

The following two dreams of the stutterer's dilemma are illustrated in Dr. Emil Gutheil's[6] authoritative book, *What Your Dreams Mean:*

1. "I am sailing on a boat through a channel, moving straight forward. These are many branches of the channel right and left. They are all obstructed. Therefore I am sailing very fast."

Association: boats going through the Panama Canal have to be stopped in their course and lifted. In this dream we see the patient's speech represented by sailing. He is avoiding intercurrent thoughts (branches) and tries to speak as quickly as possible (a very common ambition of stammerers who attempt to overcome the supposed speech difficulties by speaking quickly). The patient's association offers a very instructive picture of the disturbance of speaking: the boat has to interrupt its course and has to be lifted on to a higher level. That is, indeed, what the patient does symbolically, when stammering: he interrupts his speech and elevates his thoughts to a higher level, leaving all the oppressing (painful) thoughts below.

2. "I was on a horse going over some jumps. The first jumps were ordinary fences with wings, the next jumps were single uprights. The horse had been jumping the ordinary fences well; he also jumped the uprights, but not so well. I had an impression that there was an audience." Addition: "There was a certain danger for the horse."

In this dream the patient's jumping over fences pictures his stammering ("there was an audience"). The "uprights" symbolize his complexes, which cause him difficulties (the horse jumps them "not so well") which he cannot overcome so easily. Closer examination proved that these complexes were connected with the patient's criminal impulses against his father ("a danger for the horse").

The skill to utilize and work with dreams in the therapeutic situation is of decisive importance in the search for hidden constructive forces present in themselves. It is our job as therapist to keep open passages in their neurotic road-blocks so that they can free themselves sufficiently to utilize such constructive forces in their struggle toward health.

Specific Blockages in Stuttering

In the first hours of therapy, the patient's motivations are mixed. His constructive wish for health is blocked by his need to keep the status quo. His pride may be too great. In the case of the stutterer, his exaggerated sense of self-importance, his vanity and egocentricity, interfere with his having a real sense of self-confidence. This along with illusions of himself as the "perfect orator" in the speaking situation, have to be undermined in order that he may make less imaginary claims upon himself and others, leading ultimately to a feeling of more solid inner strength.

A major problem in the treatment of stuttering is how to encourage the stutterer to stay in and continue with the course of treatment. To quote from a recent article by Benjamin Becker,[7] "It requires courage for the patient to move forward in the therapeutic process. It is the courage of the pioneer, who is moving into unexplored territory fraught with unknown dangers with which he must cope using new and untried weapons. Although growth and change are normal phenomena of human living, transition is not easy at any stage of a person's development and more difficult if there are neurotic impediments. Patients are often gripped by pessimism about their eventual growth. Their faith in themselves and in the therapeutic process sometimes wanes . . ."

Because so many of the adult stutterers have gone from clinic to clinic, from specialist to specialist, doubts and feelings of doom become fixed in their minds. They become skeptical and cautious about any additional therapeutic attempt. Their main idea about beginning treatment is to find a quick and miraculous cure to their stuttering. They have little insight into the many other associated personality difficulties, but see their problems mainly in terms of the speaking situation. There is thus little real incentive for receiving help in the solution for their problems, and a difficult area of resistance is set up.

In working with stutterers,[8-10] it is of prime importance that this area of hopelessness be worked through before any real therapeutic work can begin. As therapist our slogan is "blockages first." We must be alert enough to discover the patient's inherent and secret desires to grow, to bring these interests into the open, and thus encourage him to be motivated by genuine self-interest. Once the stutterer is reassured that he can find a way out of his dilemma, he will on his own accord challenge struggle and anxiety, and in this way develop a basic feeling of hope and faith in his ability to develop.

A second major blockage in stuttering is that of the actual stuttering symptom. The therapist who gets involved in the hopeless struggle to remove the symptom itself and does not work with the total character structure is easily caught in a tangle of intellectual discussions on the presupposed cause-and-effect correlations of stuttering. Only by approaching the stutterer as a total suffering human being, can we hope to help him grow into a better person, and with this ultimately give up his need to stutter.

The average speaker usually experiences his speech as his own and as originating from within himself. He feels a choice of his own words or group of words, although there may be some indecision as to word pronunciation. Once he makes his decision and voluntarily chooses his words, he will have little difficulty in consummating speech. The person who stutters, however, generally experiences his speech as alien to himself and as coming from somewhere outside of himself. His dilemma in speaking is experienced not so much in terms of "what to say," but "how to say it," with all of its explicit and implicit perfectionistic claims. The therapist does well in this instance to help the stutterer become aware and hear himself as he speaks. It is also important that the stutterer be made conscious of the manner in which he speaks in groups, to see how this compares with others who don't stutter, and most crucial of all, to feel that he is essentially no different from the rest, except for his difficult speech. Once the stutterer is made aware of the neurotic usages of his speech, he will grasp the destructiveness of its implications, and in time begin to relinquish it and thus verbalize a more healthy fashion through spontaneous group interaction.

Blockages in the therapy of stuttering are also prevalent in the therapeutic relationship. The stutterer's use of magical claims on the therapist creates a formidable obstructing force. He externalizes his own feelings of magic into the therapist, and endows him with special superhuman powers impossible to attain. He sees the therapist as godlike, and someone who can magically erase his stuttering, and without the slightest effort or struggle, pull him out of his dilemma. When the therapist sees through these maneuvers, the stutterer may use his affliction, with all of its appeals, distractions and its retreats, in a desperate drive to restore his weakening defenses. But despite his show of reluctance, the stutterer secretly and truly wishes his therapist to be balanced, firm, and consistent, and if the therapist fulfills these expectations he ultimately receives the stutterer's real respect and regard, is able to give him in return a sense of security.

A final blockage in the therapy of stuttering, is the maintenance of the "Status-Quo." The stutterer's tolerance for struggle is at a low ebb, and as a result he lives in constant dread of having his protective structures invaded or removed. He is highly sensitive to criticism and fears open discussion of himself, for he cannot face his conflicts squarely or bear their related anxiety. The stutterer also fears any open display of emotions, and protects himself by hiding behind a facade of intellectualizations, evasions and rationalizations. Should these defenses in turn fail, he may resort to his stuttering, or retreat by pleading helplessness and having abused feelings, or still further, avoid the conflict entirely by resigning himself to a state of pseudo-unity. In so doing, he feels he is able to save face in at least part of the struggle.

To be effective, the therapeutic situation must give the stutterer what he most surely needs, i.e.,—a sense of belonging, an atmosphere of union and unity, a feeling of respect from others, and a controlled environment. As the therapeutic process progresses the stutterer mobilizes and utilizes many more of his constructive forces, becomes more interested in discovery "who he really is," and begins to question many of his former attitudes, feelings, and beliefs. He can feel less dependent upon the opinions of his audience, have a greater sense of self-worth, and take more responsibility when he speaks. He learns to experience his words and expressions as his own, and has the courage of stand behind his own individual assertions and convictions. The more inner strength he feels, the less inadequate will he present himself in various capacities, including that of verbal communication.

REFERENCES

1. APPEL, K. E.: Principles and practice of psychotherapy. Am. J. Psychology, 15:2, 1955.
2. REIK, T.: Listening with the Third Ear. New York, Farrar Straus, 1949, pp. 453.
3. HORNEY, K.: Neurosis and Human Growth. New York, W. W. Norton & Co., 1950.
4. RUESCH, J., AND BATESON, G.: Communication—The Social Matrix of Psychiatry. New York, W. W. Norton, 1951.
5. ——: Non-verbal language and therapy. Psychiatry, 18:323-330, 1954.
6. GUTHEIL, E. A.: What Your Dreams Mean. New York, A Premier Book. 1957.
7. BECKER, B. J.: Relatedness and alienation in group psychoanalysis. Am. J. Psychoanal., 18:152, 1958.
8. BARBARA, D. A.: Stuttering. New York, Julian Press, 1954.
9. ——: Working with the stuttering problem. J. Nerv. & Ment. Dis., 125: 329, 1957.
10. ——: Communication in stuttering. Dis. Nerv. System, 9(47):1, 1958.

The Psychotherapy of the College Student

by DANA L. FARNSWORTH, M.D.

C ONCERNS WITH the needs of emotionally disturbed college students is relatively recent in American psychiatry. Treatment and management are as yet uneven and far from adequate. Beginning at Princeton University in 1910, the development of psychiatric services in college health departments has extended until now about 100 colleges have such facilities.[1,2] Most of them consist of one part-time psychiatrist, but a few are quite extensive. The best estimates (and they are only that) suggest that 10 per cent of the students at any college are likely to need professional help for emotional problems each year. About two to three students per thousand will become ill enough to require treatment in a mental hospital.

Psychotherapy of college students differs in no fundamental way from that of persons who are not students, but the special conditions under which it may be carried out in college are of great significance. Most colleges with psychiatric services allow psychotherapy to proceed without interrupting academic studies. If a student is too disturbed to do effective work, he is usually permitted to take a medical leave of absence to receive intensive treatment. When he recovers his ability to do satisfactory work, he is permitted to resume his studies.[3]

College students are usually more receptive to seeking and accepting help than an unselected segment of people. They are above average intelligence and hence are usually able to profit from new points of view regarding their problems and to develop insight into them relatively rapidly. When they come for help, most of them are in the early stages of disability and have not yet become fixed in the use of inappropriate patterns of defense. Many students have done considerable reading or have otherwise picked up many ideas in the field of mental illness and health, and have a certain measure of sophistication about them. Their ideas may not be accurate, but as a general rule they have an awareness of the interrelatedness of physiological, social and cultural influences in producing disability, even though they may be confused about their own emotional reactions. The most gratifying feature of all is that they are often quite responsive to brief psychotherapy. Behavior which on cross-sectional examination would seem to be ominous is often quite favorably modified by brief psychotherapy. Although some of these acute episodes might subside without treatment, this should not be taken for granted; many of them can be kept within bounds by skillful management, thus avoiding unnecessary admission to a mental hospital. At best, hospitalization results in a radical change in a student's life and in his subsequent concept of himself, and should be advised only when unavoidable.

In institutions with both graduate and undergraduate divisions the psychiatrists are consulted with almost equal frequency by undergraduates and graduates, but there is a higher proportion of severe and long-standing neuroses among the latter. Motivation for improvement is nearly always strong in both groups.

In Harvard University, one of the very few educational institutions with an adequate psychiatric staff, the number of students requiring admission to a hospital during the past three years has diminished by about one-half as the size and effectiveness of the psychiatric staff has increased. The suicide rate has also fallen markedly from that prevailing prior to the last three years. There is no absolute proof of any causal relationship between these changes. We believe, however, that improved attitudes of understanding and tolerance of many people in the University toward those with emotional problems is an important factor in the reduction of the rate of hospitalization and suicide. Some students who "act out" can create much strain in the community; it can be borne with more equanimity by those affected if they know the student is receiving help, if they have confidence in the psychiatric staff, and if they know the situation will eventually be corrected. The college psychiatrist must be cautious in over-burdening the community with tolerance of behavior which is deeply disturbing to many people. The needs of the sick person and the rights of members of the community to pursue their work without interruption should both be kept in mind and a balance must be maintained between them.

The effectiveness of psychotherapy with college students depends, therefore, in large measure on the personal characteristics of the therapist himself. Students are embarrassingly quick to sense insecurity in the therapist, especially when reassurance is unwisely given. One student with early schizophrenia expressed his sentiment to an inadequate therapist by saying, "Don't make mud pies with me!" The prime requisite for the college psychiatrist is, of course, a sound knowledge of general psychiatry including the principles of psychoanalytically oriented psychotherapy since in college the latter is his most used tool. He should realize the contributions that can be made when psychiatrists, psychologists, sociologists and anthropologists work together. He should also keep in mind the biological bases of his discipline. A sure way to lose usefulness on a college campus is for the psychiatrist to retreat to the absolute privacy of one-to-one relationships with students, omitting close communication with his colleagues in other medical specialties, and with deans, counselors, leaders in student government and, when appropriate, the parents of students. It is true that the confidentiality of the physician-student relationship must be preserved, but there are many ways of doing this. The student, too, must live in a real world. He knows that if his parents know he is in treatment and ask to talk with his psychiatrist something must be done to avoid discourtesy at the very least. If the psychiatrist discusses the situation with the student, explaining what he will or will not discuss, the student will almost always give him permission to use his own judgment. If he refuses, that must be made known to the parents who will then have some awareness of the depth and complexity of their son's or daughter's emotional state. The same general principles apply to communications with deans, faculty, advisers, or others who have been involved in a student's problems.[4]

The college psychiatrist should know the ground rules regarding confidentiality—the fact that he has a duty to his patients as well as to the institution need not put him in an awkward position.[5] He should know something of the curriculum available to his students, so that he can appreciate the nature of some of the quandaries faced by them in making choices. He should be familiar with the intellectual capacity of the students as these are estimated by the admissions office or by any special group within the institution working on such problems. The rules, customs and methods of operation of the administrative board, discipline committee, academic regulations or educational policy committees, or any such group that upholds the standards of the college, should be well known to him.

A few general principles at the operational level may be found useful. One should not ask for special favors for a patient. Informing the proper official, after gaining permission, of a student's situation is usually sufficient to bring about whatever degree of flexibility is needed. In fact, a college psychiatrist should have no authority over a student (nor should any other college physician for that matter) but only the privilege of acting as a consultant to those who do—instructors, deans, and other administrators. Grades should never be changed to encourage psychotherapeutic progress; this is frequently suggested by instructors who feel deeply concerned about a troubled student and wish to help him. Although environmental manipulation of a limited sort is often useful in helping students over temporary obstacles, this should very rarely be resorted to without the full knowledge of the patient. Even a disturbed student can count on some consistency in the behavior of those with whom he is having difficulty. If their behavior changes unaccountably, even for the better, and he does not know why, he may become even more confused: his reality testing ability becomes impaired.

Brief psychotherapy, oriented to personal, social, and cultural influences affecting the student, is the core of the work of the college psychiatrist. It is his experience in this essential activity that gives him the knowledge and justification for a wider span of functions that are of significance to every one in the institution. Without being unduly presumptuous, it might be said that the successful college or university psychiatrist takes the whole institution as his patient, trying to identify those customs, procedures, or practices that interfere with the attainment of the educational goals of the institution. The fact that he adopts a clinical attitude toward the institution does not imply that he thinks it sick, but he must seek out those environmental and psychological influences which appear to be deleterious and then try to remove them. He does not assume that all the students who come to him for help in the resolution of their emotional problems suffer from neuroses or psychoses. In fact, the more frequently he can help persons connected with the college or university solve emotional conflict before the classical signs and symptoms of mental illness have become evident the better he believes he is doing his job.

College students come for help because they are failing in their work, or because they are apathetic and depressed and are getting no satisfaction from what they are doing, or again because they are burdened and perplexed in a personal relationship that is inadequate, threatening and causes them anxiety. Sexual preoccupations are, of course, of major concern to many students. Students come at the suggestion of parents, girl or boy friends, deans and other advisers, and physicians in the college health services, but nearly half of them, in the well accepted and established psychiatric services, come of their own volition.

In addition to the kinds of emotional problems likely to be encountered by any adolescent or young adult, college students have some particular stresses which seem to be heightened by the many demands made upon them. Students' progress toward maturity is delayed by attendance at college in order that they may advance after the delay to a far more effective type of living than would otherwise have been possible. It is not only their earning power that is increased by the college experience; their capacity to deal with abstractions and to appreciate more of the subtle aspects of their environment is greatly enhanced. The concepts of identity formation, crisis, and role diffusion as outlined by Erikson are of fundamental importance to all who deal with college students.[6]

If one may judge from the comments and criticisms of students concerning the kind of help they have received from college psychiatrists, they appreciate warmth, competence, and a friendly manner. Excessively non-directive techniques excite little enthusiasm and often prove ineffective. Long periods of silence may be interpreted by the therapist as favorable to intense thought, but many students are merely annoyed by them and make assumptions about the therapist that are not very favorable for subsequent progress.

Some students try to put the psychiatrist on the spot by carefully scrutinizing his technique, comparing and contrasting what he does with what they have read about psychotherapy. This habit may be temporarily annoying to the inexperienced therapist, but it soon becomes another one of the attitudes to be examined, just as one might manage a student's attempts to intellectualize his difficulties instead of working them through squarely. Students' superior intellectual capacity may often be used in expressing resistance and hostility to therapy and the therapist.

The task of the therapist is simplified if college officials do not make undue allowance for a student who is having emotional conflict—at least no more than would be given to a student suffering from any other type of disorder. The college should hold students who may be patients to the same ethical standards as it does all others. What is wrong is wrong, no matter who does it. Understanding the motive behind unacceptable or unsuitable behavior is not to be construed as condoning or excusing the behavior. Critics of psychiatry often, however, make this accusation. The therapist and student patient work together in order that the latter may achieve self-control and a sense of responsibility. If the college administrators do not insist on their usual high standards for a student in emotional conflict, the therapist is handicapped and the student may become confused—or he may falsely assume that his illness entitles him to important secondary gains.

The enforced but desirable delay in maturation represented by going to college accentuates the dependence—independence struggle common to all young people as they break away from home. They usually receive money from their parents, they must look up to their college teachers, marriage is postponed or contracted under less than favorable conditions, and they commonly have some of their cherished values stoutly questioned. Religious, political, and social views which have here-tofore been taken for granted may suddenly be quite at variance from those held by their new associates.[7] Students with strong and well inte-grated characters can usually cope successfully with these and other similar problems, but the more vulnerable ones may need professional help. Those students who have had their energies absorbed in strug-gling with earlier interpersonal conflicts may find the crises of adoles-cence and early adulthood too much for them. Timely help for these "normative crises" may spell the difference between the ability to deal with stress or a regression to neurotic or psychotic modes of coping with problems. It is highly desirable to encourage students to realize that they do not have to look upon themselves as sick before they may con-sult a psychiatrist. The presence of an emotional conflict or predicament which interferes with one's efficiency and for which no ready solution is apparent is sufficient reason for such a consultation. A corollary to this is that students who have consulted their college psychiatrist should not, therefore, type themselves as ex-patients unless they do indeed have more than transient difficulties.

Fear of failure and fear of success are both common among students. They may go to quite unusual lengths to find a rationalization for not doing well. They may put off finishing a task they have set for them-selves if they are afraid of the new responsibilities which successful completion implies. Many a graduate student has been unable to com-plete his thesis because unconsciously he wishes to prolong his relatively carefree student status, not realizing that the assumption of full re-sponsibility would be no more strenuous than what he was already en-during. Fear of examinations, occasionally reaching panic proportions, is often a way of reacting to long standing personal problems. In my experience many of these have to do with ambivalent attitudes of the patient toward authority, whether parental or other. Fear of commit-ment to any vital principle is common, but it is much more subtle than the other fears in its manifestations.

Brief psychotherapy of college students may well be one of the factors that will ultimately demonstrate whether or not preventive psychiatry is possible. Blaine[8] has outlined its main components in a volume deal-ing with emotional problems of students as encountered at Harvard University in the 1955-60 period. These components include the giving of information or correction of mistaken ideas, an opportunity for the expression of strong emotions, the development of insight and helping the patient develop better reality testing ability. The transference is utilized in building trust in the therapist by the patient who has ex-perienced much rejection and by replacement, in the person of the therapist, of a role model for the patient who has had no such adequate guide. This is a temporary device and over-dependence must be avoided. Environmental manipulation is used occasionally but with great care. Drug therapy is employed but is of relatively little use in most instances.

Preparing students who need long term psychotherapy or psychoanalysis to enter upon such treatment constructively is another important task. Psychoanalysis is impracticable in a college setting, not only because it is not often indicated at this particular stage of late adolescent development but also because of the expense and length of time which are involved. For those cases in which classical psychoanalysis is indicated it is recommended without hesitation. Psychoanalytical principles are so ingrained in the thinking of undergraduates and of most psychotherapists that brief psychotherapy which is not based on them is likely to be received with scepticism if not with disdain. No college or university is able to furnish long-term psychotherapy for all its students. Even the largest psychiatric services are able to give only emergency and diagnostic services, brief psychotherapy to those who seem most likely to receive benefit from it, and longer treatment to scholarship students or others with no financial resources who cannot obtain appropriate help in community clinics. Others are referred to private psychiatrists or public clinics. It can safely be assumed that the need for psychotherapy among college students is always greater than is apparent to college officials, including even the college psychiatrist.

REFERENCES

1. ANGELL, J. R.: Mental hygiene in colleges and universities. Mental Hygiene, 17:543-547, 1933.
2. GUNDLE, S., AND KRAFT, A.: Mental health programs in American colleges and universities. Bull. Menninger Clin., 20:57, 1956.
3. FARNSWORTH, D. L.: Mental Health in College and University. Cambridge, Harvard University Press, 1957, pp. 155-156.
4. ———: Mental Health in College and University. Cambridge, Harvard University Press, 1957, pp. 138-141.
5. ———: Concepts of Educational Psychiatry. J.A.M.A., 181:815-821, 1962.
6. ERIKSON, E. H.: Late adolescence. In: The Student and Mental Health—An International View, Funkenstein, D. H., Ed. New York, World Federation for Mental Health, 1959, pp. 74-82.
7. Group for the Advancement of Psychiatry, "Considerations on Personality Development in College Students," Report #32, New York, May 1955.
8. BLAINE, G. B., Jr.: Therapy. In: Emotional Problems of the Student, G. B. Blaine, Jr., and C. C. McArthur, Eds. New York, Appleton-Century-Crofts, 1960.

Therapy of Homosexuality

by Lawrence C. Kolb, M.D.

ONE OF THE OBSTACLES to the development of effective therapies for conditions such as homosexuality is the failure to discriminate in a sufficiently precise manner the personality structure, the sexual behaviors and the conditions under which they are elicited in the various treated patient groups and relate these patient groupings to outcome by particular therapeutic techniques. The recent report of Bieber et al. does discriminate the effectiveness of one form of treatment in two differing homosexual groups. Bieber et al, found that 29 of 106 male homosexuals became exclusively heterosexual in behavior in the course of psychoanalytic therapy; further analysis of their data showed that a significantly greater number changed from an original bisexual orientation to heterosexual. It is highly probable that the etiologic forces which establish various types of homosexual adaptation are not at all similar. If this proves to be the case one might well assume that the therapeutic technique must be varied in accordance with the specific determining influences of the particular form of sexual behavior.

That there is wide divergence in the use of the term 'homosexual' is recognized generally. Thus, one may describe as 'homosexual' an individual whose preferred method of sexual gratification is through some overt sexual act with a member of his own sex. The term is also used to designate other individuals who alternate between heterosexual and homosexual gratifications. To some the 'latent homosexual' is considered to be an individual who gains satisfaction through fantasies of the homosexual act while by others he is personified as an individual with character traits of the opposing sex, e.g., feminine traits in the male.

Kinsey and his co-workers found it necessary when analysing their reports of homosexual activity in males to scale that activity into six different groupings. Purely heterosexual men were those who had no physical contacts resulting in erotic arousal or orgasm or psychic responses to individuals of their own sex. Individuals in group 1 were rated as having only one incidental homosexual contact involving physical or psychic

131

response, the rest of their sexual activity directed toward individuals of the opposite sex. Grade 2 individuals have more than incidental homosexual experience and respond definitely to homosexual stimuli, yet their heterosexual experiences and reactions still surpass their homosexual experiences and reactions. These individuals consciously recognize their arousal by homosexual stimuli yet prefer the heterosexual. Individuals in grade 3 respond equally, both at the physical and psychic level, to contacts with members of either sex. Kinsey's grade 4 regularly have more overt activity and psychic reactions to the homosexual, while still reporting certain heterosexual activity. Individuals in grade 5 are entirely homosexual in their overt activity and their reactions to the two sexes but have incidental experiences with the opposite sex, and occasionally react psychically to individuals of the opposite sex. Grade 6 are those homosexuals who are exclusively responsive, both physically and psychically, to members of their own sex.

The structural and psychodynamic forces that determined several types of bisexual behavior were defined recently by Wiessman. He points up the super-ego demands upon the homosexual which motivate him to attempt a heterosexual solution. Wiessman also describes homosexual defense against heterosexuality that exists in some men.

A rational therapy for homosexuality requires a solid etiologic foundation. There exists no sound evidence from genetic or constitutional studies to indicate homosexual behavior in men occurs exclusive of the molding process of learning as it takes place in the developmental interactions of family and culture. The developmental thesis, initiated by Freud and elaborated further by other psychoanalysts, is supported by a mass of clinical data from which the fully relevant and specific has, perhaps, yet to be extracted. Freud saw perversions as the consequence of interactions between the inherent physical bisexuality of the individual, his psychosexual characteristics, masculine and feminine attitudes, and the types of object choice. He and others formulated the developmental characteristics of homosexuality in the following way. In the earliest stage of development, the future homosexual evolves an inordinate mother fixation which later leads to identification with the maternal object. In the selection of a sexual object he seeks a man resembling himself (narcissistic object) to love him as an object. As choices of narcissistic love objects the homosexual either desires in another male what he sees in himself, what he was (his ego ideal) or some attachment to part of himself. An unresolved oedipal conflict derives from the overstrong mother fixation from which masculine identification fails to evolve due to growth in a family environment overinfluenced by a domineering mother, derogatory to the father. The latter may be either absent, feared or unaggressive. From the maternal attachment there occurs ambivalent flight with renunciation to avoid harm by her or through fear of paternal rivalry. The psychoanalytic theory also holds that a high value is set on male genitalia with an inability to tolerate its absence in the loved one.

If consideration is limited to those males who exhibit overt homosexual behavior at some time in their life the variability is extensive in both character structure and sexual behavior. So far it has not been possible to correlate overt homosexual activity to specific personality types. In examining men in clinics, prisons and remand houses in London, P. D. Scott found that those indulging in homosexual activity represented groups of immature adults passing through a developmental phase of attraction to both sexes, as one large category; and those with severely damaged personalities, including the effeminate female impersonators, the isolated, dull, inadequate person who had been deprived of a loving relationship during his lifetime, and the resentful, antisocial individuals. He found also homosexual men with intact and well compensated personalities. In the latter group were those who adopted homosexual activity late in life. There was also a group of individuals with serious mental disturbances of psychotic type. The common personality traits of the total group of men examined were inability to reconcile deep dependent and assertive drives, a persisting procrastination in all their activities, and highly ambivalent maternal relationships.

When we examine the range of overt homosexual behavior in the male its diversity is expressed not only in relationship to the time and circumstance of its initial occurrence but also in its frequency of contact, associations with overt heterosexual behavior, types of associated fantasies, as well as preferred modes of homosexual contact.

Thus early psychoanalytic hypotheses did not make explicit those forces which lead on the one hand to overt homosexual behavior and, on the other to latent homosexuality for both of which the proposed developmental sequence is the same.

More recent psychoanalytic studies have attempted to make explicit those events which allow the overt activation of male homosexuality. As an example, Johnson and I found in certain homosexual males that the establishment of the homosexual interest and its eruption into overt form appeared to follow the sequence of events which she and Szurek had described earlier as causative for the evolution of superego lacunae in children which permitted the performance of various antisocial acts. In the case of the children, parental sanction of aberrant behavior occurred through their unconscious gratification in the act of the child. While apparently prohibiting the undesired action in their transactions with the child they communicated through innuendo, errors of omission in correcting behavior, facial expressions or other non-verbal means, including personal acting out, their tacit consent to the action.

In the investigations of the male bisexuals it was possible for Johnson and me to delineate from the anamnestic material certain family transactions which also communicated permission for homosexual acting out, thus establishing the anlage for a superego defect in this area of behavior. More recently, data which both corroborated and elaborated the former hypotheses were obtained by my colleagues and me in psychiatric and psychoanalytic investigation of five pairs of identical twins in whom one of the twin pair was overtly oriented homosexually and the other heterosexually. From this study important factors which appeared to determine development of overt sexual behavior were the prenatal fantasies of the parents with respect to the sex of the unborn child, the difficulties at parturition which were reflected in later maternal attitudes to one or the other of the twins, the presence of slight anatomical differences which allowed early identification and specific mothering toward each of the twin pair, the sexual role significance of the name given to each twin, and the role of the father in the family. Once established, early differing role expectations directed to the individuals in the twin pair led to their divergent development through family and extrafamilial transactions. When the mother desired a daughter and gave birth to male twins she sometimes identified one with a birth mark, gave him preferential treatment, and rationalized her behavior under the explanation that his physical anomaly made him less healthy. She expressed through displacement to the other twin her negative attitudes to a father whom she derogated, and this twin was forced toward the father as a source of emotional support and identification. These attitudes influenced later object relations outside the primary bond which, in turn, reinforced the evolving divergent sexual roles.

It appeared in the study that the pre-oedipal maternal identification by the twin given preferential mothering led to avoidance and repression of erotic interest in females which influenced negatively later heterosexual experimentation. Prohibitions against homosexuality seemed effective in preventing eruption of such activity, even in the face of seduction, only in the instance of that twin who had tended earlier to identify with the father, whereas prohibitions against relations with girls seemed to determine the choice of sexual object and sexual acting out in the twin fixed to the mother who eventually became homosexual.

For treatment of certain homosexuals it may be crucial to have an awareness of the possible existence of a superego defect allowing homosexual acting out and of the development precursors in family processes which established this intrapsychic error. In a series of cases it was discovered that the eruption of overt homosexual activity took place in three instances following the interdiction of homosexual interest of the son by the mother associated with her willingness to have him contact men. The inference was made that the therapist would be perceived in the transference situation as a seductive person, intent on the patient maintaining contact with him and permitting outlet only in a homosexual sphere. In such instances the therapist would be perceived in the maternal role. Also in one instance the opportunity arose of observing the initial experience of overt homosexual activity in a young man in treatment with a young psychotherapist who had expressed, through his dream life, latent homosexual ideas. When the psychotherapist made a permissive statement the patient promptly and for the first time acted out his homosexual wishes. It occurred to Johnson and me that the passive listening attitude of the psychotherapist provided a pathogenic milieu for the antisocial acting out of homosexual drives in the sense that it implicitly suggests approval of such sexual behavior as it tends to maintain the destructive permissiveness of the earlier parental relationship. Furthermore, permissive statements made by a therapist, who has failed to develop the full understanding of the psychogenic sources establishing homosexual interest and drive, may lead to the act or provide impetus to destructive acting out.

It was suggested that the therapist should intervene and interpret the relationship of the patient to him on the basis of the established relationship of the patient to the permissive parent. In such an interpretation he must indicate clearly his position is other than that of the parent, that the aim of the therapy is to strive for heterosexual adaptation and that he is unwilling to accept responsibility for the continuation of the patient's aberrant behavior. Such an interpretation is timely when the therapeutic relationship exists as a firm, dependent contact and the associative material has evolved information of the maternal interdiction of heterosexual activity as well as her permissive behavior toward homosexual contacts. At this time the therapist may interpret for the patient the psychogenesis of the homosexual acting out and suggest to him restraint of such behavior as a means of "working through." Furthermore, at the time of the original publication, it was advised that if the patient failed to meet the request for restraint arrangements should be made for the patient discontinuing treatment with that therapist and being placed in treatment with another.

It is of interest to note that Anna Freud also has indicated in the treatment of one case of homosexuality in males her technique of requesting the patients to postpone their pathological satisfaction for increasing periods as a means of intensifying the analytic work through the prohibition of homosexual acting out. In one of her patients this technique led to recovery while in another the patient was unable to tolerate the frustration of the restriction. In a sense, this position is similar to the suggestions made by S. Freud for the treatment of phobias. Judging from A. Freud's paper, on neither occasion was the request to defer homosexual activities made on the basis of psychodynamic interpretation of the genesis of the behavior. It would seem probable, however, that A. Freud's request to defer acting out may have been interpreted by one of her patients as an interdiction differing from the learning which took place earlier in life and thereby change in behavior followed with a shift in superego function. The other patient's homosexuality may have evolved on other grounds which allowed successful use of the ordinary psychoanalytic position.

Since the original therapeutic suggestion by Johnson and me, experience has suggested that strict interdiction of the homosexual acting out is likely to lead to an interruption of therapy which may not be amenable to a successful placement with another understanding psychoanalytic psychotherapist. Further consideration of the treatment plan has suggested the force of the transference dependency as a means of accomplishing the same aim. Thus, in the instance of a male bisexual patient in whom the superego defect exists as described heretofore, a similar psychodynamic interpretation may be provided for his behavior associated with a statement that the therapist does not regard his relationships with members of his own sex as the mother, and also a request that he desist from acting out as a means for promoting the treatment. Such patients will respond to this therapeutic intervention with both overt anxiety and rage as well as the defenses they have customarily used to prevent the subjective experience of these emotions. Very likely they will act out on several occasions following the interpretive statement. At this point it is possible for the therapist who has established a firm dependent therapeutic relationship with the patient to reduce the number of visits to the patient as a means of indicating the need for working through with limitation of homosexual contact in order to pursue a successful therapeutic relationship. Deprived potentially of the emotional sustenance of the therapeutic relationship, the patient then makes the effort at restraint which establishes the modus for superego growth and new identification. Several therapeutic experiences have shown that under these circumstances there occurs, following the interdiction and the restriction of visits, an evolution of heterosexual fantasies on the part of such patients and heterosexual experimentation.

Another hurdle in the course of treatment of male homosexuality is the experiment with heterosexual relations and the anxiety that may be aroused pertaining to the occurrence of impotency at the time of such contact. In the instance of the bisexual male, this problem is less formidable since the bisexual male usually succeeded in such relations in the past.

The necessity for attempting the trial of varying techniques in the case of the overt male homosexual or bisexual is evident. The wide range of behaviors which are presently classified as homosexual indicates that one must consider not only the personality structure, and particularly that of the superego, but also the balance of satisfaction obtained through homosexual and heterosexual activity in the bisexual as against the castration anxieties and fears which exist in certain men troubled by their sexual deviations. It is unlikely that a single psychotherapeutic technique may be recommended for the treatment of all overtly male homosexuals or bisexuals. Just as so many other behavioral pathologies of varying psychogenesis are expressed through a single bit of symptomatic behavior, overt homosexual behavior probably represents a single expression of a wide variety of psychogenetic forces.

REFERENCES

1. BIEBER, I. et al.: Homosexuality. A Psychoanalytic Study of Male Homosexuals. New York, Basic Books Inc., 1962.
2. KINSEY, A. C., POMEROY, W. B., AND MARTIN, C. P.: Sexual Behavior in the Human Male. Philadelphia, W. B. Saunders, 1948.
3. WEISSMAN, P.: Structural considerations in overt male bisexuality. Int. J. Psychoan., 43:159-168, 1962.
4. SCOTT, P. D.: Homosexuality, with special reference to classification. Proc. Roy. Soc. Med., 50:655-660, 1957.
5. KOLB, L. C., AND JOHNSON, A. M.: Etiology and therapy of overt homosexuality. Psychoanal. Quart., 24:506-515, 1965.
6. MESNIKOFF, A., ——, RAINER, J. D., AND CARR, A.: Intrafamilial determinants of divergent sexual behavior in twins. Am. J. Psychiat. (in press).
7. FREUD, A.: Problems of technique in adult analysis. Bull. Phil. Assn. Psychoan., 4:44-69, 1954.

Hypnotic Studies of Patients with Convulsions

by Harold Rosen, M.D.

AND

A. Earl Walker, M.D.

A S MORE AND MORE psychiatry is included in the undergraduate medical curriculum and during internship training, we may be fast approaching the time when non-psychiatrist physicians will have the necessary technical training, theoretical background and clinical experience to warrant approaching epileptic patients with hynotic techniques. At present, however, this presents serious hazards.[4, 11]

Unwise hypnosis may endanger the patient's physical and emotional health and life. In May 1960, an A.M.A. Conference on Standards on Training in Hypnosis, in which representatives from 22 medical schools participated, concluded that if the well-being of the patient is to be safeguarded, physicians who use hypnosis need work in basic psychiatry above and beyond that taught on an undergraduate level in any medical school curriculum with which the conference participants were acquainted.[2]

Mere ability to hypnotize is on a par with mere ability to press the button that starts an electroencephalogram. We expect surgeons, when they do even simple appendectomies, to have the necessary background and training to take care of whatever complications may be encountered within the abdomen. The same dictum applies, so far as hypnosis is concerned.[1] It is a specialized psychiatric procedure.[3] The physician-hypnotist should therefore have certain basic psychiatric skills at his command.[5] Whoever makes use of hypnotic techniques must acquire sufficient knowledge of psychiatry, and particularly of psychodynamics, to avoid their use in clinical situations in which hypnosis is contra-indicated.[2, 3]

Our hypnotic investigations of patients with convulsive disorders illustrate this with the sharpness of caricature. Such patients are readily hypnotizable. Of 151 studied here at The Johns Hopkins Hospital between 1948 and 1960, only 13 could not be hypnotized.

Induction techniques were extremely simple. They can be taught physicians and medical students within 15 to 30 minutes.[5, 11] We never use the word "sleep." Some patients—so-called "actor-outers"—are merely instructed to close their eyes so tight they cannot open them. Negativistic patients are told that the harder they try to keep their eyes open the tighter they will squeeze together. Still others are given suggestions to breathe deeply but comfortably; to feel relaxed or drowsy; to close their eyes or to have them grow heavy and close; and the like. This is without fanfare.

The hypnotic situation can get out of hand. Even homicidal rage may come to the fore.

With one of our patients, for whom psychomotor epilepsy was suspected, it did. During part of the psychiatric evaluation, she was instructed in a matter-of-fact voice to close her eyes, to breathe deeply but comfortably, and to state whatever it was that at the moment she was feeling or thinking, provided of course she was feeling or thinking anything. This was stated only once. We were trying to investigate fantasy formation. At this she closed her eyes, began breathing deeply and, within 20 or 30 seconds at the most, was actively hallucinating the psychiatrist as the husband she wished to kill. There was no opportunity to determine whether this was her present husband or her former one, since with one hand she had seized a heavy-based 17-pound ash tray, brandished it above her head and swung it at the psychiatrist while screaming that he was her husband whom she nevertheless quickly rehallucinated as her mother. The psychiatrist ducked and grabbed the tray—but with two hands, not one. With her left hand—the tray had been brandished by her right—she grabbed his right hand and began forcibly squeezing it as her fingers twirled around his, trying to pull his hand off the ash tray while digging her nails into his fingers. Because she was holding the tray with only one hand, it was possible to wrench it from her.

She then screamed vituperatively at the psychiatrist. He was at times her husband, whose head she intended to bash to a pulp. To quote: "And I'll pull your balls off! I'll make soup out of them! I'll feed them to my mother!" Most of the time, however, she hallucinated the psychiatrist as her mother and, again, to quote: "I'm going to bash your face in! Then I'll pull your breasts off! I'll make soup out of them for my husband!"

She ultimately became silent, fell to the floor, and started to cry while kicking her legs and beating her clenched fists up and down like a two or three-year old in a temper tantrum. After about five minutes, she began to weep again but without moving since she was now too tired to do so.

The diagnostic impression was that of an underlying schizophrenia. A competent colleague, however, who saw her in consultation a few months later, felt that she was then neither psychotic nor epileptic. His diagnosis was that of an hysterical reaction. Yet before we saw her, this patient's automobile license had been suspended because of the diagnosis of psychomotor epilepsy.

Ninety-two of our 138 hypnotized patients, it should be noted, likewise had diagnoses of organic seizures. Forty-six had psychiatric diagnoses. Both groups otherwise were indistinguishable. Both groups included (1 patients with organic syndromes who had had psychiatric diagnoses, and (2) patients with psychiatric disorder in whom organic pathology was also deemed present. The usual diagnostic criteria, both neurologic and psychiatric, require careful reconsideration and re-evaluation. The approach will be through illustrative clinical case material as follows:

PATIENTS WITH "RED HERRING" NEUROLOGICAL FINDINGS

(1) *Patients with pronounced neurological signs, who occasionally lose bowel and bladder control during attacks, may nevertheless have convulsions purely on an emotional basis.* Patients not infrequently have neurological signs.[8] In some, a one diopter unilateral idiopathic papiloedema may be present. With others, especially if on long-continued medication, the drugs may produce neurologic findings (and cause a large amount of fast activity on the EEG). Occasionally, "eager-beaver" interns may record findings that later are not clinically reproducible; and patients who have been in automobile accidents, suffered fractured skulls and been comatose for a few days, may have abnormal neurological findings although their post-traumatic convulsions are psychogenic.

One patient, who suffered a head injury as the result of an automobile accident, had after discharge what was diagnosed as psychomotor epilepsy. Attacks were not well controlled. After a few years, she was referred to us for further evaluation. The usual physical and laboratory studies were reported as normal. In addition, she was investigated on hypnotic levels.

During one session, an attack was precipitated, and then blocked, by direct hypnotic suggestion. At this she hallucinated trying to stimulate her impotent husband sexually. She spontaneously terminated the trance, explained that she now knew why she had her attacks, and added that she would rather continue having convulsions than leave her husband. She could not realize that solutions other than these were possible. She left the hospital, was attack-free for almost two months, then had another, and was again seen. During an hypnodiagnostically precipitated attack in ten times slow motion,[11] she began making, as part of her apparent epileptic seizure, forced sucking movements with her lips while she enacted the fantasy of being an infant who was at first suckling at—and then trying to bite into—her mother's nipple. Her anger, and her underlying acute almost suicidal depression, now came to the fore. She was this time able to get into a good psychotherapeutic relationship, and was therefore taken off all medication. Neurotic conflicts involving her relationship with her mother had been reprecipitated by the sexual inadequacy of her Casper Milquetoast husband. As she began to realize, while working through early material in relation to her parents, how she had contributed to his impotence, he regained a measure of potency and requested treatment for himself—and her seizures ceased. She became warmer and more feminine. This was in 1952. Treatment continued for three years. There have been no seizures since, although she and her husband are still together.

(2) *Histories can be dissimulated, confabulated or otherwise distorted and falsified.* This is especially true of the physician (or nurse) drug addict who has a convulsion. This can be a withdrawal symptom. The physician-patient may have been on demerol—and discontinued it. Occasionally, causalgia or some other type of chronic pain may be utilized as the rationalization for the drug intake. This is usually concealed. As the anamnesis is taken, a history of apparent petit mal, sometimes over a period of years, may be elicited, climaxed by what from the description seems like—and usually is—a typical grand mal affair. There may—or may not—be some EEG abnormalities which are described as minimal or moderate, typical or atypical, generalized or not well localized dysrhythmias, "consistent with a diagnosis of epilepsy." Four of our physician-patients requested pneumoencephalography, angiography and even exploratory craniotomy. Their medical knowledge is sufficient to pull the wool over their physicians' eyes—neurologists, neurosurgeons, internists and psychiatrists—for long periods of time; very intensive multi-session psychiatric evaluation frequently is a *sine qua non.*

One such patient was a 32-year old colleague who for two years, so he stated, had had infrequent petit mal (or petit mal-like) affairs for which all studies (including those for a pheochromocytoma) were negative. During the psychiatric evaluation here, marked psychopathology came to the surface. Nevertheless, diagnostically—even after months of psychiatric treatment—there was much too much that seemed to evade understanding.

He was therefore hypnotized, without letting him know that he was being hypnotized—or so it was thought. His fists spasmodically clenched and unclenched, and his jaws clamped shut. He made only one statement: he knew he had been hypnotized. He intended to "un-hypnotize" himself as fast as he could, and he wouldn't utter a single word while hypnotized. Nor did he.

The psychiatrist agreed "If some one hypnotized me," this patient was told, "the way I just hypnotized you, putting something over on me this way, I would feel the same way. But I feel that you have been putting something over on me. This may or may not be so. So if, as I think, you are taking demerol, then after leaving here and before you return next time, you will—without harming yourself or any one else—decide on psychiatric hospitalization and have the arrangements made for it."

These suggestions were effective. Two days later while in his office he had a grand mal seizure, fell against the desk, fractured a rib, saw a non-psychiatrist colleague, and put pressure on him to arrange with us for psychiatric hospitalization "for his fractured rib!" As a physician, he knew how minor the fracture was. He needed this face-saving device, then explained that he had been taking large quantities of demerol, and was therefore treated in a psychiatric hospital for several months. This was in 1956. There has been no recurrence since. He is an excellent physician.

Usually, an adequate carefully taken history will clarify, rather than complicate, the diagnostic problem. But with this patient, as with a number of other patients in this series, it concealed rather than helped. Yet the fact that it was recognized as a "red herring" was itself of prime significance. From a wider angle of approach, it told the story.

(3) *Physical symptoms, likewise, may becloud the issue.*

This can be illustrated with the sharpness of an etching by excerpts from the case history of a 21-year old divorcée with some contracture of the right gastrocnemius muscle, a marked right foot drop, a mild generalized right hemiparesis, and a mild right central facial palsy. There were other neurologic symptoms as well. Three years previously she had been in an automobile accident and had been comatose. Since her recovery, she had had more and more frequent grand mal convulsions. These at first were well controlled by anticonvulsants. However, by the time of her admission to The Johns Hopkins Hospital, she was in status epilepticus. Her convulsions were characterized by what seemed an aura (a drawing feeling in the right forehead and face with a peculiar tingling feeling which she was unable to describe but which she had learned to recognize), followed by sudden loss of consciousness and a turning on her right side with legs drawn up and arms flexed close to her body, after which she would have clonic movements, lasting from two to three minutes, in all four extremities. She would then regain consciousness and be fully alert, but the right side of her face would feel weak. At times there was tongue-biting and, rarely, urinary incontinence. Electroencephalography here revealed no definite abnormality, aside from that due to sedation. Her previous head x-rays, pneumoencephalogram and arteriogram were reviewed and considered within normal limits. Because of the difficulty in establishing a diagnosis despite multiple trephines, subcortical electrodes were implanted. Numerous recordings were made with both electrical and metrazol activation. These recordings, some made during attacks, revealed no significant abnormality. The neurosurgeon was of the opinion that her seizures were not organic.

Her history was difficult to obtain. Her mother years previously had had seizures for six months before her death from a brain tumor. This patient had then had a few mild convulsive episodes. (This was not, however, known at that time, but learned during later hypnotic interviews; she was not consciously aware of this.) Shortly after her automobile accident she married, suffered pounding headaches, and experienced convulsions. She was divorced 18 months later, and her seizures became more frequent. Eight months after the divorce she was admitted to a local hospital with practically continuous attacks. Despite electroencephalography, pneumoencephalography and left carotid angiography, no definite diagnosis was established. She had a pronounced right foot-drop which improved with a walking brace and physiotherapy. Anticonvulsants in massive dosage were prescribed. Her seizures were at first controlled, then gradually recurred, increasing in frequency and severity until she was referred to The Hopkins for study. She reached here in a status epilepticus. By the time the psychiatrist saw her there were thirty-five or more attacks a day.

She was hypnotized during the 30 to 90 second intervals between seizures and then given authoritative suggestions that the motor activity of the attack cease. It was added that whatever her movements kept her from feeling or doing she would, instead, now feel and do. This was equivalent to suggesting, first, that the attack would cease and, second, that something else on motor or sensory levels would take its place[8]. A convulsion had already started before these suggestions could be completely verbalized. Her jaws clamped together, and she twisted towards the right. She was again told that her convulsion would cease but that if other movements had to take its place, they would. At this she developed coital movements, hallucinating, as it later developed, a former sexual partner on olfactory, visual and tactile levels. This was not known at the time.

This patient's anger, as the abreaction proceeded, grew intense. She began snarling and gnashing her teeth, then rolled over, brought both hands together so that thumbs and extended index fingers were touching each other side by side; then held her index fingers pointed rigidly forward, hands between her legs so that index fingers were where a penis might be; assumed the male coital position; and, while murmuring obscene threats to her hallucinated sexual partner, engaged in movements like those of the male during intercourse.

Her fantasies about male and female in all their oral sadistic aspects later became accessible for therapeutic investigation. This had to be considered—and treated—on pregenital levels. She was emotionally much too immature for this to be considered as sexuality in the sense in which, as adults, we think of sex. She was taken off all medication, and treated psychotherapeutically on hypnotic levels in sessions lasting from three to five consecutive 50-minute hours each.

Although pronounced neurological signs were present, her attacks were psychogenic. It was almost four weeks before they disappeared completely. She nevertheless, we thought, needed further intensive psychiatric treatment. She was referred to competent colleagues in practice in the State in which she lived but did not accept the recommendation. Six months after her discharge, she was able to start on nurses' training. Two-and-a-half years later, she did have another hospitalization, this time not for convulsions but for a phobic reaction which lasted approximately three weeks. No sedatives, barbiturates, tranquilizers or anticonvulsants have since been prescribed. She has nevertheless remained completely symptom-free. There has been no seizure during the 8 years since she was treated here.

It usually is stated that trained observers—nurses and physicians with a good deal of experience with epilepsy—can when witnessing seizures state whether they are organic or not. This is just not so. The typical appearance of the attack can itself be a red herring. We have at times been misled. A noted authority on epilepsy, who saw this patient with the psychiatric consultant while she was in status, told him that her convulsions were typical, had to be organic, and could admit of no other interpretation.

A comment would seem advisable at this point. Any patient who has been comatose after having suffered a skull fracture in an automobile accident can have abnormal neurological findings and may on discharge from the hospital develop post-accident convulsions that may continue not for organic but for neurotic or psychotic reasons,[8] so that seizures although observed by competent observers can not be distinguished from convulsions organically determined.

So-called *typical* seizures can also be patterned on actual convulsions which had been witnessed, or on somatic memories of a convulsive affair previously experienced. For this reason we frequently discontinue all medication—anticonvulsants, sedatives and tranquilizers—so that the basic behavior of these patients can be observed. The case histories mentioned show why we feel this is indicated.

Such patients may even lose control of the urinary sphincter during seizures. A 34-year old patient, for instance, who was on dilantin (400-500 mg. per day) had urinary incontinence during some of her seizures, although we later determined that these were on a conversion basis. This may occur with patients whose convulsions are the monosymptomatic expression of an underlying major hysteria, schizophrenia or other condition in which the patient regresses to the bed wetting (and sometimes to the feces-soiling) stage.

A second patient, a 26-year old woman, with an eleven-year history of epilepsy, was having some three to four convulsive affairs a week. The diagnosis of grand mal (organic) epilepsy had been made on electroencephalography in another excellent teaching hospital after attacks had been witnessed by a colleague with a great deal of clinical experience in the subject. Her seizures lasted from one to two minutes, were characterized by leg twitching, tongue-biting with falling to the floor and occasional loss of sphincter control, and were followed by complete amnesia for the attack. What more could one ask for? Yet, the first seizure which he observed occurred two or three days after she had consciously felt jealous of the child she was carrying at the time. She was convinced that her husband was neglecting her. She wished for an "epileptic spell" to obtain from him the attention which she did not believe she was receiving. When she was referred here for further study our EEG tracings were not pathognomonic. Because of patellar areflexia and bilateral pupillary anomalies, an ophthalmological consultation was requested. Even in dilatation the left pupil remained slightly irregular. The ophthalmologist's impression was that of merely bilateral tonic pupils. On intensive multisession psychiatric evaluation on both hypnotic and non-hypnotic levels, the diagnostic impression was that of a personality disorder for which her convulsions were merely a symptom; an underlying schizophrenia was suspect. Loss of sphincter control, therefore, is not necessarily a differential diagnostic factor.

Summary: There seems to be a continuum, in the pathogenesis of convulsions, (1) from attacks that are directly conditioned by neurophysiologic disturbances as reflected just as directly by abnormal EEG tracings (2) to those that express outright neurotic or psychotic conflicts. Of patients with cerebral dysrhythmias, there are ten or twenty without epilepsy for each one with it. Conversely, some patients with an organic basis for their epileptic attacks may show no waking—or sleeping—cerebral dysrhythmia. When patients are investigated hypnodiagnostically or in any other way, this must be borne in mind. It is not the hypnosis or the specific investigatory technique that is important, but the clinical judgment and acumen of the investigator.[8]

PATIENTS WITH ORGANIC SYNDROMES WHO HAD BEEN GIVEN
PSYCHIATRIC DIAGNOSES

The mere fact that symptoms may disappear even spontaneously on hypnotic induction does not necessarily mean that the problem is a psychiatric one. Lack of physical and other findings, the presence of emotional disease, or the use of the convulsion to serve neurotic functions—any or all of these can be "red herrings." On the one hand, apparent organic symptoms that persist despite strong hypnotic suggestions for their disappearance may be psychogenic. On the other, motor symptoms can be blocked—and blocked completely—by hypnotic suggestion, yet this does not *per se* mean that they must be emotional and not organic.[5]

(1) *A brain tumor may be present.* This was so with four of our patients.

The first was a patient for whom all neurological and other studies yielded essentially normal results. She was therefore—on the basis of negative physical and other findings, rather than because of positive psychiatric factors—referred for psychiatric treatment. The psychiatrist elicited a wealth of psychopathology—but with competent psychiatric study this can be found in any of us. He started to treat her. He could not, however, understand her symptoms in terms of the psychopathology otherwise present. He felt uncomfortable about this, and referred her to us for hypno-diagnostic evaluation. Regressive and fantasy-evocation techniques were utilized. Symptoms were replicated on direct hypnotic suggestion. Attempts were made to integrate these into previous reaction-formation patterns conditioned by neurotic conflicts with key figures in the infantile environment as stirred up by present intra-familial and other relationships. This could not be done. Since integration of this type seemed impossible, she was re-referred to her original neurologist for re-examination: her symptoms could be, so it was stated, but did not necessarily have to be, on a neurotic basis. Since it might be several months before this could be determined through psychotherapeutic evaluation and since some intra-cranial lesions develop rapidly, neurological recheck-up was advisable.

By the time she was re-examined, signs were developing. She did have an astrocytoma. Surgical intervention was too late.

(2) *Convulsions may be masked by psychiatric symptoms:* A still more complicated and complicating "red herring" can be present in the form of convulsions that are repressed or masked as outright psychiatric symptoms develop.

In one of our patients, seizures had alternated with obvious reactive or psychotic depressive episodes, disappearing as the depression manifested itself and reappearing after the depressive episode had been treated successfully. This was a "red herring" of the worst type. She, too, had a brain tumor.

This patient was a woman in her mid-40's who, after recovery from a depressive episode for which she had had psychiatric hospitalization, experienced mild infrequent convulsive affairs while asleep. She was immediately referred for competent neurological study. This was essentially negative. Her convulsive affairs disappeared with her later rehospitalization for six months in a psychiatric hospital. On her discharge her convulsive affairs reappeared. Further neurological and other studies were again essentially negative. She was therefore referred here for combined hypno-evaluative psychiatric and neurosurgical studies. Her attacks, as we discovered on hypnotic investigation, were characterized by almost homicidal rage against both husband and mother. They were reproduced during electroencephalography. EEG tracings showed only a few muscle artifacts—and nothing else.

On hypnotic levels, her attacks could be precipitated, stopped, or blocked without difficulty. While they served obviously and readily detectable neurotic functions, all that could be said was that they channelized pronounced underlying anger. They could not be integrated into what we learned about her underlying reaction patterns. We could not understand their presence or why they had appeared *de novo*. The more usual neurological studies were therefore repeated. In time, with RISA scanning we elicited minimal findings of intracerebral pathology. A meningioma was excised. She died post-surgically.

It would seem of value at this point to recapitulate her case history, in detail, since it vividly illustrates so many of the factors involved. Her infrequent seizures were for the most part described as "mild" or "minor." They usually occurred while she was asleep. There was some slight jerking of the right leg preceded by an indescribable sensation in the head and right groin. Emphasis, by her and by her husband during history taking, was either on her depression or the problems posed in her relationship with her mother.

According to the history, she had her first attack in April 1956, at 2:00 a.m. while not fully asleep. Results of skull x-rays, electroencephalography and ventriculography were negative. She lost 35 pounds during the next four months, and then (late August) had an attack in which her leg jerked. Occasional infrequent similar attacks recurred, along with episodes of discomfort or pain starting in the right groin that, so she stated, made her draw her body to one side and caused her right leg to jerk. She was rehospitalized for further study November 1956. Spinal puncture, pneumoencephalography and electroencephalography—all yielded essentially normal results. She was nevertheless placed on dilantin and phenobarbital, but the dilantin was discontinued six months later, and equanil, thorazine and other tranquilizers were prescribed in its stead. She had crying spells with episodes of diffuse trembling. The seizures ceased, but her anxiety-depressive state became worse. She was then hospitalized six months for psychiatric care. Her depression cleared up on treatment, and she was discharged (January 1958), only a month-and-a-half later (late February) to have another mild seizure. Seizures continued at rare intervals. In one she was said to have blacked out. Some were observed, and during these she was able to talk and to answer questions.

She was rehospitalized November 1958, her condition did not improve and she was then referred here by her psychiatrist for combined psychiatric and neurosurgical study. She was hypnotized during the initial investigatory session and while hypnotized was directed to pass back through time, to the time of her first attack—and to relive it. The suggestion was effective. The toes of her right foot felt stiff; she experienced excruciating pain that radiated up her right leg and, as it became more severe, through the rest of her body to her arms; her head twisted to the right; and her leg began to jerk as the pain extended over the entire right side of her body. She therefore obviously had at least two types of seizures. The second type was induced by the direct hypnotic suggestion that she have an attack like those previously observed by some of her physicians. It began with a rather slow elevation of the right leg. There were no clonic components. As the leg was elevated with the knee almost extended and the foot in a neutral position, she was able to talk and to answer questions. Her leg remained elevated in a more or less tonic position for two to three minutes and then fell back on the couch.

When this latter attack was blocked (as it was by the direct hypnotic suggestion that it cease) she spontaneously, in slow motion, enacted kicking her husband and then having a temper tantrum, as a small child, against her mother. When, on the other hand, the first type of seizure was blocked, she just as spontaneously hallucinated (on visual, tactile, olfactory and motor behavioral levels) having just had sexual relations with her husband whom she now wished to kill because of his premature ejaculation. She was homicidally enraged at him. But as she enacted starting to beat, scratch and choke him, she found that she was clawing not him but her mother. She began screaming. She apparently had spontaneously regressed to a preschool level and gone into a temper tantrum characterized by the leg-thrusting, leg-jerking movements of her seizures. An attempt was made to block this hypnotically, but she lost contact with the hypnotist at this point. When she again came in contact, she seemed to be rehallucinating the unsatisfactory sexual relationship with her husband whom she kept tearfully imploring to bring her to orgasm, although he had lost his erection and was unable to do so. She began berating him for driving her crazy like her mother. She would rather kill herself than go into an insane asylum for ten years like her mother had. She trembled and shook, just to think of it. She dreamed about it all the time. That's what gave her the convulsions. She wasn't going to have any, any more, merely because he was impotent.

This patient's detailed case records had been obtained and abstracted in advance, but further detailed psychiatric study seemed indicated. She was hypnotized during electroencephalography, and seizures of the type described were hypnotically induced. Except for a few muscle artifacts, tracings were normal.

A detailed description of the April 1956, attack was obtained, at first on hypnotic levels, and later on non-hypnotic ones. This on hindsight, as we elicited it 2½ years after it had occurred, gave us pause. It sounded like a grand mal seizure. She had felt a "peculiar" sensation in the right knee, with electricity in her toes; her right leg had shot into the air; she screamed she was paralyzed; there was severe pain in her right leg that radiated up through her body, and she had, to quote, "passed out." According to her husband, who witnessed the attack, there were clonic movements of the foot with tongue-biting and drooling. She was unconscious for ten or fifteen minutes. Her right leg then seemed weak. Next morning she had some difficulty with its use, and there were some speech difficulties. The neurosurgical investigations were therefore continued concurrently with the psychiatric.

No abnormalities were found in the general physical examination, but on neurological examination she by this time had some slight memory impairment, right lower facial weakness, hyperactive right knee and ankle reflexes, and an extensor plantar response on the right side. A scan revealed marked increase in radioactive iodine uptake in the left paracentral region. The carotid angiogram showed a parasagittal lesion. When advised that an operation was necessary, this patient sobbed convulsively: she wished to die during the procedure, she cried, and was therefore treated psychotherapeutically on hypnotic levels daily during prolonged sessions over a two-week period, was no longer clinically depressed, and stated that she now wished to live. Her husband was highly gratified at the change in her emotional status. She was, he explained, once more her old self.

A left parasagittal meningioma was removed (January 12, 1959) under hypothermia and general anesthesia. It extended up to the sagittal sinus, from the margin of which it had to be separated. Postoperatively, however, she did not respond. The wound was re-explored the following day, but only a small amount of blood, insufficient to explain the coma, was found. She died on the sixth postoperative day. Autopsy showed lobular pneumonia on the right upper lobe with abscess formation. There was a thrombosis of the longitudinal sinus and of the transverse sinus, and an intracerebral hemorrhage of the right frontal lobe, presumably secondary to the sinus thrombosis.

Summary and Conclusions

Between 1948 and 1960, 138 patients with convulsive seizures were evaluated psychotherapeutically on hypnotic levels. They fell into two groups, depending upon whether their referral diagnoses were primarily those of organic seizures or of seizures on an emotional basis. These two groups nevertheless were otherwise indistinguishable. Referral diagnoses had little or nothing to do with whether demonstrable organic pathology was present.

Ninety-two of these patients had previously had diagnoses of organic icti. When studied psychiatrically on hypnotic levels their convulsions ceased, at least temporarily, even though in order to obtain a baseline all medication may have been withdrawn. This held true even for one patient in status epilepticus who three years previously had been in an automobile accident with resultant pronounced neurological signs, and whose convulsive affairs occasionally had involved tongue-biting and loss of bladder control, but whose seizures, nevertheless, turned out to be psychogenic.

The remaining 46 patients, who had been referred for study on the same hypnotic levels but with psychiatric diagnoses, presented comparable investigative problems. Four, for instance, had brain tumors, although all studies at first—including competent neurological examination, electro- and pneumoencephalography, angiography, etc.—elicited results within essentially normal limits, and although psychiatric examination uncovered psychopathology that made their seizures understandable on an emotional basis.

The hypnotic situation can get out of hand. According to statements of position by both the American Medical Association [1,2] and the American Psychiatric Association,[3] any physician making use of hypnotic techniques should have sufficient knowledge of psychiatry and particularly of psychodynamics to avoid its use in clinical situations where it is contraindicated or dangerous for the patient. This applies even to its use for sedation or for the relief of pain. Hypnosis is a specialized psychiatric procedure and as such is an aspect of the doctor-patient relationship.[1, 6, 7] It is to be regretted that during the past several years articles have appeared urging physicians to hypnotize patients with epilepsy, as a result of which a sizable part of our professional time has had to be devoted to helping to extricate some non-psychiatrist colleagues from the rather bad jams into which they had catapulted themselves as a result of their psychiatrically naive use of hypnotic techniques.

REFERENCES

1. American Medical Association, Council on Mental Health; Medical use of hypnosis. (Report approved by the Board of Trustees and House of Delegates of the American Medical Association, June, 1958). J.A.M.A., 168: 186-189, 1958.
2. American Medical Association, Committee on Hypnosis, Council on Mental Health: Training in medical hypnosis. (Report approved February 1960, by the Council on Mental Health, and reviewed April 1960, by the Council on Medical Education and Hospitals.) J.A.M.A., May 26, 1962.
3. American Psychiatric Association: Statement of Position Regarding Hypnosis, February 15, 1961. (Copies of this Statement are available on request from the central office of the Association, Matthew Ross, M.D., Medical Director, 1700 18th Street, N.W., Washington 9, D. C.)
4. AUERBACH, A.: Attitudes of psychiatrists to the use of hypnosis. J.A.M.A., 11:917-921, 1962.
5. BARTEMEIER, L., AND ROSEN, H.: Hypnosis in medical practice. J.A.M.A., 175:976-979, 1961.
6. British Medical Association: "Medical Use of Hypnotism: Report of the Subcommittee appointed by the Psychological Medicine Committee of the British Medical Association (and approved by the Council of the Association, April 13, 1955)." Brit. M. J. (Suppl.), 1:190-193, 1955.
7. GILL, M. M., AND BRENMAN, M.: Hypnosis and Related States. New York, International Universities Press, 1959.
8. Group for the Advancement of Psychiatry: Medical Uses of Hypnosis. New York, April, 1962.
9. MEARES, A.: A System of Medical Hypnosis. Philadelphia, W. B. Saunders Co., 1960.
10. PULVER, S. E., AND SMITH, L. A.: Teaching medical hypnosis: a pilot course at a University Medical School. Comprehensive Psychiat., 2:157-162, 1961.
11. ROSEN, H.: (a) Hypnotherapy in Clinical Psychiatry. New York, Julian Press, Inc., 1953; (b) Hypnosis in medical practice: uses and abuses. Chicago M. Soc. Bull., 62:428-436, 1959; (c) Hypnosis: applications and mis-applications. J.A.M.A., 172:683-687, 1960; (d) Hypnosis in office medical practice. M. Clin. North America, 45:1685-1691, 1961.

Psychotherapy of Schizophrenic Reactions

by Jack R. Ewalt, M.D.

Etiology

SCHIZOPHRENIA is one of the world's major health problems; it has been found to occur in every population group studied. We do not know whether it is one illness, a group of illnesses, or a form of social deviance which is erroneously classified as illness. At the present time society considers the phenomenon as an illness; psychiatrists consider it as a group of disorders with social, biological, and psychological features that are common to most, if not all, of the group. Until such time as research, accident, or divine inspiration gives us more precise information we must manage schizophrenics with the means at hand.

Space does not permit dwelling upon the social and biologic patterns present in the groups of schizophrenics; nonetheless they are present and are significant variables in all cases. Schizophrenia occurs in all cultural groups so far studied, and in all is found most often in the lower socio-economic levels of the society, although cases occur in every economic and educational group, and in 1 to 1.3 per cent of the population. To date the expression of concern with the social manifestations of the disorder in the individual patient is largely limited to working with the family and studying relations between the patient and his family.

Biologic features are undoubtedly present, but whether they are primary or secondary to anxiety resulting from the psychologic and social features is not known, even though the literature abounds with opinions on the subject. William Goldfarb believes that there are two types of schizophrenia, one of which is organic. He found varying degrees of organic pathology in his patients with childhood schizophrenia, and the more severe the organic pathology the less severe was the disruption in family patterns. The reverse also held.

Freud postulated a genetic background in neurosis as well as psychosis, but in modern times the possible effect of genetic differences is too often overlooked in planning projects for investigating fascinating clinical phenomena. Perhaps the denial is due to a fear based on faulty concepts of the role of genetic material. Physicians approaching genetics often remind one of Thurber's "The Kingfisher and the Seabee." ("Moral: You can't make anything out of cookie dough except cookies."[36]) But there is a possibility of adding nuts, raisins, spices, fruit, or oatmeal. Another quotation may express it more accurately. "The gloomy view is sometimes taken, even by experts, that there can be little chance of preventing schizophrenia by public health measures when the hereditary forces are so strong. This view is fallacious and can be refuted by pointing out that twin studies on tuberculosis show a genetic factor of precisely the same order as that shown by schizophrenia. To produce any disease, there must be a combination of genetic and environmental factors, and if the latter are sufficiently favorable then the disease will not develop, however strong the genetic loading. Rickets is another illustration of this, as Fraser Roberts has pointed out: "150 years ago it was considered hereditary; and so it is, in the sense that some people are genetically disposed to it and others genetically resistant. Yet once it was learned how to avoid the environmental factor (lack of vitamin D) the disease became preventable and disappeared."[16] And Lauretta Bender has said: "No child can develop schizophrenia unless predisposed by heredity; psychosis is precipitated by psychological crisis; the pattern of the psychosis and its defensive mechanisms are determined by psychological and environmental forces."[2] Furthermore, identification of a disorder as due to inborn metabolic error does not mean that it is hopeless. Epilepsy and diabetes are rather well controlled, and progress has been made in treating the phenylalamine defective child. The effect of environment on the genetic base is also well illustrated by the steady increase in stature of successive generations of Americans accompanying improved nutrition, although there has been no detectable change in the general genetic background of our people. In addition, the terms *genetic* and *environmental* are meaningful in a very limited sense: the gene is the environment for the molecules that form its proteins, and the cell nucleus is in turn environment for the gene; you can make your own extensions in either direction. We have a plan or blueprint for growth and development, but the plans are also a genetic-dynamic process.

Despite the fascinating byways, we must follow the main route; I wish to consider the psychological features as we presently understand them. As we review the data bear in mind that "recent anatomical and physiological studies have implied that it is the diffuse reticular core of the central nervous system which exerts a vital tonic regulatory influence on the sensory systems thereby modulating incoming sensory data in accordance with the central state of the organism or the behavioral significance of the stimulus."[3] As politicians, psychoanalysts, and clinical psychologists have long known, in a given situation we see and hear what we are prepared to perceive, and nothing more. Thus, I expend no effort in reconciling the approaches of my colleagues or even members of my staff, each of whom sees in his own approach, if not *the* way, at least some reasonable approximation of it.

Freud makes only brief references to schizophrenia, and often by comparison to neurotic phenomena. Some of his concepts of ego function and of transference phenomena (or the lack of them) reflect more of the European concept of "dementia praecox" than of dynamic psychiatry. Despite this, his concept of the basic status of ego function remains useful: "Originally, at the very beginning of mental life, the ego instincts are directed to itself and it is to some extent capable of deriving satisfaction for them on itself. This condition is known as narcissism and this potentiality for satisfaction is termed autoerotic. The outside world is at this time, generally speaking, not cathected with any interest and is indifferent for purposes of satisfaction."[9]

As psychoanalytic psychology sees it, schizophrenia is a regression to the primary or narcissistic phase. As a glib term in analytic lingo it is so familiar that some overlook the significance of this phase for understanding the patient's behavior and the implications for behavior and for treatment embodied in this view. A familiar example is the use of pseudoanalytic approaches that have as a goal the regression of the ego as it occurs, for example, in a neurosis. It is not clear to me where we hope the patient will regress to when the most primitive and undifferentiated impulses of love and aggression, those first encountered in the beginnings of the ego, so threaten the patient that he experiences the schizophrenic symptoms as the only defense he has available. Federn describes the drives as showing increased narcissistic cathexis, decreased object cathexis with ego regression, and with the repressed material becoming conscious and reality-testing becoming defective. The regression takes place before we see the patient as a schizophrenic problem. The patient's successive attempts and concomitant failures to handle anxiety with neurotic symptoms occurred before he came to us. Federn expresses it: "Topically different disturbances do not exclude each other, but one defense mechanism frequently makes all others superfluous. When with the progress of life the established set of defensive mechanisms, for example, the hysterical or obsessional, is invalidated through accumulated conflicts and frustrations, then another deeper mental disorder develops. With its characteristic defenses, compensations, compromises and reconstructions the psychosis is born."[7] Zilboorg says much the same thing; he summarizes as follows: "Having passed through the gamut of infantile neurosis—from hysteria to compulsive neurosis—and having failed, he will find but one path—away from reality, away from genitality, and back to ontogenetic as well as phylogenetic infancy which is schizophrenia."[39] And Fairburn says, "For in such cases it is usual for the final state to be reached only after all available methods of defending the personality have been exploited."[5]

The concept of schizophrenia as the best defense available to the person at the time characterizes analytic psychiatry. This is in sharp contrast to other views that consider psychosis and neurosis as distinct disease processes and not as stages in the defense of an organism under stress so great that neurotic defenses (or symptom formation) are not enough.

The acceptance as a working hypothesis that the behavior is best described as the organism's functioning at the narcissistic level and represents a regression from a more advanced stage of development should have important effects upon our approach to treatment. If such a concept is valid we should be able to make some theoretical assumptions about the schizophrenic and his behavior and should be able to check them with clinical observations. If regression is not present the expected behavior will not be found.

1. Depending upon the previous level of integration of the ego, one may expect varying degrees of ego function in the schizophrenic. Hartmann presents the concept of "conflict-free areas of ego" in the patient; Winnicott speaks of effective ego capacities in patients with extensive illness. One may expect patients who have achieved a reasonably good adjustment to have preserved many ego functions and to express the schizophrenia in a more socially acceptable way. The reverse also may be expected. In practice we do see the paranoid schizophrenic, and especially those whose illness develops in adulthood, with many well-preserved ego functions. The primitive impulses are projected and the patient preserves a considerable measure of social effectiveness. At the other extreme, the autistic child grown up shows grossly impaired ego function, often too little to work with in therapy. The hebephrenic and catatonic lie between these two insofar as age of onset and extent of ego function available for therapy are concerned.

2. One should find the repressive function poorly developed and in some instances absent, for all practical purposes. That this is a fact has been so well documented that it needs no defense. Hendrick comments: "This is the fact that one essential function of the neurotic as well as the normal ego, namely repression, is dramatically defective in schizo-

phrenia. Adequate rapport with the schizophrenic or indeed with the non-psychotic schizoid will always disclose an awareness of infantile phantasy and a consciousness of the meaning of its symbols which other adults do not possess. This defect compels him to resort to more primitive methods of defense against reality in phantasy-producing anxiety, expressing inhibition of motility and neutralization of primitive hostile drive and a retreat to profound narcissism."[18]

3. Communication will be of a primitive sort. In fact, the language and thinking are of the earliest, or most concrete form. It is true that after elaborate testing Payne and associates cast some doubts on the concept of concreteness of thinking and suggested that Norman Cameron's concept of over-inclusiveness more accurately describes the syndrome. In either view the phenomenon is seen as an attempt to express in words the earliest forms of thinking and language function. The world is as the patient perceives it. Communication is often non-verbal and its meaning original with the patient. The trick is to learn enough of the patient's language so that you can communicate with him. Here we may expect that the language function will be better preserved and communication more effective in the patient who at one time had well-developed language functions. In fact, we do observe less difficulty in language function in paranoid schizophrenics than we find in the hebephrenic type.

4. The patient will have limited tolerance to anxiety. In fact, patients translate their anxiety into hallucinations or delusions or relieve it by motor activity of a purposeless or aimless sort, a primitive type of ego defense.

5. Perception will be highly individualized, but concreteness in the language-thinking process, impaired ability to define ego boundaries, and impaired ability to bestow love on others or to receive it may be generally expected. In fact, these are often given as basic symptoms of the schizophrenic process.

Perhaps this is enough to conclude that the concept that schizophrenia represents a regression to the earliest stage of narcissism is at least a reasonable way to describe schizophrenic behavior. Can we, from this concept and other information, form theories of cause? Remember that we are presenting here only the psychological features of cause, and are refraining from discussing the biological or social aspects of etiology, all of which play a role.

The twin factors of ego regression and faulty repression make an adequate starting point. Basically the regression is a series of retreats whose purpose is to cope with the anxiety engendered by the failure of repression in the face of some combination of poor object relations and severe demands of the world in which our patient finds himself. Factual information about varying capacities for repression is scanty indeed. It is interesting to indulge in some speculation and then formulate hypotheses in relation to material in the literature. What we do know about varying strength in repression is that it is related to superego development; the degree of repression is in direct proportion with the strength of the superego. It has been observed in the sociopathic disorders that early relations between parents and child may be important as a cause of the capricious function of the superego in these persons, but the observations are neither numerous nor well documented. Hendrick, while stressing the need for investigation, gives the best theoretical formulation. "The psychotic are like the neurotic in that they also need to adapt in such a way as to avoid anxiety experiences. In contrast to the neurotic, however, their adjustments depend on the more primitive types of defense, those which normally predominate before a high degree of personality organization is attained. The most important of these less organized defenses are flight, shown in the social withdrawal of the psychotic; the simple inhibition of impulse which is very apparent in their defective capacity for normal self-assertion, and projection which is apparent in many of their delusions. These are much less highly organized defense mechanisms than repression and are derived from more primitive phases of development."[19] "In the development of the ego, the adoption and organization of patterns whose elements were originally perceived as details of other people's behavior play a very important role. We call these 'identifications'; they are reactions to emotional relations with other people and play a conspicuous role in development."[20] "It seems to me that the early identification with executant patterns of people in the environment is probably essential to the development of an ego which can deal effectively with special stresses of adult life by either normal or neurotic adaptations. The person who adapts by psychosis is one who has not adequately achieved such organization of his very early behavior patterns through identification and cannot defend himself adequately against the anxiety incident to unusual emotional stresses."[21]

Analytic research on ego development tends to support these early theoretical formulations. Hartmann, Kris, Spitz, and Erikson have made notable contributions in this area. Hartmann reminds us that Freud saw repression as a defense which presupposes the differentiation of the mental apparatus into ego and id, and goes on to say, "No satisfactory definition of the concept of ego strength and ego weakness is feasible without taking into account the nature and maturational stage of the ego apparatus which underlie intelligence, will and action."[17] Both Spitz and Erikson have postulated specific early stages in ego development, and modifications have been suggested by Benjamin and by Gifford. Spitz's formulation is as follows. In the first 2½ months there is no difference between ego and id. At 3 months smiling is the first response to the external "surround," the first step away from primary narcissism, the precursor to libidinal object. Here begins id-ego differentiation. By 6 months there is good definition of objects and the major mode of response or reaction is hitting or biting. This is normal. However, a 4-year-old who hits and bites as his primary way of relating to others is ill.

This awareness of stimuli from the environment (i.e., perception) is a first step in ego organization. The integration of object relations with the drives further establishes the ego as a structure with survival functions. You can eat the things you see, or at least some of them (and every child discovers which ones); furthermore, you can get people about you to deliver them to you. The third stage in ego organization is the development of speech or ways of communicating with others. In this final stage the "self" is finally differentiated.

Freud commented on persons who have a knack for directly understanding the unconscious—an ability assumed in fantasy by almost every budding analyst and dynamically oriented resident. "Advances in psychoanalytic experience have brought to our notice patients who have shown a direct understanding of dream symbolism of this kind to a surprising extent. They were often sufferers from dementia praecox so that for a time there was an inclination to suspect every dreamer who had this group of symbols of being a victim of that disease."[10] He makes the point that this is not so, and that some people have a special gift.

One of these is William Saroyan, who writes much more effectively on early ego function than do most psychiatrists. In the following passage a boy of about three discusses his mother's visits with his older brother. "I sometimes believed we would never see her again and I said so, but my brother said we would, probably. Then, why didn't we see my father again? He said that was different, he was dead. Even so, why didn't we see him again? He explained why. He did the best a six-year-old could do speaking to a three-year-old. He said we could never expect to see my father again, but I didn't believe that. Hadn't we just seen my mother again, after she had gone away that way? Why shouldn't we see my father again? Dead my brother said. Didn't mean a thing. Wasn't my mother dead too? Then how did we just see her again?"[30]

On the same subject Freud said: "The infant is not yet able to distinguish temporary absence from permanent loss; when he fails to see his mother . . . . . he behaves as though he would never see her again. . . . ."[11]

The problem in developing relations (or significant feelings) with others from early life on seems to be the basic issue. Poor ego structure results, repressive capacities and anxiety tolerance are poor, and psychosis follows. The problem is why this occurs in some children and not in all.

Margaret Mahler says: "We thus become increasingly aware of the enigma which confronts us. On the one hand in the face of serious insults to the mother-infant symbiotic relationship, most infants progress without severing their ties with reality. On the other hand, these atypical children, whose traumatization was not more severe, either in quality or quantity, have broken with reality, regressed and fallen back to their own devices—that is to say, regressed to the autistic state.

Obviously, some unknown factor, or combination of factors, is at work. I believe that the cardinal precipitating event in these cases of infantile psychosis is the breakdown of that highly subtle "circular process" to which Emmy Sylvester has called attention: the mutually reciprocal relationship which enables mother and infant to send out, and receive, each one's signals, a compatible, predictable interaction, as it were.

If the infant's signals do not reach the mother because he is unable to send them, or if the infant's signals are not heeded because the mother does not have the capacity to react to them, the mother-infant circular interaction pattern takes on a dangerously discordant rhythm. Gratification-frustration sequences are unpredictable, and utter disorientation as to inner tension versus gratification from an outside source obtains. Under such circumstances the infant cannot develop a capacity for confident expectation (Benedek), for basic trust (Erikson), which would enable him, from the third or fourth month on, to keep disruptive impulses toward immediate tension discharge in abeyance—a first prerequisite for the formation of ego structure."[26]

The fact that many cases are first recognized in adolescence and that some adolescent turmoil states resemble schizophrenia may also be partially understood on this basis. Helene Deutsch says that the weaker the child's ego the more he uses identification with adults in his adjustment to the adult world. But Edith Jacobson points out that until adolescence every child learns to adapt to society through the "medium of his relations and identifications with his parents and parental figures."[22] As his ego matures this identification is less essential and he develops his own autonomy. With adolescence he must largely give up his oedipal objects. If the ego has not developed its own autonomous identity the adolescent will have problems.

Our potential schizophrenic has failed to relinquish a large measure of dependency on his family, and has not developed strong oedipal feelings during childhood, so the shifts to new objects will be lacking in energy and new object relations will be tentative and ambivalent. These same ego features will offer poor support for the major shifts in superego attitude toward sexual impulses. The average adolescent becomes somewhat preoccupied with narcissistic aims, as has been pointed out by Anna Freud and also by Edith Jacobson, who says, "Trying to ward off his overpowerful instinctual strivings the adolescent may again call upon primitive impulses, such as denial, introjection, projection. Or he may use aggression in an attempt to ward off sex, or he may escape from genital to pregenital goals, from heterosexual to narcissistic-homosexual attachments and activities, and back again; from objects of his age to older persons, or even to incestuous objects, and the reverse. This is the reason why the adolescent may develop some forms of behavior which may suggest psychopathy or even psychosis."[23]

Our potential schizophrenic must rely even more on primitive defenses. The narcissistic preoccupations become predominant and the psychosis, latent since infancy, becomes manifest.

Adolf Meyer believed that "schizophrenia" (which he called *parergasia*) was a way of describing the results of a continuation of maladjustments (involving withdrawal and fantasy formation) to life situations. He believed that present behavior is the result of interaction between genetic potential and the sequence of life experiences, including family and cultural factors, encountered by each individual. His emphasis on the importance of social and family stress formed the basis and stimulus for our present concepts of social psychiatry.

One of the recent psychosocial theories advanced to explain the development of schizophrenia is the "Double Bind" theory of Bateson. As he describes it, "The first proposition from which the hypothesis is derived is that learning occurs always in one context which has formal characteristics . . . . . The hypothesis depends upon the idea that this structured context also occurs within a wider context—a meta-context, if you will—and that this sequence of contexts is an open and conceivably infinite series. The hypothesis also assumes that what occurs within the narrow context will be affected by the wider context within which this smaller one has its being. There may be incongruence or conflict between context and meta-context. The organism is then faced with the dilemma either of being wrong in the primary context or of being right for the wrong reasons or in a wrong way. This is the so-called double bind. We are investigating the hypothesis that schizophrenic communication is learned and becomes habitual as a result of a continual traumata of this kind. That's all there is to it."[1] The myth of Scylla and Charybdis provides an example of a "double bind" situation.

Each of these theories to some degree impugns the parent-child relationship, especially the transactions between the infant and the mother. We assume that the rejection is by the mother; the child's role usually is not mentioned, although Sylvester, Mahler, and William Saroyan are exceptions to this. The following passage from Saroyan describes two seven-year-old boys in an orphanage. "The two who cried had nobody. That's the way I figured it. They might actually have had a mother somewhere or a father or a brother or a sister, but I figured they had nobody. They were entirely alone. They were so alone they couldn't wait for the lights out to let themselves go. It happens to kids in big families even. Surrounded by love even, some kids are entirely alone, and it hurts, it makes them cry in the dark, God love and protect them."[31]

The effect on a child of separation and deprivation of mother love has been repeatedly documented by Spitz, by Anna Freud, by Bowlby on children and by Harlow on monkeys. The observation in the human studies is on the infant and young child during and immediately following the deprivations. The disastrous effect is apparent and takes the form of profound disturbance of total body function. The physical aspects are severe enough to cause death in some instances, and the mental aspects result in the "autistic," the "atypical," or the schizophrenic child.

More hazardous or speculative but moving observations of relationship between the schizophrenic reactions in adolescents and adults and deviant family constellations have repeatedly been reported. Bearing in mind the hazards of conclusions based on correlations, we will mention some of the studies dealing with the "schizophrenogenic mother" or "schizophrenogenic family."

Lidz and his group have studied the schizophrenic family intensely; their work can be summarized by the observation that when investigated *intensely* no observed schizophrenic patient came from a reasonably well-integrated family.

Fairburn states: "The type of mother who is specially prone to provoke such a regression is the mother who fails to convince her child by spontaneous and genuine expressions of affection that she herself loves him as a person. Both possessive and indifferent mothers fall in this category."[6] These studies make observations only on the sick, and not on a total population sample.

Schofield and Balian made a study of the life histories of some so-called normal persons (from hospital staff, business, and industry) and compared them with schizophrenic histories. (There were about 150 plus in each sample.) The study involved 35 major aspects of early history and adjustment; 37 per cent (or 13) aspects revealed no reliable difference, 22 per cent (or 5) showed greater pathology in the normal group (e.g., more poverty, invalidism in childhood home, poorer hetero-sexual adjustment, a more ritualistic attitude toward religion, and an unreliably greater frequency of divorce in childhood homes). The schizo-phrenic group showed unfavorable relationship with both parents, poor attitudes toward achievements in school, less success in occupation, fewer satisfactions from occupation, a lack of social adeptness, narrow interests, limited aspirations, vague life plans, and a lack of initative. They conclude: "The notion that any single circumstance, deprivation or trauma contributes uniformly and inevitably to the etiology of schizo-phrenia is called into serious question."[32] They suggest that it is the total life pattern of experience that is of significance, and in so doing again remind one of the teachings of Adolf Meyer.

In the Midtown study Langner has shown that the incidence of broken homes is higher among the well than the mentally ill. Neverthe-less, their data seemed to show that the child's concept of his parents' attitudes toward him and his feeling for his parents is of importance in determining his future mental state, and that a feeling of rejection is associated with increased mental morbidity.

Whatever the reasons, schizophrenia exists; to borrow a phrase from Bridgeman, we must do the best we can with the information at hand. For purposes of organization and instruction we will confine the balance of this discussion to the psychotherapy of schizophrenia, but this is only one facet on the total social, psychological, and in some instances biological approach needed to get the job done.

THERAPY

Freud warns that the goal of treatment is to help the patient and not to demonstrate how clever the doctor is, an admonition phrased in larger context by Osler. Each physician must develop his own style or approach, but detailed observation of "styles" of psychotherapy suggests that the differences are more apparent than actual. The therapist approaches the patient in view of his own character and experience. We can outline a basic set of "do's" and "don'ts," leaving to the individual and his teachers the development of his unique way of "doing" and "don'ting."

1. A first principle is to remember that we don't cure the patient. We seek to aid nature's spontaneous healing process (or trend to homo-geneity) by suitable method.

2. Do not undermine the present defense, i.e., the psychosis, until you and the patient are established in therapy, so that he can use the therapeutic situation to work off anxiety. During the first phase (Semrad's "Denial" phase and Searle's "Out of contact" phase) drugs may be helpful for control of anxiety; once they are started they should be continued until the patient is in good therapeutic relationship. Federn says: "Every psychotic who is not feebleminded has enough intelligence to grasp and accept the explanation of his own mechanisms. His mental disease brings him nearer to intuition and understanding; normal persons, laymen and psychiatrists alike, have much greater resistance because of the logical, emotional and ego components."[8] The situation is often encountered in supervision in which a therapist-trainee prevents his patient from presenting important unconscious material by interruptions or diverting questions. The therapist-trainee usually (but not always) recognizes his intervention after it is pointed out by the supervisor or, on occasion, by the patient.

3. Deal with the current situation first. Because repression is faulty the symptoms may be of the here and now; dealing with the present situation permits adequate exposition of primitive material, repressed in the normal and neurotic. On this subject Fromm-Reichmann says: "One danger implied in over-rating the significance of free associations is the possibility that the therapist may fail to pay close enough attention to apparently inconsequential factual events in the current lives of patients."[13] "The investigation of a patient's current interpersonal relations should never be neglected. It is important for the psychiatrist to press for their recital because they are an important source of information for uncovering ego-defenses and security operations and the motivating anxiety behind them."[14]

4. Do not dwell too long on the patient's hallucinations, delusions, and other symptoms. Pursuit of the details of the delusions and unusual experiences, fascinating as they may be, can be antitherapeutic. Kahn comments: "Instead of transference readiness they [borderline-schizophrenics] tend to provoke or seduce the analyst into a tantalizing relation to their material . . . Instead of communication, there is exhibition of psychic contents."[24] These disturbances have been described as restitutional, and they may indeed have some such function, but my experience leads me to believe that they are principally a method of defense. They express symbolically the primitive impulses which the schizophrenic patient cannot repress, and thus enable him to control them. In therapy patients will hallucinate or show other symptoms when you push into areas that produce anxiety. Too much attention focused on the mani-

festations of defense (the content disturbance) strengthens them, rather than encouraging understanding.

5. Establish working relations with the patient. This is done by accepting his behavior as his solution or way of handling the anxiety induced by his primitive fantasies. Learn to understand the meaning of his behavior. In conversation work with the healthy areas of his ego. Examine with him his feelings and attitudes about the treatment situation, and about you. This makes possible further clarification of the terms of treatment. Anny Katan notes that with children "verbalization of feeling leads to an increased mastery of the ego."[25] The same applies to schizophrenic patients. Many psychiatrists underestimate the amount of socially useful ego function retained by very sick patients. We should utilize the patient's rational functions and aid him in extending them.

6. Do not probe for "deeper material." The patient is fully regressed in some aspects of his attitude toward you in the treatment hour. Historical data about feelings and traumatic events will be produced as he can tolerate them.

7. Be tolerant of verbal expressions of primitive material. Savage says: "One therapist remarked to his somewhat startled colleague, 'I never have counter-transference problems in my schizophrenic patients.' He had carefully dissected the libidinal implications of the patients' hallucinations and delusions and could describe them in a manner vaguely reminiscent of an autopsy report. He had completely ignored the I-thou relationship. He changed the subject when questions of intimacy and dependency appeared."[27] "If the analyst cannot identify with the patient he will encounter difficulties, but identification in turn leads to other difficulties . . . . . the analyst then experiences the patient's intense anxieties, fears, rages, lusts and conflicts as his own, and unless he faces these problems and deals with them directly he may resort to controlling devices to allay the patient's anxiety and his own—such as excessive tenderness or other devices similar to those employed by the patient's parents, or he may resort to primitive defenses similar to those used by the patient, especially paranoid defenses."[28]

8. Do not act out with the patient and do indicate by attitude and by discussion that his behavior is to be controlled within his abilities. "Identification in counter-transference is bothersome and projective. Introspective identification means in operational terms experiencing what the patient experiences, while projective identification is equivalent to living precariously through the patient, particularly gratifying one's impulses through the patient's activities. When projective identification occurs the counter-transference problems are more subtle. The patient will act out the unconscious conflicts and impulses of the analyst in the

same way that disturbed children act out the unconscious conflicts and impulses of the parents. It is this propensity of schizophrenics and their analysts that makes essential the close cooperation of analyst and either the hospital's staff or the family. . . . . I am intrigued with how repeatedly the schizophrenic children provoke their parents into behavior which an analyst would consider pathogenic. I am also intrigued by the fact that they provoke the staff, including myself, into reacting the same way."[29]

9. Do not make premature demands for "dynamic" material, or for improved behavior in social or work situations. Such demands are made, as a rule, to satisfy some omnipotence fantasies of the therapist or to elicit certain satisfactions which would be more appropriately pursued outside therapy. This tendency, very real in the insecure and in the anxious neophyte, can be partially controlled by trying to understand the patient's behavior in the particular hour or on that specific day and the feelings he has about the day's events and about you. My own objection to the use of an administrator in the treatment of schizophrenics is that the therapist may relegate to him the significant material of the day's events while himself pursuing, in practically unending pseudoanalytic conversation, what he considers the "deeper and the significant material." Such a procedure causes the patient to defend himself further against the therapist, whom he correctly perceives as sharing with him real problems in reality testing.

10. Don't give advice. Fromm-Reichmann says: "In the long run, the patient appreciates it if the psychiatrist does not comply with his request for direct practical advice no matter how much he may be pressing the doctor for it at the time. His innate tendency toward health, growth and maturation will eventually be greater than his time-bound wish for the type of help and advice that may interfere with his motivation toward health and independence."[15] One may ask a patient to postpone a decision of importance pending discussion of its meaning for the patient, but the final choice must be the patient's, unless the act is so self-destructive as to warrant emergency intervention (and this seldom is the case).

11. Be aware of the patient's distress signals, so that you do not inadvertently stumble into areas too sensitive to tolerate probing. Sullivan discusses this point at length: "Success in therapy and in research is basically dependent on the physician's skill in handling the movements of anxiety in the patient."[34] "The effectiveness of the psychiatrist as a worker in clinical research is in large measure a matter of his acquaintance with and facile recall of the security operations—the efforts to escape or to minimize anxiety—which he himself once lived and which

now are being paralleled in the performance of the patient. His effectiveness increases in the measure that he is able correctly to foresee the anxiety-provoking aspects of his efforts in investigation and thus adjust his intervention toward optimum efficiency—with or without calling out anxiety in the patient but striving to learn from each instance of unexpected sensitivity so that he does not twice evoke severe anxiety because he has forgotten what he has observed."[35] In brief, if you push the patient too hard or awkwardly he gets more psychotic, commits suicide, or, if you are lucky, quits treatment.

12. Avoid use of the couch, free associations, and an analytic approach in the early phases of treatment. Although exceptional situations may occur, in general I am wary of such procedures and suspicious of the motives behind their employment. It is difficult to endure constant scrutiny during therapy sessions by a patient who may be hostile or suspicious and who will look for signs of rejection. A casual glance at one's watch or scratching may be interpreted as boredom (and the patient is often correct in his assumption). But, in my experience, if you can tolerate it face-to-face therapy more quickly establishes rapport and helps establish ego boundaries. Some analysts use the couch with certain schizophrenic patients—Semrad, for example, does this. Boyer also comments on experiments in using an almost classical analytic technique. For best work with schizophrenia you must be a real person. Undoubtedly, you will be a transference figure as the patient improves, but first you must be you, and you must be available on demand. Patients may manipulate for extra time, but especially in the early phases it is better to err on the side of being "used" until you and the patient have a firm working relationship and have worked out the therapy situation and the meaning of extra appointments. Patients, even very confused ones, can understand the realities of a physician's life. While they may be distressed by the limitations of time, intelligence, or social graces represented by the personal reality of the therapist, they usually can learn to accept them when they are honestly presented, and especially when they are discussed without too much defensiveness occasioned by the therapist's insecurity or by countertransference.

13. Start with two preconceptions. (1) The patient has had earlier unfortunate experiences with people and he may not emotionally embrace you with the full measure of trust your energy and interest deserve. (He may guess that his demands interfere with your analytic hour, supervision hour, or pressing professional or social engagements.) Give him time to decide how satisfactory you are as a giving figure when he is not better than number four on the time priority list. (2) You and the patient will have trouble in communication. He will use simple,

concrete language at times, and much of what he "says" will be on a nonverbal level. You may ask what he means when you don't understand patient. The patient will think he does understand what you mean by words and gestures, and will not ask for clarification, since this is part of his perceptual disturbance. But his interpretation may be far from your original conscious intent. Or you may not think you "said" anything with your gestures, but they may have said a great deal to the patient. (And you may later discover that the patient was reading your unconscious and was substantially correct in his reading.) Therefore you must speak in simple, concrete terms. Do not use allusions, trick phrases, or indirect inferences. For example, if a previously disheveled female patient enters your office with hair carefully styled, and you feel that a comment is indicated, say, "Your hair looks nice" or, "You look pretty with your hair done that way." Do not say, "My, you look nice today," or. "You must be expecting important visitors," because you leave too much room for the patient's personal interpretation of your remarks. The same principle applies to use of names. Patients should be called Miss Jones, Mr. Smith, etc., until you know the meaning of your use of their given name or nickname. In an attempt to be informal you may be "infantizing" or depreciating them.

14. Schizophrenic patients seem to be very much aware of material in you that is unconscious for you. If a patient is too long evasive or distrustful, check your own feelings for the patient. Often you will find that the patient frightens, bores, or annoys you or in some way is a burden to you. But the patient senses it first, and may overinterpret. You may have worries and preoccupations which have no reference to the patient, but he may believe that you are rejecting him because your attention wanders a bit.

15. Be patient about silence. Study the patient for nonverbal clues. You may once or twice in the hour suggest that you may understand him more easily if he will talk to you, but you cannot be sure what his silence means. If he seems very angry or very sad for some time (i.e., most of the hour) you may offer the observation, but don't dig or harass him. Make a game of what you can see from watching him—it will keep you awake and you may learn something. Freud said: "He that has eyes to see and ears to hear may convince himself that no mortal can keep a secret. If his lips are silent, he chatters with his fingertips; betrayal oozes out of him at every pore."[12]

16. Arrange for supporting person or persons outside the therapy hour. Federn stressed the importance of this and reported that mother, sister, or brother were most often suitable and father and spouse less often so. He further stated that work with patient without work with the family

was futile. (This is all pre-World War II, I might add.) Ozzie Simmons'
work with discharged schizophrenics shows that the family of birth is
more tolerant of residual symptoms than is the spouse. Paul and others
have evidence that unresolved family conflict of a subtle sort may
prevent complete rehabilitation of the patient.

17. As you establish working relations with the patient, or when you
are "in business" (to quote Semrad) the primitive material will manifest
itself. If you can tolerate it without undue anxiety (and barring, or the
part of the therapist, seductive behavior or some personal misfortune
such as illness or death) the patient finds it possible to explore his
feelings about you, the hospital, his family, and other significant figures
in his life. He in time finds that he can express feelings and that the
feelings can be controlled. Finally the primitive impulses are repressed
and sublimated. In the process the patient may experiment with
infantile, juvenile, and adolescent ways of behavior and expression. He
may experiment with obsessive, depressive, hysterical, and sociopathic
defenses. He will try your patience and bait you. He will find rationalizations for terminating treatment. He may even have a severe relapse
to test you and his family, or to protest if you are too hostile, too
awkward, or too ebulliently investigative in your approach. He may
run away. But, on the other hand, he may get well.

Criteria of Improvement

And what are the implications of "getting well"? Two types of
adaptation may be discussed.

First, there is the patient who begins to perceive his primitive impulses
as less than magical, represses them, and successfully sublimates. This
result may occur less often than we think or wish, but it is the goal of
treatment. Establishment of firm emotional ties to some dependable
person who is also a skilled therapist (or who is becoming one with
supervision) is basic. The family's ambivalent attitudes and wishes to
keep the patient dependent and to destroy him must be worked through
with the family.

The second type of result occurs in the patient who manages to
isolate or socialize his symptoms by a process of learning, so that he
seems to recover. This type of therapy, called "brief" or "support"
therapy, is the preferred treatment in dealing with many schizophrenic
patients. Patients so treated learn to lean on some person or ritual if
their anxiety is too great. Perhaps relief may be obtained through
fantasy of dream-like character. At times I receive a letter, small gift, or
phone call from some former schizophrenic patient. Apparently I am

supporting such patients from afar. I always answer promptly and appropriately because I suspect that I have, unknown to me, been magically murdered or eaten in fantasy and the purpose of the communication is to check up, to make sure that I still exist; my answer helps to redefine ego boundaries and reality.

The question may be asked, Does treatment help? What about spontaneous remissions? Hastings reports 29 per cent "spontaneous" recovery in schizophrenia. Other reports range from 25 to 80 per cent, but the meaning of remission varies and is usually not clearly defined. I believe that we can learn much from spontaneous remissions, but the phenomenon is difficult to study because patients do not wish to return and if they do the study may produce a relapse.

It is interesting to speculate on how "spontaneous" these remissions are and how many patients received effective but accidental treatment. A few cases will illustrate this point.

Mrs. X, a stabilized schizophrenic on a chronic ward (she had been there for 12 years) in a country state hospital was made custodian of a new electric iron. The iron was a gift from a volunteer for the ladies to press their clothing. The patient began a steady improvement, the first in 12 years, and was discharged in a few weeks. A second patient asked for custody of the iron and she also improved and was discharged. (Alas, No. 3 is still there, as far as I know.)

Spontaneous remission? Technically, yes. But let us probe the situation a little. In terms of chronic backward society a cigarette, a pair of used shoes, or a second-hand coat have a value that few can imagine. A new iron, a gift motivated simply by concern and love of mankind, may have an impact on some patients not unlike the gift of a new sports car for the young among us. Furthermore, the salaried personnel expressed confidence in the patient, a type of caring, by giving this magnificent thing into her custody. The esteem of her colleagues increased and she became busy scheduling their use of the iron and supervising its proper maintenance. She improved and the overworked staff had the skill to note this, to increase her responsibility, and to let her go at the proper time. Now how can we evalutae the spontaneity? What would the patient say to these speculations if she could or would answer? And what meeting of internal and external transactions coincided with the appearance of the iron? And finally, exactly what prompted the volunteer to give that ward an iron? Here is another case.

Mrs. Y, an attractive thin blonde in her 30's was referred by a gynecologist because she was paranoid. The patient was a well-organized, intelligent paranoid schizophrenic whose disturbance was of a few years' duration. She said that she was made nervous by her persecutions and that Dr. L. told her that I could cure her in a visit or two. She came twice. I made the standard opening gambits in what seemed destined to be a long, tough case. She called and cancelled her third appointment, saying that she was well and would not need to come. We agreed that she would call if she felt it necessary. I thought I had made some technical error and that she was politely withdrawing from treatment. I next heard of her about 10 years later when she consulted one of my colleagues in another city for some advice. She told him that she was consulting a psychiatrist because previously one had cured her of a serious illness. She then told him of her paranoid symptoms and her recovery after two visits. He called me to ask about her and then examined her carefully. A little rigid, perhaps, but well-defended, bright, active, in charge of her house—and no schizophrenic or paranoid, or so he said, Now it may be that I burped at the correct pitch or that by unconscious or subliminal communication I effected a cure. If so, the treatment is not repeatable, and I must call it "spontaneous." On the other hand Dr. L. had a blind faith in my abilities. He was handsome, strong, warm, and in their fantasy a father, lover or both (and safely so) to many women in town. He referred cases well, and as a rule I found his cases easier than most because I had the semi-divine blessing on my efforts. I would have had to be fumbling indeed to rend the web of illusion spun by Dr. L. But who can say exactly what the specific element was that brought success?

Señorita Z., a thin, noisy, hebephrenic daughter of a powerful and wealthy family of Mexican descent and culture remained in the hospital with some member of her family in constant attendance. During the examination we used sedatives (this was in the pretranquilizer era) and physician and nurse gave support to patient and relatives. In about two weeks the family reported the patient sufficiently improved to go home. To me and to the nurses she seemed no different from what she had been like at the time of admission. Now, Mexicans are probably the kindest people in the world insofar as friends are concerned, and I thought the talk of improvement was to spare my feelings and was not a statement of the family's reason for leaving us. We parted friends, and I expected them to bring her back within the hour. They did not; but many months later one of their friends brought a sick relative to me on the recommendation of the Z. family because we had so effectively treated Senorita Z. They assured me that she had recovered. What recovery means to them I don't know, but I am confident that the warm supporting family, and not my efforts alone, provided the therapy. Yet we would call it a spontaneous remission.

Too often patients are treated without the therapist's having a specific sequence of goals and adequate theoretical model to guide his efforts. Platitudes about "relationships," "transactions," "transference," etc., have no meaning except in some conceptual framework. In treating psychotic persons there are enough difficulties because of the patient's confusion; there is chaos unless the therapist has specific goals and a map for getting there.

REFERENCES

1. BATESON, G.: Minimal requirements for a theory of schizophrenia. Arch. Gen. Psychiat., 2:477-491, 1960.
2. BENDER, L.: Childhood schizophrenia. Psychiat. Quart., 27: 663, 1953.
3. CHAMBERS, W. W., LEVITT, M., CARRERAS, M., AND LIU, C. N.: Central determination of sensory processes. Science, 132:1489, 1960.

4. COHEN, L. A.: Neck mechanisms on body orientation. J. Neurophysiol., 1, 1961.
5. EWALT, J. R., et al.: Fever Therapy Technique. New York, Paul B. Hoeber, 1939.
6. ——: Mental Health Administration. Springfield, Ill., Charles C Thomas, 1956.
7. FEDERN, P.: Ego Psychology and the Psychoses. New York, Basic Books, Inc., 1952, p. 129.
8. Ibid., p. 124.
9. FREUD, S.: Instincts and their Vicissitudes. In: Collected Papers, Vol. IV. London, Hogarth Press, and the Institute of Psychoanalysis, 1925, pp. 77-78.
10. ——: The Interpretation of Dreams. Part II. In The Standard Edition of the Complete Psychological Works of Sigmund Freud. Vol. V. (1900-1901). London, The Hogarth Press, and the Institute of Psychoanalysis, 1953, p. 351.
11. ——: Collected Papers. London, Hogarth Press, etc.
12. ——: Fragment of an Analysis of a Case of Hysteria. In Collected Papers, Vol. IV. London, Hogarth Press, and the Institute of Psychoanalysis, 1925, p. 94.
13. FROMM-REICHMANN, F.: Principles of Intensive Psychotherapy. Chicago, University of Chicago Press, 1950, p. 73.
14. Ibid.
15. Ibid., p. 209.
16. HARE, E. H.: The Epidemiology of Mental Illness. Roy. Soc. Promotion Health J., July-August, 1959.
17. HARTMANN, H.: Ego Psychology and the Problem of Adaptation. New York, International Universities Press, 1958, p. 107.
18. HENDRICK, I.: Dream resistance in schizophrenia. J. Am. Psychoan. Assoc., 6:672, 1958.
19. ——: The contributions of psychoanalysis to the study of psychosis. J.A.M.A., 113:918, 1939.
20. Ibid.
21. Ibid.
22. JACOBSON, E.: Adolescent Moods and the Remodeling of Psychic Structures in Adolescence. The Psychoanalytic Study of the Child. Vol. 16. New York, International Universities Press, 1961, p. 168.
23. Ibid., p. 172.
24. KAHN, M.: Clinical aspects of the schizoid personality: affects and technique. Internat. J. Psychoan., 41:430-437, 1960.
25. KATAN, A.: Some thoughts about the role of verbalization in early childhood. Psychoanal. Study Child, 16:184-188, 1961.
26. MAHLER, M.: On sadness and grief in infancy and childhood. Psychoanal. Study Child, 16:340-341, 1961.
27. SAVAGE, C.: Counter-transference in therapy with schizophrenics. Psychiatry, 24:53, 1961.
28. Ibid.
29. Ibid.
30. SAROYAN, W.: Here Comes, There Goes, You Know Who. New York, Simon and Schuster, 1961.

31. Ibid.
32. SCHOFIELD, W., AND BALIAN, L.: A comparative study of the personal histories of schizophrenic and non-psychiatric patients. J. Abnormal & Soc. Psychol., 59:216-225, 1959.
33. SEMRAD, E.: Personal communication.
34. SULLIVAN, H. S.: Therapeutic investigations in schizophrenia. Psychiatry, 10:121-125, 1947.
35. Ibid., p. 121.
36. THURBER, J.: Further Fables for Our Times. New York, Simon and Schuster, 1956.
37. ZILBOORG, G.: Deeper layers of schizophrenic psychosis. Am. J. Psychiat., 11:493-518, 1931.

PART V

CHILDHOOD AND ADOLESCENCE

Children of the Kibbutz: Clinical Observations

by MORDECAI KAFFMAN, M.D.

F OR MORE THAN fifty years Israel's communal settlements (in Hebrew, Kibbutz; plural, Kibbutzim) have been carrying out a unique program in child-rearing. By now the number of adult Kibbutz born "sabras" (namely, youngsters born and raised in the Kibbutz) amounts to several thousand functioning members of the Kibbutz Movement.

KIBBUTZ UPBRINGING

In the great majority of the cases, the Kibbutz child is brought up from birth until the age of about 18 in separate children's homes. It stays within the framework of a stable peer age group. First, there is the Infants House, then the Toddlers House, the Pre-Nursery and Nursery School, the Primary School and finally the High School. A steady trend to increase daily child-parent contact can be noticed at present. Considerable emphasis has been laid upon mother-child closeness throughout the first year of life. During the first half-year, at least, the usual maternal activities such as feeding, cleaning, handling, and fondling the baby are mainly performed by the mother. Later, the trained nurse and the different types of educators gradually take over complete care of the child (e.g., feeding, toilet-training, discipline areas, social interaction, etc.) except for the daily time spent by the child with its parents. Daily, in the two or three hour interval between the parents' return from work and the child's bedtime, the child stays in the parents' room. Often enough, whenever the parents' work schedule makes it possible, young children meet their parents on additional occasions for

171

shorter contacts. On rest days, the child spends practically the whole day with its parents. Both father and mother are equally active in sharing their time with the children.

From this brief description, the following significant differences between the Kibbutz system of education and the traditional Western family can be set down: the transfer of several parental functions to other consistent adult figures; the early and stable peer group whose importance for the child steadily increases, commencing with the second year of life; the equally active roles assumed by father and mother in the child-parent relationship; the nightly separation, with different dwellings for children and parents—the children's night watch woman being the only adult close to the child during the night hours.

CHARACTERISTICS OF PARENT-CHILD RELATIONSHIP

A common belief held by outsiders is to assume that the emotional ties between the Kibbutz child and its parents differ substantially or are less intense than in the regular family situation. Despite the crucial role of nurses and educators, regarding both quality of tasks and amount of time spent with the child, the parents, nevertheless, constitute for the child the most important figures in its life.

A very interesting variant is that of those Kibbutz children and their parents who for various reasons (training purposes, financial or educational missions abroad, and the like) transfer temporarily from the Kibbutz environment to a conventional family life, and return to the Kibbutz after two or three years. The writer's clinical experience, based on a close follow-up of six Kibbutz families with this experience whose members were seen and interviewed in both life situations, shows that no significant difference can be observed regarding the nature of the emotional attachment. In both environments the Kibbutz parents continue to be the most important love-objects, and no outstanding change in the quality and characteristics of the parent-child interaction can be detected. In the Kibbutz, as in the traditional family situation, the parents constitute the child's most decisive and stable object of emotional attachment.

Undoubtedly, the transfer from Kibbutz to regular family life and vice-versa involves varying degrees of readjustment and stress reactions in the whole family. The change in either direction may be accompanied by symptoms of emotional disturbance related to the environmental shift but no substantial modification in the nature of the child-parent relationship, emotional closeness and mutual love was noticeable either by the clinical observer or by the parents themselves.

Frequency of Emotional Disturbances

Whether the Kibbutz system of education is apt to engender a higher or lower percentage of emotional disturbances at different age-levels, as compared with the conventional family pattern, is an oft debated issue. Since very meager comparative data are available, it is rather difficult to contrast symptoms and behavior of Kibbutz children with those of "normal controls." In an attempt to help obtain an answer to this question, a survey was conducted by the writer[1] on the frequency and intensity of a wide range of behavior problems in a representative sample of 403 Kibbutz children up to 12 years of age. This study yielded no evidence of a greater incidence of behavior problems or deviant behavior characteristics among Kibbutz children. Symptoms such as excessive or inhibited aggression, temper tantrums, enuresis, rhythmic motor habits, tics, speech problems, night fears, and learning problems seemed either to match the usual figures in samples of unselected groups of children or appeared even less frequently. Only thumbsucking, a habit which for various theoretic reasons Kibbutz parents and educators permit at any age, appeared to be much more prominent among Kibbutz children beyond the preschool age. In sharp contrast to this high incidence of thumbsucking, a low incidence of eating problems was found in Kibbutz children. Nevertheless, a disproportionately large number of Kibbutz children were referred for professional guidance for parent and teacher guidance, supervision of child treatment carried out by special educators, or different forms of psychotherapy for children and parents. Statistically, these were granted by the Oranim Child Guidance Clinic of the Kibbutzim in 1962 to 4 per cent of the total Kibbutz child population under its care.* Different surveys[2] give rather contradictory figures on the proportion of non-Kibbutz children in need of the advice and care of child guidance specialists, with figures ranging from 1 to 40 per cent. It would appear that a high proportion of emotional problems is better tolerated in rural areas and in poor urban districts than in middle-class urban centers.

For the present, the Kibbutz is one of the few places in the world in which accurate epidemiologic figures on Mental Health can be obtained without too complicated a setup. In the case of Kibbutz children, the developmental history, behavior characteristics and problems of each child can be accurately traced from infancy to youth through the re-

---

*This Clinic was set up to help emotionally disturbed children in a population of about 20,000 children and adolescents, up to the age of 17, raised in 130 Kibbutzim affiliated with two large Kibbutz Federations, the Kibbutz Artzi and Kibbutz Meuchad.

corded observation of nurses and teachers, parents' cooperation, medical records, and additional available data. The high rate of population stability in the average well established Kibbutz constitutes a supplementary asset in this respect. Furthermore, most of the Kibbutzim have created a special Advisory Committee in which experienced educators take notice of the referrals of parents, nurses or teachers with regard to emotional problems of children and seek ways to handle them suitably.

The writer, acting as a Consultant Child Psychiatrist, has had the opportunity to follow closely, for several years, the total child population of several Kibbutzim. A strikingly constant annual proportion of children in need of help because of emotional disturbances has been observed—the rate being 12-15 per cent of the total sample. Surely enough, this seemingly high figure embraces all kind of diagnostic possibilities from minor reactive behavior problems to severe internalized emotional disorders. On the other hand, we cannot minimize the fact that trained nurses and educators considered the symptoms sufficiently serious to require the advice of an expert. Although psychiatric advice or treatment for Kibbutz children is sought at all age levels, a more marked pressure is felt from the age of 4 to 10.

It is the writer's belief that 12-15 per cent of emotionally disturbed children is not exceptional in view of the ample opportunities in the Kibbutz framework for detecting problems. Experienced nurses and teachers observe closely the child in an experimental life situation which renders possible not only to them but to the parents a constant evaluation of the child as compared with other children of his peer-group. Any deviation from "normal standards" can be checked more easily under these circumstances. If the conclusion is reached that the child shows abnormal behavior characteristics, advice will be sought to help the child and his significant environmental figures—parents, nurse, teacher, and sometimes peer-group—to find a suitable solution.

Therefore, a combination of three positive factors seems to explain the apparently high figure of referrals of emotionally disturbed Kibbutz children. First, the possibility of early detection being increased by permanent comparison with "normal standards"; second, the existence of available advisory and clinical agencies which have been established in order to help the emotionally disabled Kibbutz child; thirdly, advice and therapeutic help are accessible to the total group of Kibbutz children without any exception or discrimination regarding social status, financial possibilities or diagnostic categories.

CHARACTERISTICS OF KIBBUTZ PSYCHOPATHOLOGY

The issue has been raised whether a specific or a prevalent form of child psychopathology related to the Kibbutz system of upbringing can be detected. Diagnostic and therapeutic work with 1,783 emotionally disturbed children referred to the Child Clinic of the Kibbutzim in the course of the past seven years has failed to reveal any separate clinical entity that could be recognized as a specific or prevalent "Kibbutz syndrome." Diagnostic categories are the usual ones tabulated for children raised in the Western traditional family. The different types of conduct and behavior disorders: the varied forms of psychoneuroses, personality disorders, childhood psychoses and organic conditions—all these diagnostic entities have been recognized among Kibbutz children and youngsters. In a parallel way, all the usual types of child-parent relationship, both normal and abnormal, can easily be found in the Kibbutz environment.

Throughout the year 1962, the writer conducted psychiatric examinations of 93 seriously disturbed Kibbutz children referred to the Child Clinic of the Kibbutzim either because of the initially severe symptomatology or because of the failure of previous attempts at treatment. Beyond any doubt, these cases constituted a representative sample of the distribution of the most serious psychopathology to be found among Kibbutz children. The age distribution seemed to indicate a low incidence of severe disturbances among preschool children as seen in the following figures:

Age	Percentage
Preschool age (below 6 years)	4
Primary School (from 6 to 12½ years)	56
High School (from 12½ to 18 years)	40

Almost three quarters of the referrals (72 per cent) were boys, a sex difference that has been generally noticed at all age levels. Table 1 shows the diagnostic classification of these 93 severely disturbed children.

TABLE 1.—*Diagnostic Distribution of 93 Severely Disturbed Kibbutz Children Age Range: 3½ to 18*

Diagnosis	N	Percentage
Primary behavior disorders	6	6
Neurotic traits	19	20
Psychoneurotic disorders	12	13
Personality trait disturbance	3	3
Sociopathic personality	4	4
Borderline psychosis	7	8
Overt psychosis	6	6
Diffuse brain damage	20	22
Idiopathic mental deficiency	7	8
Psychosomatic illness	3	3
Miscellaneous conditions	6	6

Behavior Disorders, Preneurotic and Psychoneurotic Reactions

Altogether 25 children were diagnosed as having behavior disorders of reactive nature. In all the cases there was a clear-cut connection between the behavioral reaction and an impaired child-parent relationship. The emotional conflict is externalized with some degree of acting out, although it might also have reached a stage of partial internalization. In 12 other cases an organized psychoneurosis with a structured, fixated pattern due to an internalized conflict was recognized.

The prevailing symptoms lacked specificity and could be found in children raised elsewhere. A relatively frequent cluster of symptoms present in one third of the children with an externalized or preneurotic conflict included enuresis, excessive fears, and hyperaggressiveness or inhibition of aggression. For the neurotic group the prevalent symptoms were a sense of inferiority, insecurity, inhibitory anxiety and stuttering.

Learning problems were also seen both in the group with primary behavior disorders (4 children) and in the group of neurotic children (4 children). Altogether 23 children out of the total group of 93 have been referred with the specific complaint of learning difficulties. Therefore, the diagnosis of an emotional learning block in which the emotional problem is primary and the learning difficulty is symptomatic was made in 36 per cent of the cases of learning disabilities. In the remaining cases (64 per cent) the learning disability was due to faulty brain functioning related to diffuse brain damage or to mild types of mental deficiency.

Out of the total group of 36 children with behavior disorders, neurotic traits and psychoneurosis in only 2 children were eating problems mentioned among the referral problems. This is a negligible incidence as compared with the usual figures in Child Guidance Clinics.

Sociopathic Personality Disturbance

This diagnostic category constitutes a rare finding among Kibbutz children. Out of four boys, aged 14 to 18 with antisocial behavior, two were clinically considered as having an underlying ambulatory schizophrenic process, so that it was only in the remaining two cases that the diagnosis seemed to be unquestionable. All of them showed impulsiveness, shallow interpersonal relationship and lack of anxiety or guilt reactions. In all four instances, we found an ineffective, submissive or absent father along with a close-binding and overpermissive mother; often both parents encouraged the child's antisocial behavior as a disguised way of expressing disconformity with the Kibbutz way of life. No overt form of rejection directed at the child was found to be associated with the development of the disturbance. The most obvious finding was the extreme parental overindulgence with constant yielding to wishes and demands of the child. On the other hand, the group and the educational framework were characterized by obvious abnormal conditions of development. For a variety of objective reasons, the child moved from his original group of peer ages to an alien group and frequently changed his nurses and teachers. The educational handling was mostly lenient and inconsistent, fitting into the permissive parental approach. Therefore, very slim chances remained for positive identification with a stable, self-assertive father-substitute figure.

According to the writer's clinical experience with both Kibbutz and urban children, the former show a seemingly decreased symptom severity and a lower incidence of sociopathic disturbances.

Overt Psychosis and Borderline Disorders

The group of 13 psychotic Kibbutz children seemed to be rather heterogenous as to clinical symptomatology, course, and eventual etiopathogenic factors. Only one case, a girl 10 years old was considered a "typical" instance of childhood psychosis. There was also a boy, 3½ years old, with a characteristic syndrome of primary infantile autism in which diffuse brain damage was strongly suspected. Four additional cases categorized as overtly psychotic were adolescents with an acute schizophrenic episode or a chronic schizophrenic pattern all of them fitting into the clinical picture of adult schizophrenia.

Among the remaining seven children diagnosed as borderline cases or schizophrenic adjustment, there were three associated with diffuse brain damage and two already mentioned in which the differential diagnosis with sociopathic personality was not possible in view of the mixed symptomatology.

In this psychotic group of 13 Kibbutz children, sex distribution was approximately the same, unlike all the other diagnostic categories in which there was definite male preponderance.

Diffuse Brain Damage

A relatively high percentage of brain-damaged children were included in the total sample: 20 out of 93 children. The diagnosis was established on the basis of combined positive findings. Prenatal and neonatal pathogenic factors were considered along with the developmental and clinical history, psychological and psychiatric evaluation, neurological and encephalographic examination. The sex ratio was strikingly higher for boys, the proportion being 8:1. It might be worth emphasizing that most of the cases (12 out of 20 children) showed, in addition to the common psychological symptoms which are a direct result of brain injury, a superimposed reactive emotional disturbance. The symptoms which were the result of secondary reaction ranged clinically from behavior disorders to psychotic-like behavior. The high percentage and severity of the emotional secondary reactions constitutes a rather disappointing fact. Despite strenuous efforts to provide the brain-damage child with a normal environment along with early individual and specialized care a large percentage of cases in the Kibbutz do not escape the fate of serious reactive emotional disturbances.

Comparative Psychopathology of Kibbutz
and Urban Children

When the disturbed Kibbutz children here described were compared with a group of 50 emotionally disturbed urban children referred to the Haifa Kupat Holim Mental Clinic the former seemed to exhibit a lesser severity of the clinical symptoms in the parallel diagnostic groups. There is also a lower incidence of sociopathic disturbances among Kibbutz children. As indicated, this clinical difference derives partly from the earlier detection and treatment of child emotional disorders in Kibbutz facilities. An additional explanation seems to be the buffer influence of the multiple object—relationship (parents, age-mates group, nurses and teachers) to neutralize or attenuate any single pathogenic factor in the child's interpersonal experience. It appears that gratifying multiple relationship with stable objects might serve as a supportive influence to counterbalance an eventual pathogenic conflict. The emotional health of the child seems to depend to a lesser degree on the exclusive influence and vicissitudes of the child-parent relationship.

In order to substantiate this hypothesis the writer has compared the emotional reaction and behavior disturbances of two groups of ten Kibbutz children and four control children, who at an early age lost or were deprived of either their mother or father. The follow-up of these children showed a substantial difference. The impact of parental deprivation and incidence of emotional disturbances were by far more severe in the control group. The Kibbutz children seemed to have a more balanced reaction to the trauma of a temporary or permanent separation from one of the parents.

Undoubtedly, there are still other reasons to explain the less severe emotional pathology of Kibbutz children. Direct group pressure on the "deviant parent" and individual tendency toward conformity with Kibbutz-approved standards of child-care will help to attenuate obvious parental pathogenic handling of the child. It is almost impossible to think of an overpunitive or a neglecting Kibbutz parent who would not feel a very strong social pressure to modify detrimental practices. On the other hand, beyond any doubt the symptomatology of the Kibbutz emotionally disturbed child is also influenced by values and goals of his own age group which are at the same time an expression of the remarkably high degree of adult moral standards in the Kibbutz.

THE THERAPEUTIC APPROACH

The solid core of the therapeutic program adopted at the "Oranim" Child Clinic of the Kibbutzim for children in emotional conflict is that every Kibbutz child is entitled to receive therapeutic assistance. However, even after constant expansion of the clinical services, there is still a wide gap between this aim and the concrete possibilities at hand, mainly because of the limited number of available trained therapists. No rigidly orthodox plan of treatment can succeed in supplying ways of dealing with the emotional problems of a large number of children, amounting annually to more than one thousand, for whom some form of treatment is sought. New methods must be tried and modified on a trial and error basis.

The Clinic works in close cooperation with auxiliary personnel attached to each Kibbutz. Mostly these "field workers" are Kibbutz members with educational experience who have been selected and trained to supply specific help to the child in emotional conflict. At present there are about 70 of these special educators. They attend regular training courses and receive systematic supervision. The special educator carries the bulk of the management of child emotional problems which are considered as being of a reactive or preinternalized nature. He is in regular contact with the child and his significant object attachments.

Usually, the child is seen in the play therapy room of his own Kibbutz two to three times a week, but it is not rare for the child to be treated on a more intensive schedule. The special educator makes use of the recognized child therapeutic techniques in order to achieve insight into the more conscious conflicts, with deliberate efforts to lead the child and its significant environment to a readjustment, goal modification and full use of potential possibilities. There is no attempt to go into unconscious conflicts, so that essentially the special educator makes use of a variety of relationship therapy with re-educative goals. Experience seems to show that this kind of therapy is apt to be quite successful in the reactive preinternalized type of disorders. Clinical results can be favorably compared with those achieved by other forms of insight therapy with reconstructive goals.

Although we do not assume that a clear-cut boundary can be drawn between internalized and reactive conflict in the child, the present trend is to refer to the Clinic the child in which the pathologic process seems to be fixated and internalized. Therefore, the most seriously disturbed children are seen not in their own Kibbutz but at the Central Clinic. A routine procedure is undertaken for clinical diagnosis, psychodynamic evaluation and therapeutic recommendations. The procedure includes separate interviews for parents and teachers, together with psychological and psychiatric examinations of the child. Treatment is not centered in the child but in the total constellation constituted by the child and significant object figures, generally both parents and the main educator. An eclectic philosophy of treatment utilizes every helpful method: guidance and counseling; environmental manipulation; individual, family, or group insight psychotherapy, combined drug therapy, etc., etc. The needs of the individual case and the available therapeutic facilities, rather than a rigid theoretical approach, dictate the plan of treatment for the child and his environment.

REFERENCES

1. KAFFMAN, M.: Evaluation of emotional disturbance in 403 Israeli Kibbutz children. Am. J. Psychol., 117:732, 1961.
2. BUCKLE, D., AND LEBOVICI, S.: Child guidance centres. World Health Organization, Monograph Series N° 40, Geneva, 1960.

Developments in the Isolation Therapy
of Behavior Disorders of Children

by RICHARD L. COHEN, M.D.

> "When one is a stranger to oneself then one is estranged from others too. If one is out of touch with oneself, then one cannot touch others. How often in a large city, shaking hands with my friends, I have felt the wilderness stretching between us. Both of us were wandering in arid wastes, having lost the springs that nourished us—or having found them dry. Only when one is connected to one's own core is one connected to others, I am beginning to discover. And, for me, the core, the inner spring, can best be refound through solitude."
>
> *Anne Morrow Lindbergh—*
> *Gift From the Sea*

THE HOSPITAL MANAGEMENT of children with severe character disorders presents many problems. Among the more difficult are those having to do with (1) the development of appropriate therapeutic relationships with the patient in which his dependent status as a child is recognized, and (2) containment of destructive acting out.

Early in the development of our own inpatient program in 1958 we began to experience massive resistances to treatment in the group of character disordered children which comprised about one-half of our patient population. These resistances assumed many forms including active efforts at manipulation, rejection of daily care, destructive and provocative behavior and mobilizing of antisocial peer group forces to resist adult authority. We decided that these major obstacles to treatment required the application of equally powerful intervention techniques.

Coincidentally, at this time we began to become familiar with the work of Heron et al.,[5] Lilly,[8] Azima et al.,[1] Solomon et al.,[11] and others,[3,4,9,10,12] all of whom were studying and observing various aspects of isolation and sensory deprivation as they affected behavior.*

*For excellent, more recent reviews of the clinical implications of sensory deprivation and isolation, the reader is referred to Kubzansky[6] and Kubzansky and Leiderman.[7]

It occurred to us that several aspects of this work were applicable to the therapeutic dilemma with which we were struggling in our own treatment program and we began to devise a technique for isolation and sensory deprivation with which we have had considerable success. It is the intent of this paper to describe this procedure briefly, to give some idea as to its rationale, to indicate some of the results we have obtained and to discuss the significance of these.

DESCRIPTION OF TREATMENT PROCEDURE AND RATIONALE

Perhaps it is important to emphasize first that this procedure is not one in which "isolation" and "sensory deprivation" are carried out literally. In essence, there is really selective control of relationships and stimuli to which the child is exposed according to the need of treatment at any given time. In other words, the isolation and sensory deprivation are relative and not absolute.

As has already been suggested, this technique was originally conceived as a way to deal with crises of extreme acting out accompanied by high degrees of resistance to care and treatment and denial of dependent need. The sensory deprivation aspects were not seen as too significant at the outset.

At first the primary aims were:

1. To remove the child from destructive peer resources which were providing channels for resistance to adult care and authority.

2. To demonstrate, through total environmental control, the ineffectiveness of fantasies of omnipotence and magical thinking which seem to occur universally in character disorders.

3. To provide maximum possible opportunity for use of psychotherapy (undiluted by non-crucial relationships) through heightened anxiety and forced introspection.

4. To insure the physical security of the child and the group.

In order to effect these aims, the following procedures were instituted:

1. The child was placed continuously in an isolation room in which there was subdued or relatively no light and in which sound was dampened as much as possible.

2. The child was permitted no furniture except a mattress and sheets.

3. The child was permitted no toys or other play objects.

4. Staff contacts consisted of at least hourly visits, from one to three psychotherapy hours per day carried out in the isolation room, contact with the case worker and the child's parents as indicated, and careful pediatric and nursing observation.

Many refinements of this technique have been built in as we have learned more concerning the powerful resources in children for defense and resistance and the breadth of potential of the method. For instance, we began to develop greater emphasis, not only on critical control of interpersonal contact, but, in general, the amount and kind of sensory stimulation which was permitted. These had to be controlled through careful examination by the group of a child's defenses and maturity level at any given point. For instance, one important area of sensory input to which we paid increasing attention was that which allowed temporal orientation. The degree to which children were able to cling to even vague or fragmentary reality anchors in order to keep track of time and the events which were occurring outside of the isolation room was amazing.* We began to manipulate meal times and personal hygiene routines, to create disorientation by refusing to become fixed to any particular schedule or the role of the psychotherapist,[2] and to introduce the parents into the isolation room for controlled interaction at crucial points in the child's development.

The Treatment Process

We have used this procedure only in selected situations. The shortest period which has been required for its completion has been 2 months, and the longest 24 weeks, with the average stay in isolation being about 3 months. To date, we have been through this experience 6 times and in each instance a definite pattern has emerged, not only to the treatment process itself but to the development of the child's personality during his stay in isolation.[2] The latter comprised 5 stages:

1. A period of initial panic during which there is precipitous exposure of underlying fears, a sense of decompensation, accompanied by extreme anxiety because of the child's inability to use adults appropriately.

Case Illustration

Peter, age 10, had been alternately obsequious, ingratiating and highly seductive on one hand and covertly rebellious and undermining of authority on the other. During his previous 12 months in the unit he had made little or no progress in his adjustment and in his relationships with the staff or his parents. He had never been known to display any signs of overt anxiety since admission.

His first 24 hours in isolation proved tremendously stressful for him. Although he made no effort to get out of the room, he verbalized panic at being alone. As long as some adult was with him, he was relatively comfortable although

---

*One child learned to identify the sound of the bread truck which came at approximately the same time each morning. In this way, he could gain a sense of the sequence of other events occurring in the unit.

most of the conversation revolved around pleas for the staff member to remain. When he was alone, he shrieked and sobbed in terror, banged on the door or called for various staff people by name. He refused food unless someone remained while he ate. He complained of vague aches and pains and of inability to sleep. Although we had never noted any expression of self-concern or need previously, he could now say that he was "scared something terrible was going to happen to him." He could not elaborate on this. He kept asking to see the other children and for information about what was going on in the unit. He grasped desperately at reality landmarks by which he could maintain orientation (time, day of week, staff members on duty) but none of these questions were answered for him. It was suggested to him that he was not really alone, that we were as available to him as ever, even more so, perhaps and that, in fact, he had been alone for years but had been avoiding coming to grips with this. His therapist made the comment that the source of his terror lay inside of himself and that he could not escape it by being with other people.

2. The second period is one during which there is recompensation of defenses. The child holds desperately to reality anchors and fights off any yielding to the inner process of isolation. There is a heightened expression of angry, omnipotent demand.

Within forty-eight hours, Peter had reconstructed his defenses quite well. He no longer talked about his fears of being alone and when this was raised with him, he shrugged it off. He was the Peter of old. If anything he reached new heights in his efforts to (1) be removed from isolation (2) extract information which would serve to orient him (3) receive special foods, playthings and other individual attentions. When seductiveness failed he resorted to angry, omnipotent commands, threats and innuendoes of the consequences for all of us if we would not comply. He seemed never to be anxious or depressed. He sat and sang to himself quietly for long periods or held imaginary conversations with himself concerning what he would do to all of us for depriving him so. He asked for no one and seemed interested in seeing no one whether staff or family. He slept soundly and ate well. With his therapist he was cocky and glib.

3. A loosening of personality organization culminating in dramatic exposures of the child's sickest state. There is a living out in symbolic forms of the destructive aspects of the parent-child relationships frequently accompanied by hallucinatory experiences or nightmares of the mother coming into the room or out of the radiator or through the window. During this period there also is a more clear cut emergence of the child's defective self image.

By the end of two weeks, Peter's defenses began to decompensate. Without orienting stimuli and without constant opportunity to manipulate objects and people, his former modes of coping with his depressed feelings proved inadequate. He cried frequently, not about being in isolation but simply because he felt miserable. He said he was no good and could not believe that anyone liked him. He became more and more introspective.

On one occasion he screeched in terror that someone, "a woman," had been in the room with him and that she had tried to kill him.

On another occasion he asked for a child care worker who had left the unit six months previously. He insisted she was still around and that she come to see him.

He resorted to more primitive forms of self-comforting. He rocked and he sucked on his fingers or his blanket.

The most significant area of work in therapy revolved around his projections that the therapist also saw him as worthless and unlovable and that the deprivation which he had been experiencing was the outward manifestation of his therapist's wish to withhold from him.

4. This is usually followed by an intensification of resistance, the maintenance of an amazing sameness for days and even weeks. The child may even be able to verbalize his feeling that "It's too hard; now I know what I have to do and I know I can't do it. I give up." Often, however, this is simply acted out and is sometimes accompanied by a total yielding to the isolation experience. In essence, the child is saying "this is the womb and here I stay." One child added to this "Here I die."

Peter began to become comfortable in isolation for the first time. The staff became aware of his almost total yielding to the security of the setting. He found little ways to occupy his time. Although he was not permitted playthings, he became quite creative in improvising things to play with out of bits of cardboard from a cereal box or bits of yarn which he would tease from a sweater or blanket. He was polite and matter-of-fact to the staff. He displayed no anxiety. He made no effort to get out of the room. He was highly organized and cooperative around procedures.

We found that Peter was not sealed over during this time. In fact, he was able to discuss clearly and with some appropriate feeling the trouble he had with his parents and peers and how this had made him feel about himself. He doubted his capacity to do anything about it, however and seemed resigned to spending the rest of his life in isolation.

In retrospect, as we have reviewed Peter's and the other children's courses in isolation it would appear that he was mobilizing his resources for the final move in treatment; but at the time, there was much discouragement in the staff because it seemed that our hopes for this technique might be unfounded.

5. Finally, there is a period of significant therapeutic intervention during which the parents, and the mother figure especially, may be introduced into the child's regressed existence in a different way. The child yields up old defenses. His behavior, although more primitive, is more direct in relation to the mother and there is an intense expression of dependency need on the adult figures. In a controlled fashion the child's violent affects in relation to the mother may be given expression during periods of direct interaction with the latter. Following this one sees a reorganization through which a new social tie to the mother takes place. In effect, it is during this period that the child loses his fear of being alone and, as one child put it, "now I can be by myself." One mother, following an especially dramatic hour

during which her 8-year old daughter lay in her lap in an infantile fashion fondling her mother's breast, said "I became a mother today." Another child in retrospect said about this period "I was born in that room."

After several weeks during which Peter seemed to live in limbo in the womb-like state of the isolation room, there began to appear a subtle and gradual shift in his attitude about himself. He was more clear that no one was really forcing him to change; that for the first time in his life, the way in which he would use his resources was a decision he would make for himself. He became interested in more frequent and direct contact with his parents. He was able to share his fear with his therapist that his parents would not be able to bear the angry negative feelings he had about them and that they would not be able to see and to meet his hungry infantile demands on them.

Finally, with the parent's caseworker always present as a buffer, he began to experiment with more direct expressions of feeling with his parents. Although he began with his father with whom the risks were less, after a few sessions, he gradually moved toward his mother. He shared with his therapist that he wanted to know if they were any different. In essence, he seemed to be trying to find out whether they could see him and hear him as being separate from themselves and having his own identity. If they could, then he was ready to explore getting close to them again. Although he was not able to do this in an age-appropriate way, when he was convinced that they had begun to see him as a real child, he began to seek out closeness with them in ways which suggested that he was returning to the point where his emotional tie to them had been ruptured. At this time, Peter had achieved maximum benefit from isolation.

It is important to emphasize once more that this is a phase of the total therapy. The child is not "cured" when he leaves the isolation room, nor is he ready to return home. A fairly intensive period of treatment continues during which the gains with the parents must be consolidated and built upon. The whole staff is involved in a process of resocialization of a child who was not only anti-social originally but who now displays many regressive elements in his behavior. We find it characteristic of the children during this post-isolation period to be very hungry for socializing and ego-building experiences. They gulp down new school work avidly. They want to learn to shop and to swim and "get along with regular kids". The post isolation period has lasted in our cases from about 10 to 20 weeks.

DISCUSSION

This encapsulated picture of one child's progress through isolation varies, of course, from child to child but we have been able to trace the basic pattern through six different isolation experiences to date. We view this process as being implemented in the physical and social context of isolation through the child's interaction with three basic human forces:

1. *The psychotherapist.* We believe that the role of the therapist is somewhat different in this experience than in the conventional therapeutic procedure. The active transference toward the therapist which is so basic in conventional psychotherapy as it embodies primarily the child's conception of and attitudes toward the parent figures is less essential in isolation. Only in one instance where the child's mother was deceased and he was the ward of a social agency was it necessary to carry out the process as described in phase three of the treatment process, through direct use of the transference relationship. In other instances, the child was able to work through his feelings about the parent figures in the direct security and protection of the isolation room with the parents themselves. Of course, considerable support is necessary from the therapist in order to do this. We viewed the main task of the therapist, however, to be that of preparation of the child for giving up of his defective self image.

2. *The child care staff.* It became the primary task of the child care staff to deal with omnipotent and narcissistic defenses through total control of the child's environment. The activities of the staff serve to develop acute awareness in the child of his deep conflict over dependency by exposing the nature and intent of his demands on other people.

3. *The case worker.* We used the case worker as a kind mediator and buffer between child and parents in order gradually to allow a reciprocal expression of violent affects, to communicate increasing acceptance on the part of the changing parent toward the child and the retraction of projections on the child which occasioned conflicted and ambivalent care in the first place.

Results

In all instances, the children who were involved in this treatment procedure, after the relatively brief period of resocialization following isolation were sufficiently improved to be discharged either to their homes or to social agency type residences. These children were sent to us originally with extremely guarded prognoses and with a history of treatment failures in a variety of settings over several years. Follow-up information now extending over 2½ years indicates that all of them are still in the community. No child has required re-hospitalization in ours or any other psychiatric hospital. All children are attending school, although some require special private school settings.

It is not sufficient to speak of the child in assessing results. It is our conviction that this reintegrating experience had such a powerful impact on the total family constellation that each of these families has continued to operate at a much higher level of maturity as a group, and that the other siblings in the family have profited considerably from the rather dramatic changes which have occurred in most parents.

It is also important to point out that the nature of the deprivation which is inherent in this treatment procedure is such that, in most instances, it came to represent to the parents,* whether consciously or unconsciously, the expression of their own unresolved hostile impulses toward the child. The working through of the rather violent affects associated with enforcing this level of deprivation and recognizing that the child is being provided an opportunity for true autonomy for the first time in his life proved to be a powerful maturational stimulant for all parents.

REFERENCES

1. AZIMA, H., et al.: Effects of partial perception isolation in mentally disturbed individuals. Dis. Nerv. Syst., 17:117, 1956.
2. CHARNY, I. W.: Patterns of regression and reorganization in the isolation treatment of children. J. Child Psychol. Psychiat., in press.
3. GIBBY, R. G., et al.: Therapeutic changes in psychiatric patients following partial sensory deprivation. Arch. Gen. Psychiat., 3:33, 1960.
4. GLYNN, E.: The therapeutic use of seclusion in an adolescent pavillion. J. Hillside Hosp., 6:156, 1957.
5. HERON, W., et al.: Cognitive effects of decrease variation to sensory environment. Am. Psychol., 8:366, 1953.
6. KUBZANSKY, P. E.: The Effects of Reduced Environmental Stimulation on Human Behavior: A Review in the Manipulation of Human Behavior. Bidermand and Zimmer, Ed. New York, Wiley & Sons, 1961.
7. ——, AND LEIDERMAN, P. H.: Sensory Deprivation: An Overview in Sensory Deprivation. Solomon and others, Ed. Cambridge, Harvard Univ. Press, 1961.
8. LILLY, J. C.: Mental Effects of Reduction of Ordinary Levels of Physical Stimuli on Intact, Healthy Persons; Psychiatric Research Reports, No. 5, American Psychiatric Association, June 1956.
9. MORSE, W. C., AND WINEMAN, D.: The therapeutic use of social isolation in a camp for ego disturbed boys J. Soc. Issues, 13:1, 1957.
10. SHURLEY, J. T.: Profound experimental sensory isolation. Am. J. Psychiat., 117:539, 1960.
11. SOLOMON, P., et al.: Sensory deprivation. A review. Am. J. Psychiat., 114:357, 1957.
12. WEXLER, D., et al.: Sensory deprivation: a technique for studying the psychiatric aspects of stress. Arch. Gen. Psychiat., 79:225, 1958.

---

*This area became the most difficult for the staff itself to deal with. These children had all provoked much anger in the staff so that feelings of guilt could easily be exposed by the child's accusations of deprivation unless these had been worked through first in supervision. The success of the procedure depends to a large extent on the capacity of the adults to view this as more realistic giving to the child and as a catalytic force for further growth and development.

The Therapy of Adolescent Offenders

by Nicholas G. Frignito, M.D. and
Carlton W. Orchinik, Ph.D.

The Mask of Maturity

DELINQUENT BOYS detach themselves abruptly from parent and family figures in contrast with the more orderly separation and gradual withdrawal found in the more conforming youngster.[1] There are often especially facilitating circumstances that result in such precipitous flight from family. Extreme dependency concealed by a mask of maturity is regularly found. The parents create unrealistic pictures of maturity by viewing it as a state totally independent of parents and free of anxiety and tension. The ideal is the person who achieves an all pervasive confidence and serene competence in managing his life problems. He is jealous in defending honor, quick in quarrel and seeks reputation in face of all adversaries; violence is taken for granted. He is perhaps typified as a lone cowboy or a gunman wholly without family, able to drift into any situation and emerge uninvolved, safe and victorious.[2] The attractiveness of the cowboy and underworld motion pictures for many non-delinquents and adults may incidentally betray the unresolved fascination for such an ideal.

Flight into delinquency may also be implemented by the threat of succumbing to strong dependency and attachment to parent. Such masculinity and independence from parental supervision may have been emphasized or foisted on the child while dependent needs remain pitifully unmet. The child as a result acquires higher dependence on peers.[3] Some parents may be erratically indulgent, even smothering during the pre-school years only to relinquish their ties abruptly with the beginning of school or as soon as sexual differentiation is clearly established. In other instances there are repeated early separations.[4] The child as a result assumes the manners of aggressive adult even during childhood years while basic capacity for independence is limited.

DEFIANCE OF TRADITION

In adolescence the hasty, headlong flight from parental attachment and supervision into the no-man's land of pseudo-maturity is frequently characterized by affinity for an older boy who typifies the fearless and invincible, and by affiliation with a formal or informal gang. Tradition and custom are defied in the changed interests, attire and attachments that separate the adolescent from his parents and also from their surrogates, teachers and the world of adults. Strong passions consistent with the conception of manliness are at times authentically demonstrated, perhaps more so than at any other time in life. Because of changed ego boundaries in the company of his associates, the adolescent can at times enjoy new feelings of freedom and independence without being enveloped by anxiety.

Having tried to break with tradition, he is also closer to the expression of unfettered impulse. Original ideas, intellectual curiosity and accomplishment may be based upon constructive use of intellectual freedom, but the delinquent is not often so inclined. Energy is used to support ideals and codes native to the peer group or to some fictional adult heroes. There is a rush to fill the need created by the combined impact of separation from parents and by the nascent energies of the age that seeks affection and security to overcome the loneliness.

Defensive aggression is used to deny anxiety at being uprooted and without a realistic ideal to emulate. Delinquents and other adolescents all too frequently feel themselves excluded from the world of adults. This is partly because grownups do reject adolescent participation in adult life, and often because the adolescent himself feels he can not measure up to the mistaken conception of maturity that he holds.

FALSE PICTURES OF ADULT LIFE

Adolescence perhaps always requires a realistic redefinition of the role and life of grownups. It is a period of transition when the emergent adult sees more clearly that the ideal of childhood is not likely to be entirely satisfied. Greater ambivalence must be tolerated. People must be accepted for what they are and one need not be in despair castigating himself for failing to live up to a heroic perfection. The delinquent is infuriated by weakness, by those who are infirm and effeminate. He stubbornly seeks to maintain a front of bravado. In his world of such strong feelings there is little room for moderation and little tolerance for doubt and uncertainty. Identification with a female figure is the threatened alternative after the destruction of the unrealistic manly image. Aggressive and assaultive acts are frequently frantic attempts to ward off this threat of losing one's identity.

GROUP THERAPY OF THE DELINQUENT

To alleviate these precipitous adolescent reactions, we have employed Group Therapy as the method of choice in the rehabilitation programs at the County Court of Philadelphia. Among the advantages of the group method are:

1. Group members serve in various roles and relationships to each other. This helps to point up areas of difficulty.

2. Because the delinquent acts in a socially deviant manner, the group experience comes closer to the social nature of the adolescent personality problems.

3. Group conditions and processes are especially advantageous in improving social skills and communication.

4. Communication verbally is in contrast with other forms of acting out which the adolescent more habitually employs.

5. The group increases the security of the individual when he feels threatened by adult authority.

6. The group allows clearer delineation of defenses and irrational processes.[5] At the same time self-critical, inhibiting self-conscious tendencies decline so that the delinquent verbalizes these attitudes more openly.

7. The group enhances opportunity to form and modify identifications. It allows members to observe and study models with whom they can selectively identify.

8. The adolescent can experience more guided social interaction with opportunities to achieve greater self-understanding.

Let us examine some of the processes and conditions of therapy in the Court setting.

Incorporating Custom and Tradition

The apprehended delinquent on probation is an unwilling member of the Therapeutic Group, but is ordered by the Court to attend the group sessions. To meet some of the problems of social estrangement and departure from parental authoritarian control and his break with tradition and custom, we attempt to restore his continuity with the community by developing routine traditional procedures and ritual. These formal procedures tend to cut down excessive tension caused by a relatively unstructured therapeutic setting. For example, in many instances a large group of probationers is assigned to Therapeutic Groups in a public ceremony conducted by the Judge, at times with outside dignitaries also addressing the group. Both parents and probationers are present and the court hearing opens with the pledge of allegiance.

Another procedure is routinizing membership in the group itself. When a new group meets, the members each take personality tests. After this, the new members interview and introduce each other to the group. Members then sign an attendance book on leaving. Thereafter on entering and leaving the session, this signing in and out occurs. At the end of each session, the therapist stands at the door, shakes hands with each member and says "I'll see you next week". In time the group participants reply in similar fashion although they begin by sheepishly muttering something under their breath. The handshake becomes more formalized and the limp hand soon becomes a firm grip in accord with established custom. In this way we have sought to provide ego support and to foster ties to conventional adult life. We try to lessen estrangement between the adolescent and adult by introducing a degree of general conformity of procedures to which both subscribe.

Increasing Group Cohesiveness

Another traditionalized procedure is the introduction and acceptance of a new member to the already established group. The prospective candidate having been assigned to the group by the Judge must now be accepted by the members who are given the privilege of admitting or rejecting him. When he appears before the group, he is interviewed by all the members who may ply him with questions "Where do you live?" "What school do you go to?" "Who are your friends?" "Do you know Frank, who lives out your way?" "Do you belong to a gang?" Indifference to the prospective members is discouraged. The group then discusses accepting him. They bring up the matter of the Judge's reaction if he is not accepted, and at times threaten to pose their authority against the Court. That this is not an act of rivalry with the Judge is brought out as well as the fact that the group has the same goals as the Judge—that of helping the prospective member. Oftentimes such observations occur spontaneously in the group. After the member is accepted, and he usually is, he returns to the group and receives the congratulations of the members. He takes his test, and then signs the attendance book on leaving.

Imitation of such social customs is an initial step in the program to advance the delinquent's social conformity. Independent activity, decision making and compliance with traditional procedure are here involved. Admission of a new member is also an important source of discussion. Out of it comes a number of significant interactions that are repeatedly referred to in ensuing therapeutic sessions: Meeting strangers, reaction to people who are different, getting to know people, acquiring feelings of empathy are all issues that may at one time or another be related to this experience.

This procedure is designed to encourage members to share in self-affirming roles. It aims to increase group cohesiveness by providing some status and recognition of each person's views and worth; it seeks to encourage and stimulate more cooperative effort in solving a problem.

Changing Relationships within the Group

Freedom of expression is a principle of the group and there is an initial period of testing out. Anxiety, hostility and power struggles are involved. The therapist may be shown a variety of discourtesies. Remarks directed toward denying the significance of the group, remonstrance about attendance, limited participation, private conversations, open expressions of boredom and fatigue, among other things, all challenge or show disrespect for the therapist or his authority. Freedom to speak freely is interpreted as license to such behavior. The members probe for weakness in the armor of the therapist to determine if his manner and indications of strength are genuine, or if he is to be ridiculed or pounced upon for his inadequacies. Tension is sustained by the group therapist at the appropriate level by supplying supports and controls when the tensions become excessive or uncontrolled and by encouraging spontaneity when tensions are too well dampened.

Under such conditions the therapist must also build his friendly but authoritarian relationship. The limits of the provocations must be imposed by general rules. Behavior in the room in which therapy is held is governed by the rules of the building. Private discussions during the group sessions by one or two members are discouraged or brought out into the open for all others to hear. Thoughts expressed as words, not assaultive or physical actions are permitted. This distinction between such words and other actions is an important one for the delinquent and for all acting out disorders. It is during this phase that the therapist may hear complaints about parents, police, the court and teachers. While he is attempting to secure his position as a friendly person, the group therapist is also frustrating the adolescent expectations of retaliation for the aggressive remarks that are frequently levelled at the authority figure.

One immediate objective of the group therapist is to build an image which the adolescent can respect. The therapist partly accomplishes this by the following procedures and conditions:

(1) Failing to be controlled or manipulated.

(2) Demonstrating ability or authority through legal powers and superior knowledge.

(3) Maintaining fearless personal integrity.

(4) Demonstrating social competence.

(5) Being unmoved by threats or derogations.

Even the administration of the initial test creates an aura of knowledge about the therapist. As a powerful figure, he duplicates by analogy or reactivates the cherished omnipotent ego ideal who remains in complete control of himself—a most challenging problem for the adolescent with his intense drives. This view of the therapist's power, capability and competence is further developed when the adolescent receives the assurance that the therapist is trained, understands and knows what is taking place in adolescence. The therapist may offer various astute observations based upon minimal clues or take up topics for discussion that reveal adolescent problems even though he may not apply any insight to a particular group member at this point. A topic that is embarrassing may enhance group interests and cohesiveness.[6] Strength is also derived from acknowledged authority to decide when the boy is ready to terminate and from power to enforce attendance at these sessions. Favorable intercession on behalf of a boy with parent, teacher or Judge also demonstrates this unusual capacity and augments the image of the therapist. Dependency is enhanced in this way: it is easier to trust and rely on a strong figure than on a weak one.

Strengthening Identification with the Therapist

Whether one deals with structured situations, such as prearranged discussions, dramatic presentation or spontaneously recurring conflict and anxiety in the group, the therapist as group leader retains an intellectually and emotionally imposing position. Among adolescents, the extent of power attributed to the therapist includes ability to read minds, capacity to hypnotize or control the mind and total fearlessness. Ambivalence toward him is lurking at all times, but the therapist remains a hero figure, who can potentially satisfy desires and who offers the hope of resolving personal problems as well.

Group procedures frustrate adolescent expectations. The sessions are not as controlled as the classroom, although questions and answers and other structured programs may be employed to hold down some of the anxieties. The group strains to secure the regularity and order of the familiar, and to place the authority figure in a more conventional role. At first imitation of the therapist is fluid and subject to rapid ebbs. It is enhanced by the delinquent's dependency, anxiety and attributes of omnipotence attached to the group leader.

Elementary identification with the therapist may be observed when in the group sessions a boy aligns himself with what he believes is the moral, conventional or conforming side of an issue. Ability to stand in opposition to the group on an ethical issue may be based on strength borrowed from the therapist as well as on a dependent desire to secure the therapist's good will.

Other behavior changes include dressing up for the session, bringing in a popular record for discussion or a sample of handicraft work done in school or as a hobby. Even though this imitative effort is not sustained in other outside behavior—it may even be regarded as a way to "con" the therapist—there is the desire at least within the group to confirm to the high standards seen in the therapist as well as a wish to gain his direct approval. At the same time, there is the pull to remain tied to peer group standards. This conflict is resolved by changing quickly after the group session so as to meet peer group expectations. It is at this point that the matter of self-consistency is appropriately brought up by contrasting and comparing behavior carried· out while being watched by authorities and behavior while being on one's own or with a group of associates.

Ego support is also provided by taking up various topics that are especially troublesome in adolescence. Anxiety, guilt, embarrassment, feelings of being subordinate and the like under a variety of social conditions may be discussed. These themes are useful in revealing the patterns of the delinquent's attitudes and behavior. The question of self-consistency may be here examined by looking at these topics and comparing them with behavior observed in the group relationships. As the therapist reveals his understanding of these issues, he further demonstrates his omniscience.

Humanization of Heroes

For more substantial progress to occur, humanization of adults and heroes must take place. Some of these human qualities are already being introduced as the therapist takes an interest in and tries to understand the delinquent. They also demonstrated in the therapist's reasonable attitudes. Thus simultaneously with the growth of the picture of symbolized strength, control and power are indications of more considerate qualities. Even though the humanitarian aspects are demonstrated by the therapist almost from the beginning of these group sessions, confronting the adolescent with softer qualities of sympathy and cordiality comes only after the therapist is established as a strong figure comparable to the fictional ideal.

Opportunities to reappraise heroes also occur as the adolescent attacks teachers, parents and the police. Authority figures may be rejected because they do not satisfy dependent wants. They may be considered unworthy of emulation because they do not achieve omnipotent perfection. Underlying this attack may be the feeling that identification with strong figures is impossible because of the adolescent's own inadequacies. The delinquent is frequently fearful of demonstrating qualities other than those reflecting aggression and violence. The problem centers around the delinquent's intolerance of ambivalence with its attendant anxieties. Many delinquent acts, particularly aggression against the weak and the inadequate, occur because the delinquent can not stand seeing anything that falls short of expected masculinity.

The therapist also acknowledges various inadequacies when he says "I was not considerate of your feelings" or "I did not understand you", or when he fails to protest critical comments made by members about how he is conducting the therapy. These criticisms and attacks are tied in with the unrealistic picture of heroes that the adolescent holds. They are also used to make reconstructive interpretations about the delinquent's own past ideals. In explaining the various human qualities and the other relevant insights, the way is clear for accepting individuals as they are. As criticism is levelled at the therapist who is capable of standing this social threat or withdrawal of love, the adolescent is in a better position owing to partial identification with the therapist to accept more realistic self-appraisal and criticism. As ability to tolerate ambivalence toward others including the therapist increases, he can approve those human characteristics which are valued while recognizing the fact that flaws are also present.

Supporting Efforts to Help Others

Having introduced these corrective influences regarding adults and having reduced defensive sensitivity to criticism, the therapist continues to foster and extend identification with an authority figure. Since criticism has already been made about the way the therapist conducted the group, the therapist now asks for specific recommendations to improve procedures and to help others. He supports the suggestions and efforts of the adolescents to help each other. He affords group members greater opportunities to serve in the capacity of group leader. He encourages them to use rational processes to help work out difficulties that arise in the interpersonal relationships of the group and in discussion about problems occurring outside. The result is that the adolescent assumes a more adult role of responsibility and takes more interest in aiding others to work out their problems.

REFERENCES

1. FREUD, A.: Adolescence. In The Psychoanalytic Study of the Child. Vol. XIII. New York, International Universities Press, 1958, pp. 255-278.

2. ALEXANDER, F.: The Don Quixote of America, The News-Letter, Vol. VII, No. I, 1937; In The Scope of Psychoanalysis Selected Papers of Franz Alexander—1921-1961. New York, Basic Books, 1961.

3. McCORD, W., McCORD, J., AND VERDEN, P.: Familial and behavioral correlates of dependency in children. Child Development, 33: 313-326, 1962.

4. BENNETT, I.: Delinquent and Neurotic Children. New York, Basic Books, 1960.

5. KOTKOV, B.: Power factors in psychotherapy groups. Psychoanal. & Psychoanal. Rev., 48:68-77, 1961.

6. CARTWRIGHT, D., AND ZANDER, A.: Group cohesiveness: Introduction. Chapter 3 in D. Cartwright and A. Zander (Eds.) Group Dynamics Research and Theory—2nd Ed. Evanston, Row Peterson and Co., 1960.

Community Therapy of Child Delinquents

by SELWYN BRODY, M.D.

R ESIDENTIAL TREATMENT, while utilized as an expedient for defeated families, and for authorities to dispose of delinquent youths, actually represents the community's last resort, in many cases, for these individuals to receive treatment. On the other hand, it is a unique facility for psychiatrist and delinquents to be brought together in this special milieu for an extended period.

SELECTION

The psychiatrist in the screening process helps to select youths likely to benefit from residential treatment. He attempts to determine aspects of treatability and reversibility of the delinquent process. In this connection, we have begun to interview the family at intake. However, eloquent psychodynamics do not guarantee prediction, and experience has shown that individuals "weeded out" as not worthy of treatment may prove to be more responsive than those who had impressed the consultant favorably.

Faced with an ever increasing number of candidates from the juvenile courts, the administration has set the following criteria in keeping with the *limitations* of residential treatment goals:

No murderers or others with a history of extreme violence, or suicidal tendencies are acceptable; fire-setters, overt sex "maniacs" or deviants, overt psychotics, mental defectives are excluded; those with central nervous system disease, such as epilepsy—and those over 15 years of age are finally eliminated. There is the more pressing requirement that the youths on application have at least the semblance of a family which can be involved in the critical need for family therapy and to whom the youth can be returned upon discharge. (In lieu of a family, Children's Village has set up a program of foster homes and group homes in the community. For a period of as long as five years after these children have been discharged from in-treatment, they are given an extension of all of the supervisory and clinical services they received at the residential center.)

DIAGNOSIS

If the problem of diagnosis is prodigious in the entire field of mental and emotional disorders, it is multiplied in the province of delinquency. From our clinical and psychological studies, conviction grows that delinquents rarely suffer from mild emotional disorders. Unfortunately, there are few in whom we have confirmed a benign diagnosis of transient adjustment reaction of adolescence, or psychoneurosis.

In contrast with the psychic structure of the patient with psychosomatic or organic disorders, where the ego is dominated by the need to control destructive impulses towards others,[1] the delinquency syndrome expresses a life preservative function for the release of intolerable tensions.[2] The form of the sickness represents the only way by which the majority of the delinquent youths can discharge destructive impulses and tensions outwards against others, and actually the only means through which they can ever get help.

Such a youth has never attained a healthful organization for the outlet of his aggressive drives and reactions to frustration. Nor has he reached the state of ego-superego functioning defined as the psychoneurotic solution. But by the delinquent method for the disposition of aggressive drives he protects his ego against mental and tissue breakdown.

There is an urgent diagnostic need to understand the interaction between delinquency and psychosis or depression.[3] The current screening process favors an increased number of younger, so-called "unsuccessful" delinquents. These are disturbed adolescents who are more borderline or psychotic[4] than delinquent. Their roots are sick, their foundation poor, although occasionally presenting an appearance which may be deceptively attractive. This type is not the casehardened, "normal" delinquent. The veneer of defiance and self-confidence is thin. They may be mumblers or non-verbalizers. They are mostly aimless and joyless and without friends. Few are from organized gangs; rather they are truants who have committed minor crimes alone or in small groups. This lonely, unappealing "failure" often is dull, with severe learning problems. His self-esteem is minimal.

THERAPY

Treatment is the reason-for-being of the residential institution. Here we are challenged by formidable problems. One cannot be intimidated by the authoritative views on the *unanalyzability of the delinquent patient,* but must search for other parameters. According to Greenwood, there are a number of children in residential treatment for whom individual psychotherapy is not appropriate.[5] Frequently after having experienced the total therapeutic climate of the residential center, such a child might be considered for individual treatment. For practical purposes, the residential population must be roughly divided into three groups. Actually, sharp lines do not stand up to scrutiny and overlapping makes statistical figures not too useful.

(1) The first group consists of those in whom a favorable response to environmental and individual therapy occurs. Superego development and reaction formation are essential factors in their progress. Improved behavior contributes to a better self-image. The youth becomes able to feel more worth while in his own as well as in our minds. Follow-up studies would determine the permanence of improvement.

(2) The "unsuccessful" delinquent, who is accessible to adults and on whom "a dent can be made", is considered available for therapy. But he may regress, when he feels pressure towards yielding the dependence he has never had consistently gratified. In such instances he may reveal a whining, sticky behavior—or panicky withdrawal. If he is not penalized by transfer to a mental hospital, two years of therapy may be only a beginning.

Some of these borderline or schizoid delinquents vacillate between withdrawal and clinging to an attached adult. Their negativistic behavior and mood is related to realistic progress and to positive feelings in the therapist. Basically, these patients can tolerate only a minimum of successful emotional attachment or communication of positive feelings. Some will use regression for an immense need to tear down hated parent figures.

(3) The so-called "normal delinquent" troubles the milieu far less. He is a "treatment rejector,"[6] who feels above and beyond needing help. He is pseudo-mature, controlled, and his masculine self-image precludes confiding in therapists. He derives a certain satisfaction out of "playing it cool" for time, adroitly adjusting to the residential structure. On him "no dent has been made." One can only hope that two or three years of residential containment will rub off on his ego surface. This could aid in improved superficial functioning, even if the basic personality is unchanged. However, the evidence indicates that his psychopathy is strengthened by his two years of successful manipulation of the staff, which more often than not has unwittingly played into his hands. Consequently he is the one most likely to make the front pages with capital crimes. The limited goal of containment is seriously questioned.[7]

The paucity of *teachable methods* contributes to the treatment dilemma for juvenile delinquency. It must be emphasized: *no one knows what cures delinquency.* Exponents of reliance upon milieu for progress are warned by Redl[8] against naive overexpectations. For individual therapy, it is equally magical to depend on psychoanalytical formulations.[9-11]

Eissler contends, "With delinquencies the technique of free association cannot be applied since they will not obey the rule," and Josselyn, "Even modification of analytic technique is rarely serviceable in the treatment of adolescents."

Epstein has observed that boys who have not responded to individual treatment by caseworkers have been formed into groups, from which they obtained marked benefit.[12] And Slavson has reported boys who, after experiencing in the group universalization and reduction of guilt, ventilation of feelings, discharge of hostility, and by having been accepted, have sought out the group therapist for individual talks.[13]

Hendrickson, discussing the treatment of hospitalized adolescents supports the writer's emphasis on the value of the individualized treatment. "Therapy of the adolescent is a highly interpersonal process. Adult relationship is seen as the best means of understanding the processes of therapy with patients in this age range. This is also the most useful framework in which to study the psychology of adolescence generally, as we rarely have an opportunity to observe them directly except in relation to ourselves."[7]

Sometimes the therapist's most reliable ally is the patient himself. Beneath the smoke and noise lie the youngster's unconscious ego ideals, his wish to like, respect, trust others and his desire for reciprocal treatment. In building a relationship we sometimes have to act as a frustrating, depriving disciplinarian. Actually, the disturbed adolescent can initially find great comfort in regarding his therapist as an unreasonable tyrant.[7]

We may learn also from the work of Weinrib,[14] who states, "In confronting the ego of the impulsive adolescent we seem to impress him that we are strong and helpful, and we can help him learn control over his frightening but tempting impulses." Weinrib claims that unwilling youths have thereby become involved in a meaningful therapeutic relationship.

Limitations and Treatment Fitting the Individual

Reality factors and psychologically negative considerations force us to fit our goals to existing limitations. We have yet to develop a conveyor line product, whether by milieu or by individual psychotherapy on delinquents. The time honored need to make treatment fit the patient is attenuated if not lost. The important consideration is that many of these youths *are* treatable. And despite the fact that there are "no well-established treatment procedures in this field," we can draw upon methods of treating disturbed ego functions. Some modifications I have found to be effective in therapy and teaching include:

(1) *Supportive therapy* with emphasis on warmth and positive relationship has the widest application.

(2) *Reinforcement of defenses* based on the principle of joining forces with the delinquent. Through this technique, the attempt is made to help him outgrow his symptomatic defenses.

In one case, treated individually once a week for a period of three years, there was dramatic redirection of a blustering, bullying exterior to the underlying personality of a shy, weak, self-conscious boy. In quietly standing his ground, the therapist gradually was able to uncover (and reinforce) the patient's basic motivations, which hardly could have been observed as a defense. Beneath the shouted abusiveness, the patient's wish to be better controlled was his essential goal. The therapist chose to join forces with this fundamental wish, rather than with the more obvious outwardly expressed wish, his overt defense, his apparent desire to be a "bigshot."

Case Illustration

A. N. was a 15 year old boy on admission to residential treatment. The final court charge was that of exposing himself, in mutual masturbation with other boys, on a rooftop in full view of neighbors. A previous charge arose from his dialing of random telephone numbers. When a woman answered he would make obscene sexual propositions. The last call occurred when a woman on the other end of the line agreed to meet him in her car. She had set a trap for him and at the appointed place he was terrified to find not only a lady, but a policeman. The woman he had called was the wife of a policeman. They forced the boy into the car and drove to an old graveyard where the policeman made him get out, drew his revolver and forced him to his knees. Only as the panicked boy cried and begged for mercy did the couple relent and then brought the charge against him.

His homosexuality had been initiated by a grocer who at first had plied him with candy and fruit when he was 13. He had reached the second term of high school although his school work had shown deterioration from earlier years, when he had actually been at the top of his class. He recalled the onset of conduct troubles, stealing kitchen matches from home and selling them for pennies to his second-grade classmates, who would set small fires. When the teacher had caught him, his father was summoned by the principal. The father's response was mockery of the school for not recognizing his son's enterprise.

The father, a large, handsome man was 40 at the time of the boy's admission, had himself been an inmate of the same residence a quarter of a century ago. He had continued to be in financial and gambling jams and seemed always on the verge of imprisonment. The mother was an immature woman, who overprotected the boy. The boy often said he did not know which to turn to, or who was worse. He had no respect for either; though he was more ashamed of his father he expected to follow his father's footsteps.

Before admission the father had made one of his sporadic efforts to discipline the boy and in the scuffle the boy threw his father so violently against the wall that he had sustained a dislocated fracture of the elbow. The boy felt very remorseful over this incident. He, too, was well-developed, nearly six feet and weighed 180. He was immediately chosen for the football squad, but was unable to qualify for the varsity team until several months of therapy had helped him to overcome his timidity towards aggressive contact with his opponents.

His general attitude towards treatment was one of attempted intimidation, and of constant derogation of the therapist and psychiatry in general. He loudly proclaimed no need for therapy and "as a real man" he could solve his own problems. The initial sessions were marked by patient's storming out of the office and slamming the door whenever he felt the therapist stand up to, question or frustrate his blandishments and demands.

This deprived, hostile boy had the frustration tolerance of a sensitive and hurt two-year-old child. And yet, the therapist's quiet refusal to "budge an inch" when being on the receiving end of the verbal attacks acted as a frustration, not of the attacks themselves, but of their efficacy. When patient had had his fill of being allowed to verbalize his rebellion against the very treatment itself: "Give me a *rush* job—I have no time for this nonsense—I am no psycho, etc.,"—all in the loudest, rudest tones; when he learned that no acting out was permitted, only verbal behavior, he reacted to the reality frustration of his attempt to be a "big shot." He could come to the end of his bluff and get down to his real need for a more positive relationship, and reveal his deeper wish to have better control of himself. It was the therapist's recognition of this deeper need and his "joining forces" with it that enabled patient to come to treatment with expression of his mass of fears regarding his appearance, his intelligence, his sanity, etc. He shed his swagger and began to talk about his family life and his inner feelings.

(3) *The Technique of reflecting negative patterns*[2] encourages the ego to discharge hostility verbally.[15] One of the most difficult problems is that of the non-verbalizing delinquents. Occasionally such dreary youths can be helped by the therapist's mirroring his silence.

One such patient said, "Why don't you ask me questions?" The reply, "When I did ask you, you didn't answer anyway, so why don't we both just be quiet? Didn't you ever sit quietly with your parents?" This evoked an interesting line of conversation and enhanced the therapeutic relationship.

Another boy, who mumbled and whimpered, was echoed[16] by a kind of mocking of his negative behavior. He finally became angry. He overcame his ineffectual exterior and related that he was an expert at building model airplanes. He said he could even spell Mississippi.

Another boy who said he was no good at making friends, no good at reading, no good at sports, the therapist remarked, "You're good at getting people discouraged." The boy's smiling response was, "You'll have to be *very* good not to quit on *me*."

The techniques of *reinforcement of defenses* and *reflecting negative patterns* are specialized extensions of ego-strengthening procedures, advocated by Spotnitz.[17] They augment the therapist's devices for treating the delinquent when a positive relationship cannot be sustained.

(4) In the treatment of these youths, there is an *induced delinquency* syndrome in which delinquency patterns are aroused in the

therapist.[18] When this induced delinquency is effectively exploited by the patient, his deviant behavior is enhanced. When successfully conducted by the therapist, he defeats the delinquent at his own game; the result is control of delinquency, reminiscent of Aichorn's method, particularly as elaborated by Noshpitz.[19] Intensive research is required for the exploration of this technique.

(5) The currently intense interest of psychiatry in the family is reflected in the residential centers.[20] Therapists are being assigned to treatment of the family of the residents. Without treatment of the family, improvement of the juvenile delinquent has, upon occasion, contributed to destructive relapse of parental delinquency.

(6) Group psychotherapy is being expanded as a useful tool, but the principal therapeutic factor is the interaction of the residential community as a whole. The relationships of boy to boy and staff member to staff member, as well as to each boy, help to create healthier contacts for each boy with each area of the center.

REFERENCES

1. BRODY, S.: Psychological factors associated with disseminated lupus erythematosus and effects of cortisone and ACTH. Psych. Quart., 30:54, 1956.
2. GLOVER, E.: Functional Group of Delinquent Disorders. On the Early Development of Mind. New York, Intl. Univ. Press, 1956, Chapter 25, p. 379.
3. TOOLAN, J. M.: Depression in children and adolescents. Am. J. Orthop., 32: 404, 1962.
4. BURKS, H. L., AND HARRISON, S. J.: Aggressive behavior as a means of avoiding depression. Am. J. Orthop., 32:416, 1962.
5. GREENWOOD, E. D.: The role of psychotherapy in residential treatment. Am. J. Orthop., 25:692, 1955.
6. BRODY, S.: Syndrome of the treatment rejecting patient. Presented at APA Meeting, San Francisco, 1958. To be published.
7. HENDRICKSON, W. J., et al.: Psychotherapy with hospitalized adolescents. Am. J. Psychol., 116:527, 1959.
8. REDL, F.: The concept of a therapeutic milieu. Am. J. Orthop., 29:721, 1959.
9. EISSLER, K. R.: Problems of technique in the psychotherapy of adolescents from psychoanalytic study of the child, 13:223, 1958.
10. ——: Effect of the structure of the ego on psychoanalytic technique. J. Psa. Assn., 1:104, 1950.
11. JOSSELYN, I. M.: Psychotherapy of adolescents at the level of private practice. Psychotherapy of the Adolescent, Balser, Ed. New York, Intl. Univ. Press, p. 32.
12. EPSTEIN, N., AND SLAVSON, S. R.: Breakthrough in group treatment of hardened delinquent adolescent boys. Int. J. Group Psych., 12:199, 1962.
13. SLAVSON, S. R.: Patterns of acting out of a transference neurosis by an adolescent boy. Int. J. Group Psych., 12:211, 1962.

14. WEINRIB, J.: Impulsivity in the Adolescent and Its Therapeutic Management. Paper No. 102; p. 109 Summaries of Papers. A.P.A. Annual Meeting, 1959.

15. FRAIBERG, S.: A therapeutic approach to reactive ego disturbances in children in placement. Am. J. Orthop., 32:18, 1962.

16. SPOTNITZ, H., et al.: Ego reinforcement in the schizophrenic child. Am. J. Orthop., 26:146, 1956.

17. ———: The narcissistic defense in schizophrenia. Psychoanal. & Psychoanal. Rev., 48:24, 1961-62.

18. SEARLES, H. F.: The effort to drive the other person crazy—an element in the etiology and psychotherapy of schizophrenia. Brit. J. M. Psychol., 32:1-18, 1959.

19. NOSHPITZ, J.: Opening phase in the psychotherapy of adolescents with character disorders. Bull. Menn. Clin., 21:153, 1957.

20. ACKERMAN, N. W.: The Psychodynamics of Family Life. New York, Basic Books, 1959.

PART VI

THE FAMILY

Family Diagnosis and Therapy

by Nathan W. Ackerman, M.D.

FOR MANY PSYCHIATRISTS schooled and trained along established paths of theory and practice, and oriented to the one-to-one relationship of doctor and patient, a method of diagnosis and therapy for the whole family signifies a radical departure from tradition. It constitutes a major shift from an exclusive focus on the manifestations of mental illness in the individual to a system of diagnosis and treatment directed to the family unit as the matrix of health. It is still relatively crude, exploratory and experimental, but is a fluid, evolving procedure.

In the purview of history, the effort to diagnose, treat, and prevent personality disorders through a family approach is propelled by several converging forces: (1) the revolutionary transformation of the family pattern, induced by social change; (2) the recognition of the principle of contagion in emotional disturbance, and the intimate connection between social and mental disorder; (3) the greater appreciation of the limitations of the conventional procedures of diagnosis, treatment and prevention that are restricted to the individual patient; and (4) specific new developments in the behavioral sciences which include a range of studies in ego psychology, small group dynamics, social psychology, anthropology and communication. Such developments, rapidly unfolding on the contemporary scene, bring a rising pressure for a method of study and therapeutic intervention in the family group as a living entity.

It is self-evident that the course and outcome of illness rest not alone on the content of unconscious disturbance, but also on the resources that can be mobilized to counteract the core of pathogenic experience. A more expanded understanding of the relations between inner and outer experience would illuminate the mechanisms of coping with conflict. It would shed light on operations of defense, homeostatic control, and on the learning and growth processes of personality.

Almost always, in discussions of contemporary mental health services, the tendency is to leap to what appears, at first glance, to be the practical side of the problem, the chronic disproportion between the limitations of available mental health facilities and the ever-mounting demand for them. Always the same outcry: more hospitals, clinics, psychiatrists, psychologists, social workers and expanded resources for professional training. But surely the quantitative insufficiency in mental health services in the present day community is not the only issue. We must face other questions. Do the conventional therapeutic procedures really cure? Are they appropriate and specific to the disorders characteristic of our time and culture? Are the goals of therapy linked to the goals of prevention? If not, why not? It is in relation to such questions that we must examine the implications of the concepts of family diagnosis and family psychotherapy.

At the family level, the procedures of diagnosis and treatment are interdependent activities. On the one hand, diagnostic judgment determines the clarity and appropriateness of the choice of therapeutic goals and the specificity of the techniques of family psychotherapy. On the other hand, it is the therapeutically oriented family interview that is itself the pathway to diagnosis.

The goals of family therapy are therefore: (1) to alleviate emotional distress and disablement and to promote the level of health, both in the family group and in its individual members; (2) to strengthen the individual against destructive forces, both within him and surrounding him in the family environment; (3) to strengthen the integrative capacity of the family. This calls for a continuous effort to enhance the homeostatic balance of both the family and the individual. It means the introduction of those influences that favorably alter the balance of forces, as between those tendencies that maintain effective health in family living and those that move toward breakdown and illness. It also signifies a concern with the level at which the family members complement one another's emotional needs, buttress one another's defenses and how this, in turn, affects the balancing and harmonizing of essential family functions.

Until now, we cannot be said to have developed a true psychotherapy of the family group, but rather only feeble and ersatz gestures in this direction. By the qualifying term 'true,' we mean a specific method of intervention that influences the family as an organismic whole, based on systematic diagnosis of family development and behavior, focused on distortion of interactional patterns, coping with the interplay between interpersonal and intrapersonal conflict, and pointing its techniques toward the relations between the emotional functioning of the family as a unit and the emotional development and destiny of any one member.

Individual therapy, or even therapy of family pairs, while exerting certain partial effects on family relations, does not of itself signify a true family therapy. Such forms of treatment concern themselves only minimally with the health functioning of the family as a whole; the effect on family relationships is indirect, secondary and non-specific. Such therapy may help or harm family relationships. It may bring family members closer together or, paradoxically, it may intensify the trend toward alienation among them. By contrast, a true family psychotherapy points its corrective influence not toward the isolated individual, but rather to the family and the relations of the family with its members.

The rationale for this method of intervention can be summed up as follows: it is a natural level of therapeutic participation in human distress. It approaches troubled persons in their usual habitat, the family and home. It defines human conflicts and disablements not in isolation, but rather in the matrix of significant relationships, the day by day intimate interchange among family members. It gives recognition to the principle that the experiences of family participation play a potent part in making or breaking the mental health of its members. These experiences may precipitate an illness, may fixate a member in illness, may reward him for staying ill, or, by contrast, motivate him for recovery.

These principles are strongly documented by clinical observation. Their validity rests on a basic axiom: mental illness by its very nature is a contagious and communicable type of disorder. The seeds of mental breakdown are passed from person to person, from one generation to the next. They exert their influence within the mind of one individual and also move between the multiple minds of family members. Over the stretch of time, the center of pathogenic conflict experience may move from one part of the family to another. It is in this sense that the chain of family relations constitutes a kind of conveyor belt of disturbance, a carrier of pathogenic foci. The contagious influence is transmitted across time and also across space. In fact, it is the organizational pattern of the family group that determines in great part how each member asserts his emotional need and which of his defenses against anxiety become operable or inoperable. To achieve his objective, the family therapist must pursue the following aims:

(1) Help the family achieve a more clear definition of the real content of conflict. The first step, in this sense, is to stir a greater accuracy of perception and a lessening of the confusion of interpretation of family conflict.

(2) Counteract inappropriate displacements of conflict.

(3) Neutralize the irrational prejudices and scapegoating that are

involved in the displacement of conflict. The effort here is to put the conflict back where it came from in family role relationships, that is, to reattach it to its original source and attempt to work it out there, so as to counteract the trend toward prejudicial assault and disparagement of any one member.

(4) Relieve an excessive load of conflict on one victimized part of the family, either an individual or family pair.

(5) Lift concealed interpersonal conflicts to the level of interpersonal relations, where they may be coped with more effectively.

(6) Activate an improved quality of emotional complementarity in family role relationships.

(7) Replace the lacks in the patterns of family interaction through the appropriate and selective use of the therapist's personality. This means a discriminating injection of healthy elements of emotional interaction to replace sick ones, as the alignments in family relationships shift.

In family life, disorder of emotional communication can be a serious problem. At one pole, there is the type of family in which the members hardly communicate at all; the group is fragmented and the members are alienated from one another. At the opposite pole, there is the type of family whose members have abundant contact, but they battle one another continuously in a destructive way. The distrust and the hostility are fierce. There is a strong tendency to deny and displace the blame and guilt. The members of the group argue about the wrong matters or about trivialities, and they make scapegoats of one another. Loss of emotional control is a constant threat; now and then, there may even be an outbreak of physical violence. In such families, periods of acute chaos are not uncommon, or the family alternates between phases of murderous silence and explosions of uncontrolled fighting.

In dealing with the emotional problems of family groups, the clinician fulfills the part of a parent or grandparent. He is interested; he is actively involved. He uses his therapeutic self in a special way. He activates an increasingly correct definition of the important areas of family conflict. He confronts the members with these conflicts. He elaborates their expressions, their harmful consequences, not merely for one individual, but for all members. He elucidates the failing and injurious results of the family's habitual ways of coping with these conflicts, and shares with the members his view of the deviant and destructive efforts at control and defense. He stirs an awakening to other avenues of possible solution, or at least compensation of conflict. Whenever needed, he injects into the hopper of family discussion more appropriate and fitting images of family relations, with the corresponding healthier kinds of emotion.

The role of the family therapist, therefore, is an active, open, forthright one. In this situation, there can be no question of therapeutic anonymity; the therapist cannot hide his face nor can he be merely a passive listener. He pitches in with the family, implementing the emotional elements which are missing in family interaction. He acts as a kind of catalyst or chemical reagent dissolving the barriers to communication, stirring the interactional processes among the family members, shaking up the elements and promoting a realignment of family relationships toward health. He follows the movement of the center of sickness-producing disturbance from one part of the family to another. In so doing, he engages the family members in a process of working through of the elements of conflict. The core of pathogenic conflict may shift about from the mother-child pair to the husband-wife pair, and, at times, it may become concentrated in one member, such as a child, who often becomes the pawn of conflict between the parents. As the central conflict moves about from one place in the family group to another, the therapist follows along, stirring selective support now to one part of the family, now to another. He may call pointed attention to facial expressions, body postures, movements, etc.; by these means, he hopes to expand and sharpen the perception of relevant conflict experience. With discretionary use of these subverbal aspects of intercommunication, the therapist is enabled to challenge unreal and impossible demands, fruitless, vindictive forms of blaming and omnipotent destructive invasions of one member by another. Step by step, the therapist is able to activate awareness of new avenues of sharing, new kinds of intimacy, new levels of identification, and mobilize a realignment of emotional relationships toward health.

The therapist initiates the procedure of family therapy in a simple, casual manner. Regardless of the presenting complaint and regardless of which member of the group is tagged with the label of the "sick one", the therapist invites the whole family to come in and talk it over. He avoids any lengthy or complicated explanations of the family interview. He simply asks them all to join in a family conference. This approach generally brings an optimal response.

In troubled families, there is awareness of the multiplicity of disturbance and also of the contagion of such disturbance. The members know very well that the whole family is in a state of disorder. They are, therefore, receptive to a clinical approach which gives an honest recognition to this principle.

As soon as the members become invested in the live events of the family interview, they show an increasing desire to participate and they then quickly lose their initial self-consciousness and restraint. The threat of personal exposure becomes less frightening, and the fundamental urge to be understood and helped becomes increasingly important. Family psychotherapy may be the method of choice; it may be the sole method, or it may be used in conjunction with individual or other therapies. On principle, family therapy has a wide range of applicability, but must, of course, be flexibly modified to accommodate different conditions. It can be helpful in those psychiatric disorders in which intrapsychic conflict is not the major problem, or where the disturbance is not of long standing. For optimal progress, all members of the family unit should be involved.

Family therapy can be of substantial value for disturbances at all periods of the life cycle—childhood, adolescence, adulthood, and old age. It is, of course, especially potent in disturbances involving the relations of the child with his family.

No method of psychotherapy is comprehensive and total; each exerts selective and differential effects on different components of human disturbance. To set one therapy in competition with another is naive and unsound. One must recognize that each psychotherapeutic method is characterized by specific strengths, but also by certain weaknesses and limitations. By way of generalization, one might say that psychoanalysis has a favored access to unconscious mental mechanisms and is useful in the resolution of those components of emotional disorder that have their origin in entrenched forms of childhood conflicts. Group psychotherapy, in turn, holds the power to modify character traits and ego defense operations. In turn, family psychotherapy possesses certain unique potentials of its own, not apparent in the other methods of therapy. The selective features of each of these methods derive from the special social structuring of the therapeutic interview. From this point of view, the application of family therapy does not preclude the use of other forms of treatment. Within this context, it is useful to think of individual therapy with specific family members, where clinically indicated, as being an auxiliary to the psychotherapy of the whole family.

Psychotherapy of Families of Hospitalized Patients

by Stephen Fleck, M.D.

C LINICAL INTEREST in the patient's family has a long history, and yet systematic consideration and investigation of family functions and problems have been sparse, scattered, and vari-disciplinal. The physician has traditionally assumed the care of all members of a family but has not concerned himself particularly with the function of the family as a group or the interrelational processes in it, and usually receives no training in family dynamics or family oriented services. He is considered the diagnostician and manager of contagious agents, usually biological or physiochemical in nature, which he may encounter in the family group, and when consulted may advise on cohabital practices. The physician also has habitually supported all family members during the "crises" of birth and death and more recently rendered some premarital services, but not routinely marital guidance or counselling with regard to emotional or mental health issues of family life.

The behavioral scientists have focussed on family composition, structure, and its sociocultural characteristics as an institution. Most of these inquiries have been topical, comparative and statistical rather than directed to all dimensions of family interrelatedness.[3,22]

The legal profession has established a large body of knowledge on the contractual aspects of family life although in recent years interest in the emotional and psychological sphere of intrafamilial relationships has resulted in law school courses on this topic as well as in ancillary court services. [17,40]

The social work profession has a tradition of family-oriented service, but in recent decades has concentrated on individual casework, group therapy and community organization in training and practice.[28]

All disciplines have often dealt with the family in oversimplified concepts. For instance, it is a fond platitude to state that the family is the keystone of society, or that the changes in family composition and "stability," at least in Western society during this century, are the source of many if not all social ills and evils.[2] Obviously the family can be viewed as the keystone of society, but its structure, composition and social role are also the outcome of a long history of behavioral patterns, mores, and beliefs, all of them characteristic for a culture over generations. The family as a social institution and the culture in which it exists, therefore, have developed and changed together in a circular and reactive fashion. There is better evidence that the family is the keystone of personality in the sense that in most societies the family is the prime and certainly the initial transmitter and teacher of the cultural mores and instrumentalities. We know now that if the family performs this task inadequately or in a fashion too deviant from the cultural norm, the offspring in such a family are handicapped and may be harmed in their personality development.[3,10,22,29,33]

Although Freud presented us with incisive insights as to how the dynamics of family relationships can be precipitated in the form of personality traits, his clinical focus remained strictly individual. Indeed, the techniques he innovated for the study of personality have hampered the clinical consideration of the family as a whole, let alone the direct observation and treatment of this group.[25] Of course, it is preferable methodologically to study interpersonal processes and problems and their treatment in a two-person field instead of in complex groups. Simultaneously the spectacular success of bacteriological medicine has led psychiatrists, like all physicians, to hope despite ample evidence to the contrary that all diseases will fit the particular mode of pathological events characteristic of infectious disease and that mental disorders will yield to similar treatment approaches, i.e., therapies in which emotional and interpersonal factors are of minimal importance. Although few physicians would disagree with Dubos' statement that "all important pathological disorders are the summation of a multiplicity of interplays of internal and external environment," or with similar assertations of the multifactorial determination and causation of biological processes, medicine in general and even psychiatry continue to be practiced much of the time as if disease came about through simple cause-and-effect mechanisms.[8]

Like treatment, most psychiatric research has focused either on the difficulties of the individual, whether these are conceived primarily as psychological or biological, or recently on large populations such as hospitals or a community. In the absence of well defined "normal dynamics of family life" epidemiological and other investigators of mental disturbances have been reluctant to undertake family studies. But a "healthy family" is no more definable even for a particular subculture than a scientific definition of health is possible. Both terms refer to goals and ideals rather than to fixed states and both, to requote Dubos, are a function of an equilibrium between internal and external forces of a very complex nature. Such methodological difficulties must not deter us from studying the dynamic effects of interpersonal relationships, and to establish (or disprove) the coexistence of particular intrafamilial processes and personality features in the adult who has emerged from the family group. Because the paramedical professions have emulated our focus on the individual, very little attention was paid to this immediate social environment in which an individual develops, before the past ten to fifteen years. Yet the family is the obvious and crucial link between an individual and his society, and adequate understanding of the family's impact upon and role in the development of the individual and his psychosocial adjustment is overdue despite the methodological difficulties. Focusing on the family as the clinical unit for treatment is thus a logical extension of family research and a clinical implementation of social psychiatry.

Family therapy with psychiatric in- and out-patients and their families in our era was probably first practiced by Midelfort.[27] Ackerman[1] has been the pioneer in child psychiatry and many centers are experimenting now more or less systematically with conjoint family treatment and its evaluation, whether the patient is a child or an adult.[20,31,32,39] Families with a hospitalized psychotic member have also been treated, and Bowen and his colleagues at the National Institute of Mental Health took the daring and imaginative approach of hospitalizing the entire family.[4,5]

In our own approach based on earlier family studies, we have focused less on technical problems of treatment than on realizable goals to improve functioning of the family as a group and of its members as individuals.[7,11,12] In general this is the goal of family treatment.

Some of the important givens and principles of therapy with the family unit which prevail regardless of particular techniques may be listed briefly:

Unlike other treatment groups family therapy starts with only one designated patient and the family has to learn that all of them constitute the clinical unit; as a group the family has a biologically and culturally predetermined life span independent of treatment effects; there are four role parameters in the family according to the divisions into two generations and two sexes respectively; the family differs further from other treatment groups by virtue of its pre-existence as an intensely interrelated group with an idiosyncratic pre-existing communication pattern; family therapy need not be office-bound, and at least during emergencies it may take place in the home.

THE FAMILY AND THE MENTAL HOSPITAL PATIENT

Admission to a hospital for psychiatric reasons occurs at a point of crisis which involves a group and not only the designated patient, and such crises actually arise from interpersonal situations more often than from a change in a disease process confined to one individual.[11,12,15,21,30,36,37] The nature of the crisis varies. Family physicians have long recognized that any illness in the family disturbs all members and that they may need assistance or at least reassurance and, furthermore, that the attitude of family members may be an important consideration in the course and treatment of chronic illnesses such as tuberculosis or cardiac and rheumatic diseases. Chronic disability of one individual in a family group can play an important role in the life of the family, and may become essential in a family's equilibrium. This is not uncommon in families containing psychiatric patients.[16,19,26,33,34] Disturbed family interaction with one member as the fulcrum may constitute an equilibrium for that family and the imbalance created by this member's hospitalization causes additional stress for all concerned, more so if hospitalization occurs for psychiatric reasons.

Another type of crisis is hospitalization as a step in a family's efforts to exclude and reject a patient. This contingency must be ascertained and dealt with even if such rejection is masked by defensive behavior which on the surface may appear as distress and suffering caused by the patient's institutionalization.[11] If admission was precipitated by a shift in the family dynamics dictated by factors not primarily involved in the patient's illness or familial relations, the family members remaining outside the hospital have to achieve a new balance of forces, a process in which the hospital should participate helpfully. If such helpful participation is denied or refused, the new equilibrium may exclude the patient for good, which may not be desirable for the patient. Or the family, particularly parents of a patient, find separation from the patient intolerable and he is removed from the institution regardless of his welfare. In general all these situations can be assessed and diagnosed better if the family is seen as a group with the patient included if possible.[7,11,36,38]

Thus at the time of hospital admission the family as a unit usually needs attention and often therapeutic assistance, and some relatively long-range decisions about the service rendered to the family have to be made in at least a tentative way. Can or should the family manage with but cursory contact incident to the admission procedure and the regular visiting patterns established by the hospital, or are regular therapeutic meetings with them indicated? Will such therapeutic work aim at a young patient's emancipation from the family or is the family to be prepared for reintegration of the patient with the family group? Such considerations must be raised immediately and preliminary plans to meet them must be made, especially if a short period of hospitalization is envisioned. The chances are slim that one decision can meet all pertinent considerations constructively. For instance, while it might be clear that the family should learn to live without the patient and the patient to live apart, implementation of this goal in treatment may be postponed because observation of the family as a group may be necessary to an understanding of the problems involved before the patient can be helped very much in individual therapy. Another family may be unable to tolerate immediate confrontation with the advice for permanent separation. Yet in other instances one may give the weaning process priority and forego the advantage of information that could be obtained by seeing the entire family as a group in order not to promote the slightest degree of hope in the family that reunification will be advisable or possible.[7,11,23,24]

A preliminary decision as to whether or not the patient is to be reunited with the family should, therefore, be made actively and as early as possible, as it obviously will influence the composition of the family group to be treated as well as the issues to be focused on during therapy.

As the family becomes familiar with the hospital routines, and the staff with the family, therapeutic issues shift more to the patient's daily existence, the extent or frequency of visits, but also to the deeper levels of competitive alignments and divisions in the family, to their ambivalent diadic attachments and defensive maneuvers which become thus recognizable. These disturbances can be illuminated through family group discussions, and some of these intrafamilial conflicts are found to range from incestuous involvement to overt rejection and from extreme jealousies to symbiotic blurring of ego boundaries between a parent and a child. Viewed as role conflicts they constitute marked deviation from the culturally accepted behavior for parents and children or for males and females, respectively. [1,10,13,23,24,26,31]

All these conflicts are more discernible and treatable in the group; however, flexibility is in order. On occasion only the parents are seen, or only one parent if the circumstances require it. In other families the inclusion or exclusion of a patient's children must be carefully weighed. Similarly the composition of the therapy group on the staff side should not be standard but designated to meet each family's need at a particular time. Most often one therapist will meet with the family, but the individual therapist of the patient or of any other family member can be included in some or all of the meetings. The indications for this are found in the need for support of one member or another, the possible advantage of therapists who are involved with the same family sharing information openly, minimization of scapegoating of one member, and dilution of transference intensity to one leader.[11,33,35] A different kind of team work from the traditional clinic pattern with fixed professional roles is required. Each professional, nurse, social worker, psychologist or psychiatrist, has his contribution to make (and ideally the referring physician also), but how the job is divided for a particular patient and his family should be determined by their needs and secondarily by the demands on and commitments of the staff team to the service or hospital as a whole.[7,12,18]

Another form of family treatment which incidentally saves professional manpower, is the establishment of groups of families or parents, or combinations of them. In such groups there is often transference to an image "the hospital" as if it were a person and the therapist can deal with this phenomenon in ways to help families grow and overcome unrealistic dependency needs.[7,11]

It is in the process of disposition that family treatment is most crucial and pays the most important dividends. We have already referred to the essentiality, if necessary through treatment, of preparing some families for permanent separation from the patient or him for emancipation from the family circle. If the patient is to be reunited with his family, psychotherapeutic evaluation of this social context is at least as important as that of the ward environment. Rehabilitation of the mental patient is an empty phrase unless professional care is extended to those areas where the patient has to cope with his readjustment and reintegration into his prehospitalization circumstances, and therapeutic concern with the family must start with admission of the patient. Community services for rehabilitation with respect to occupational and physical medicine are by and large available.[14,16,36] But most psychiatric patients return to a home and a family, and procedures for extending therapeutic assistance into this situation are not standardized in practice, and left to whatever agency happens to become concerned, and rarely has the personnel in such agencies been trained systematically in family treatment.

Public health nurses deal with the family as a unit more often than any other professional people, but most social workers and psychiatrists are oriented toward the individual, and their group experiences have been mostly with patients gathered into a group on the basis of diagnosis or therapeutic goals, whereas family therapy must deal with a group sui generis. It is therefore as important in the training experience of all mental health specialists to deal with such "unselected" groups as the family or similar groups of patients in the hospital who live in one unit as it is to learn psychotherapy and group therapy in the traditional sense. Many of the techniques and principles are similar, and some of the important differences have been listed. Most important are skills and proficiency in meeting a family group on an unscheduled basis in an emergency or crisis because in this procedure lies one of the important preventive opportunities. The psychiatric emergency home care program has proved its worth in The Netherlands and elsewhere. It is our clear obligation to see to it that treatment services which focus on the family as the clinical unit be instituted and rendered on the highest level of professional competence, both in emergencies and as a routine mental hospital practice.[6,9,11,30,36]

REFERENCES

1. ACKERMAN, N. W.: The Psychodynamics of Family Life. New York, Basic Books, 1958.
2. ———: Adolescent problems: A symptom of family disorder. Fam. Proc., 1: 202-213, 1962.
3. BELL, N. W., AND VOGEL, E. F.: Toward a framework for functional analysis of family behavior. In: A Modern Introduction to the Family. Bell, N. W. and Vogel, E. F. Eds. Glencoe, Ill., The Free Press, 1960.
4. BOWEN, M.: The family as the unit of study and treatment. Am. J. Orthopsychiat., 31:40-60, 1961.
5. BRODEY, W.: Some family operations and schizophrenia. Arch. Gen. Psychiat., 1:379-402, 1959.
6. DAVIS, E. D.: Continuity of Nursing Care. Presented to the Mental Health Nurse Consultants at the annual meeting of the A.P.A. Miami Beach, Florida, Oct. 13, 1962.
7. DETRE, T., et al.: An experimental approach to the treatment of the acutely ill psychiatric patient in a general hospital. Conn. Med., 25:613-619, 1961.
8. DUBOS, R.: Mirage of Health: Utopias, Progress and Biological Change. New York, Harper, 1959.
9. ELDRED, D. M., et al.: The rehabilitation of the mentally ill—the Vermont story. Am. J. Publ. Health, 52:39-46, 1962.
10. FLECK, S.: Family dynamics and origin of schizophrenia. Psychosomat. Med., 22:333-443, 1960.
11. ———: Psychiatric hospitalization as a family experience. Forest Hospital Publ., 1:29-37, 1962.
12. ———, et al.: Interaction between hospital staff and families. Psychiatry, 20: 343-350, 1957.
13. ———, et al.: The intrafamilial environment of the schizophrenic patient. Incestuous and homosexual problems. In: Individual and Familial Dynamics. Jules H. Masserman, Ed. New York, Grune & Stratton, 1959.
14. GERTY, F. J.: Address at A.M.A. Conference on Mental Health and Illness, Chicago, Ill. Oct. 6, 1962.
15. GREENBLATT, M., et al. (Eds.): The Patient in the Mental Hospital. Glencoe, Ill., The Free Press, 1957.
16. HAGGERTY, R. J.: Family medicine. J. M. Educ., 37:531-580, 1962.
17. HARPER, F.: Family Problems. New York, Bobbs-Merril, 1962.
18. HOLZBERG, J.: The historical traditions of the state hospitals as a force of resistance to the team. Am. Orthopsychiat., 30:87-94, 1960.
19. HUBBARD, J. P.: Observation of the family in the home. J. M. Educ., 28: 26-30, 1953.
20. JACKSON, D. D., AND WEAKLAND, J. H.: Conjoint family therapy. Psychiatry, 24:30-45, 1961.

21. KLEIN, D. C., AND LINDEMANN, E.: Preventive intervention in individual and family crisis situations. In: Prevention of Mental Disorders in Children, Gerald Caplan, Ed. New York, Basic Books, 1961.

22. KLUCKHOHN, C.: Variations in the human family. In: A Modern Introduction to the Family. Bell, N. W. and Vogel, E. F. Eds. Glencoe, Ill., The Free Press, 1960.

23. LIDZ, R. W., AND LIDZ, T.: Therapeutic considerations arising from the intense symbiotic needs of schizophrenic patients. In: Psychotherapy with Schizophrenics. Brody, E. and Redlich, F. Eds. New York, Internat. Univ. Press, 1952.

24. LIDZ, T., et al.: The intrafamilial environment of schizophrenic patients: The transmission of irrationality. Arch. Neurol. & Psychiat., 79:305-316, 1958.

25. ———: The relevance of family studies to psychoanalytic theory. J. Nerv. & Ment. Dis., 135:105-112, 1962.

26. ———, AND FLECK, S., II.: Schizophrenia, human integration, and the role of the family. In: The Etiology of Schizophrenia. Jackson, D. Ed. New York, Basic Books, 1960.

27. MIDELFORT, C. F.: The Family in Psychotherapy. New York, McGraw-Hill Co., Inc., 1957.

28. NORTON, N.: Unpublished data.

29. PARSONS, T.: Social structure and development of personality. Psychiatry, 21:321-340, 1958.

30. QUERIDO, A.: Early diagnosis and treatment services. In: The Elements of a Community Mental Health Program. New York, Millbank Memorial Fund, 1956.

31. SCHEFLEN, A. E.: A Psychotherapy of Schizophrenia: Direct Analysis. Springfield, Ill., Charles C Thomas, 1961.

32. SERRANO, A. C., et al.: Adolescent maladjustment and family dynamics. Am. J. Psychiat., 118: 897-901, 1962.

33. SPIEGEL, J. P.: The resolution of role conflicts within the family. Psychiatry, 20:1-16, 1957.

34. TOWNE, R., et al.: Schizophrenia and the marital family: Accommodations to symbiosis. Fam. Proc., 1:304-318, 1962.

35. VOGEL, E., AND BELL, N. W.: The emotionally disturbed child as the family scapegoat. In: A Modern Introduction to the Family. Bell, N. W. and Vogel, E. Eds. Glencoe, Ill., The Free Press, 1960.

36. WARNER, S. L., AND BULLOCK, S.: The Philadelphia Program for home psychiatric evaluations, precare and involuntary hospitalization. Am. Publ. Health, 52:29-38, 1962.

37. WOOD, E. C., RAKUSIN, J., AND MORSE, E.: Interpersonal aspects of psychiatric hospitalization. I. The admission. Arch. Gen. Psychiat., 3:632-641, 1960.

38. ———, ———, AND ———: Interpersonal aspects of psychiatric hospitalization. Arch. Gen. Psychiat., 6:39-45, 1962.

39. WYNNE, L., et al.: Pseudo-mutuality in the family relations of schizophrenics. Psychiatry, 21:205-220, 1958.

40. ZIMMERMAN, C. F., AND FRAMPTON, M. F.: The Family and Society. New York, Nostrandt Co., 1935.

PART VII

GROUP THERAPY

Group Psychotherapy in Child Guidance Clinics

by Joseph J. Geller, M.D.

W E MAY CONSIDER group psychotherapy to be the definitely applied, purposeful use of group interaction processes, by professional personnel, to effect psychotherapy. It is the use of these processes in the child guidance clinic with which this paper will deal.

GENERAL THERAPEUTIC PRINCIPLES

There are several basic principles upon which child psychotherapy may be based. First, there is relationship therapy in which the emphasis is on facilitating emotional growth and development of ego strength through the use of appropriately designed relationship situations between therapist and child. Second, there may be insight therapy through the use of guidance and learning principles for development of insights into emotional difficulties. Third, there may be insight therapy through analysis and synthesis of intrapsychic phenomena. One of these three is usually the basic principle for therapeutic operations in a given child guidance clinic with elements of the other two techniques being used to a minor extent. In this paper, the primary emphasis will be on group psychotherapy of an analytic, insight-developing nature.

In this type of therapy, certain basic phenomena are involved. The establishment of communication among the patients in the group and between patients and therapist is essential. Catharsis of emotional feelings is encouraged. Confrontation, for patients, with the defense mechanisms they use and the personality factors they possess occurs. For children particularly, the development of moral standards and ethical values is a useful part of the therapy. As these and other therapeutic phenomena occur, it is expected that the consequent development of insight and emotional growth will result in a healthily functioning personality in the youngster being treated.

When using group psychotherapy it is worthwhile to plan some time for individual sessions for the members of the therapy group. The two treatment modalities, individual psychotherapy and group psychotherapy, used together afford an enriched psychotherapeutic situation which is broader and more useful than either applied alone.

Children's Therapy Groups

Two principle types of therapy groups are available for use with children: activity-therapy and insight-therapy groups. Activity-therapy groups are an extension of recreational and craft activities. Here we have groups of eight to ten children. Youngsters from six to nine might comprise one age range and possibly nine to twelve or thirteen another grouping. In operation, various types of activity are encouraged, e.g., model building, plastic material usage and wood working. The leader or therapist encourages the children in the activity. Emphasis is on the broad element of performance. The development of emotional catharsis is expected and encouraged. There is seldom a specific focusing on a given child's individual problems; rather the trend is to foster freedom of feeling and expression in an atmosphere of general acceptance. Emotional reactions appear as frustrations develop, and anger and hostility are definitely expressed. There are ego satisfactions in working at a constructive task as well as in being able to finish an object for which recognition will be given. Security is engendered from being part of a stable, on-going group situation and there is loss of fear of overt emotional expression.

The insight type of children's group therapy differs from the foregoing activity groups in that it more nearly approximates an analytic type of therapy. Efforts are made to achieve specifically directed and deep therapeutic results.

Age ranges for this type of group are as follows. One set of groupings would be for children up to the age of six. In this age range both boys and girls could be in the same group. The groups would be small in size, consisting of two or three children. The next age range would be ages six to eight, of just one sex, and would consist of from three to five children. A third age range would be eight to twelve, one sex and with four to six children present.

In all of these groups, play therapy would be the modality of expression and communication. As in individual play therapy, definite and purposeful procedures would be used to develop in the child awareness of his feelings and conflictual material.

Selection for these insight-therapy groups would be based primarily on the ability of a given child to communicate adequately with others in the group. The precise psychiatric diagnosis would not be nearly as relevant for assignment to a specific group as the child's level of emotional development, the nature of his communications systems and his behavior. It would be feasible, for example, to combine in one group a schizophrenic child who was functioning at an immature level with another child who was younger but whose emotional development approximated that of the emotionally retarded, schizophrenic child. Neither would the degree of illness be an essential criterion for grouping as long as emotional levels were sufficiently similar to make interests and type of symbol systems similar within the same group. A heterogeneous grouping, with one schizophrenic child, one or more behavior disorders, and one or more children with neuroses can constitute a good, working therapy group.

It should be noted that these are therapy groups of relatively small size as compared with adult therapy groups. This small size has been found essential in children's groups in the latency period age range. When larger groups are attempted defensiveness interferes significantly with therapy.

The task of the therapist in analytically based group psychotherapy consists of using the dynamics of group interaction to perform the basic therapeutic functions of psychoanalytic therapy. Assuming familiarity and experience with these basic functions, necessary modifications of one's individual therapy techniques are needed to make them operable in the group milieu. For example, confrontation, dream interpretation, interpretation of transferences, analysis of behavior in the group and material reported from outside are used freely. In addition, adjustment by the therapist to the phenomena of the group situation that are qualitatively new for him is necessary.

A unique feature of children's therapy groups is the combination of activity and discussion that goes on. One approach is to have an unplanned mixture of activity and discussion during a given time period, such as an hour, of the group's operation. Others prefer to have a specifically planned discussion phase and a separate activity phase. For example, there may be first a planned period for discussion, followed by an activity phase. The activity phase becomes an acting out period for material just discussed, and facilitates a tapering off of anxieties that have been aroused during the discussion period. As a rule, time limitations for activity and discussion phases are smaller than the total time used with adult groups. That is, about 20 to 30 minutes for a discussion phase followed by 20 to 30 minutes of activity would be considered average, whereas with adult groups much longer times are useful. In general, an unplanned mixture of activity and discussion is applicable for groups under age eight, for less disturbed youngsters and for therapy groups where significant improvement has begun. The division into separate discussion and activity phases is needed for groups of more severely disturbed children.

In therapy groups with children it is necessary that some of the disciplinary features of the classroom situation be developed, unlike the situation in unstructured adult groups. Limit setting is necessary with children to maintain a degree of integrity and continuity of on-going themes, as well as specifically to help the youngsters learn about limits. Children cannot be expected to develop principles of democratic behavior on a purely spontaneous basis. Limit setting is especially necessary in the discussion phase of the group psychotherapy. Such rules as no sustained physical fighting, not taking things physically from one another, no actual destructiveness of property and similar common sense limits are advisable. The therapist must be alert to prevent too much interruption yet must avoid destroying spontaneity. Association and flights of fancy are essential but must not get to the point of chaotic and rambling disorder. Ideas should be pursued to some significant point without obsessionally carrying every concept to full closure. In the activity phase, relaxation of limits is possible. Even here some direction and focussing may be useful and total permissiveness is not indicated. A high degree of skill and sensitivity in these and other important aspects of group psychotherapy develop with experience and on-going training.

A word of caution, however, is in order. The therapist needs to be careful not to overburden the group situation with rules. In this case, obsessional values may develop and lack of freedom of expression is apt to result. Sometimes rules are promulgated to relieve the insecurities of the therapist rather for the primary benefit of the therapy situation.

The development of a group ego is encouraged with the children's group more so than with adult groups. The therapist facilitates such development actively but unobtrusively. The resultant solidarity affords support, and enhances and develops the self respect of the group members. In addition to its therapeutic value, a healthy group ego helps prevent material from "leaking" out of the group back to schoolroom situations or, possibly, to the parents where injudicious use might be made of material from the group.

With children's groups, it is frequently necessary for the therapist to stimulate either activity or discussion. One does not allow long silences as with an adult group. The material should be appropriate to the specific group and to the situation at hand. One needs to stimulate discussion (or activity, as the case may be) without arousing negativism or encouraging dependency. Here, the skill of the therapist in working with children again comes into play.

Therapy groups such as these are ideally held a minimum of once weekly; twice weekly is suggested where time and staff facilities make this possible. In general, these therapy groups are best carried on in conjunction with some degree of individual therapy. With children who are still in the first months of therapy, a minimum of once weekly individual sessions is indicated. The individual session in this case need be only a half hour in duration rather than the usual hour period. As therapy continues, some of the children may do adequately with fewer individual sessions. As warranted, extra individual sessions may be added during periods of stress or when therapy is moving fairly rapidly.

For those guidance clinics which treat twelve to sixteen year olds it should be pointed out that activity or play therapy groups are not used in this age range. Here, discussion type group therapy is advisable. Six to eight youngsters comprise the optimal group. It is usually necessary to have one grouping of twelve to fourteen year old youngsters and another fourteen to sixteen. Experience has shown that in the twelve to fourteen year range, groups of one sex are best. In the fourteen to sixteen year range, whether to have groups of the same sex, or to mix sex groups, depends on the individual therapist. There are both advantages and disadvantages for either possibility. Thus, each therapist needs to work out for himself which of the two he finds most useful.

Adult Psychotherapy Groups in the Child Guidance Clinic

It is a basic principle in child guidance to offer therapy to one or both parents when children are being treated. This may be done at the guidance level or it may be done at a level of definitive personal psychotherapy for the adult. In treating the adults, it is advantageous to utilize group psychotherapy to achieve the desired goals. In addition to being used for definitive psychotherapy, group methods have been adapted to some of the other aspects of working with the adults involved in the processes of the child guidance clinic. Thus, as long waiting lists have developed in connection with the work of the child guidance clinic, it has been found helpful to develop pre-intake groups and post-intake groups.

A pre-intake group consists of groups of parents seen before formal intake procedures have been possible. These people are afforded a forum for discussion, an opportunity to ask questions, and are given orientation and support immediately following the initial contact with the clinic. In operating such groups, fifteen to twenty people are a workable size and meetings of two hours duration once a month are held. The therapist focuses discussion on common problems parents have. Considerable latitude is allowed to encourage the parents to bring in any specific problems they have in connection with the child who is awaiting workup. Such group work with these people relieves some of their anxiety while awaiting formal workup. In addition to being thus helpful to the parents, the sessions are useful to the staff. The worker who conducts the pre-intake group obtains information about the people in the group which is of use during the intake process. Occasionally it becomes apparent during these sessions that the child guidance clinic is not the appropriate resource for the given family situation, so that re-referral can be carried out even before the intake process has occurred. As a rule, such groups go on for from three to six monthly meetings for a given family, by which time actual intake processes begin.

The post-intake groups, as the name implies, are made up of the adult(s) in those family situations where therapy has been recommended following the intake staffing but where a waiting period is necessary until therapeutic time is available. These groups are more therapeutic in content than the pre-intake groups since therapy has already been decided upon. They, too, are held once monthly for two hour sessions. Often, unfortunately, they continue longer than the pre-intake groups since the wait for treatment is apt to be a lengthy one. The primary function of such groups is to maintain contact for and with the family and clinic staff. This results in a more humanistic and therapeutically useful relationship than is likely with hit and miss waiting periods that may occur without this post-intake group arrangement.

There are rewards in using these post-intake groups over and beyond mere exigency. Thus, this beginning of therapy makes the parent even more amenable to ultimate individual or group therapy when the actual therapy for these adults can begin. Further, the workers can continue to learn about the patient, to help determine the type of therapeutic regime when time becomes available. Judgments made in the intake process can be validated or modified depending on the actual findings in the quasi-therapeutic situation that the post-intake group represents. It is possible, too, for the patients themselves to develop some awareness of what is involved in therapy and get some real insights into the nature of their children's problems. Rarely a family situation may even resolve itself with the modicum of help received from this post-intake group session so that more definitive therapy may not be necessary.

When actual treatment for the parents becomes possible, group therapy should be considered as a significant treatment modality. It is possible, of course, to work with parents exclusively in terms of how they may best help their children during the child's therapy. When this type of guidance approach is the predominant one, groups composed of married couples are set up. It is also useful gradually to work parents into being in therapy in their own right albeit in conjunction with their children's therapy. When this is done groups in which the husband and wife are not in the same group with each other are more worthwhile.

The same criteria and methods of operation that would be used in any adult group psychotherapy apply to the work being done with adults coming to the child guidance clinic with their children. Thus, selection for such groups would be based upon ability to communicate rather than on criteria of psychodynamics, homogeneity of symptoms, or similar factors. Unlike working with a children's group, age range is not very pertinent. Two important criteria in selection of adults are these: first, the members of a given group should not be too disparate in social level nor in intellectual development. It has been found that when the range in a group of either of these factors is too wide, the ethical and moral values of the people involved are noticeably strange to each other. Similarly, symbol systems and abstract conceptualizations of people in markedly different social and intellectual ranges are sufficiently far apart to make communication difficult. Hence, for efficiency and effectiveness of therapy group operation some degree of homogeneity of social level and intelligence range is useful.

The second important criterion for selection is ability and motivation to communicate. Thus, a highly anxious or depressed person would not do too well in a group at least so long as the anxiety or depression continued to be acute. Similarly, a person not motivated to a communication type of therapy would do as poorly in a group as in individual psychoanalytic therapy. Essentially, though, these factors, social and intellectual range on the one hand and communication motivation, on the other, are broad and general.

There are some negative qualities to be avoided in placing people in a given therapy group: e.g., severe, persistent monopolizing, or repeated attacks of acute anxiety or depression. Also to be avoided are patients who act out neurotic behavior in a compulsive way such that group exposure will exaggerate these tendencies to the point of making life difficult for themselves.

In actual operation, then, if there are no reasons to eliminate people from a group, the heterogeneous mixture afforded by the usual run of parents coming to a child guidance clinic can be used to make up a given therapy group.

The size for such groups, being run along analytic-insight lines, is eight or nine patients. These groups meet once a week for one and a half to two hours at a time. One may expect adequate benefit to be achieved in twelve to eighteen months for the usual type of problem. On occasion, as the child's therapy may finish, an adult who has gotten fairly deeply into therapy in his own right may be transferred to an adult therapy situation when no longer eligible to be carried in a child guidance unit.

Some individual therapy sessions are essential for a given patient's therapeutic regime to be most effective. For patients with no previous psychotherapy, individual sessions several times a month are important. As therapy proceeds, or for patients who have had some prior psycho-therapeutic exposure, a once monthly individual session may be adequate. Even this regime, however, should be flexible. From time to time, acute anxiety situations may develop which necessitate weekly or even more frequent individual sessions for brief periods of one or two weeks. It is important for therapy that time for these individual therapy sessions be available. When defense systems are interfered with, therapeutic gain is increased if one can work immediately with the problems and prevent the patient's anxiety from causing re-repression of material.

The question of changing groups may arise. There might be a change from a group of couples (where a guidance orientation process is going on) to a mixed group (where an analytic-insight therapy is being used). Another type of change might be from one mixed group to another when, for a therapeutic reason, such a change is warranted: e.g., the patient has made the group a kind of new family unit which he uses as an escape from the reality of his daily life. Shifting him to a different group could help interrupt such a dependency transference.

It is seen then, that the treatment regime for parents in a child guidance clinic would parallel closely that of adult treatment facilities. It is worth re-emphasizing that this phase of the child guidance program may be one of affording to the parent treatment in his own right, or it may, at a more superficial level, have the parent come mainly for orientation and help in handling the child who is the primary focus of treatment.

Problems Incident to a Group Psychotherapy Program in a Child Guidance Clinic

It is essential that the professional worker doing group psychotherapy have initially a sound basis in his profession and then adequate training in group psychotherapy. It is also important that supervision be available for those participating in the group psychotherapy program. The supervision may be conducted with the usual one-to-one supervisor-therapist relationship. It is even more worthwhile to have therapists supervised as a group thus affording each worker a chance to compare his own work with that being done by others. In addition, the group interaction phenomena that occur in the group of workers are useful to illustrate phenomena of group psychotherapy itself in a most graphic, cogent and immediate form.

There are certain other problems that arise after the plans for training and supervision have been dealt with. It is the general experience that when group psychotherapy methods are newly introduced into a child guidance setting, persistent resistances to acceptance of the methods develop on the part of staff members. One needs to start working on such resistances prior to the onset of the group psychotherapy program, and during the supervisory sessions as group psychotherapy actually goes on. It may be a matter of several years from the onset of a group psychotherapy program before a given staff may feel fully comfortable about utilizing group psychotherapy processes. Common resistances that arise are as follows. The thought of "diluting" the therapeutic relationship between worker and the family members, with consequent weakening of results, is one. The concept of the loss of confidentiality if personal problems are discussed amongst a group of people is another. The possibility of losing control of a therapy situation in a group setting is a third. The possibility of patients traumatizing rather than helping each other is still another. Rational though some of these points may be, they seldom appear to have a serious or destructive effect in actual group psychotherapy. They serve to cover the general insecurity involved in beginning any new process as well as specific insecurities of therapists unfamiliar with or inexperienced in group psychotherapy methods.

In addition to resistance phenomena, other defensive aspects of staff personalities may appear when beginning (and during) group psychotherapy. Unresolved aspects of competitiveness may be seen. Accentuation of needs for dependency or control may develop. The group and individual supervision, sensitively and adequately handled, helps work through many of these problems much as in the individual supervisory relationship.

The problem of lay and professional relations may also appear in child guidance clinics which utilize a group therapy system. Thus, both the public, and professional groups outside of the clinic may have defenses about and resistance to group psychotherapy. These could adversely influence attitudes in the community toward the clinic. In recent years, as group psychotherapy has become more well known and generally respected and accepted, problems of this nature are disappearing.

One may find resistance to entering into group psychotherapy amongst the patients. Here, once the members of staff have developed secure feelings about group psychotherapy for themselves, professional skills come into play. One is dealing with resistance to psychotherapy in general rather than resistance to group psychotherapy itself and the usual professional skills to handle this rather common problem are used.

Summary

Group psychotherapy is a worthwhile treatment modality for the child guidance clinic. It is used both for the children who are the primary focus of the clinic, and the significant adults in the child's immediate environment. It is not a production line method of achieving extensive expansion of clinic treatment facilities. Although with its use there can be a minimal increase in patient load, its noteworthy impact is in affording the patient a greater reactivity potential, a qualitatively richer therapeutic experience and a broader, more substantial gain than without its use.

Group Therapy As Primary Treatment in an Outpatient Setting*

by Arthur P. Burdon, M.D.

AND

William Ryan, Ph.D.

T HIS CHAPTER is a description of some of the methods and techniques of group psychotherapy which the authors and their associates evolved as a result of a research effort to test psychoanalytically oriented, small-group psychotherapy as the primary treatment modality. The psychiatric outpatient department of the Mount Auburn Hospital, a community general hospital in Cambridge, Massachusetts, was converted into a group therapy treatment center for the handling of all applicants for psychiatric treatment.[1,2,3] In order to test the outer limits of the application of group therapy on a community level, the staff deliberately made no attempt to prejudge an applying patient as unsuitable for a group treatment during the six-month trial period. Furthermore, without regard to divergencies in age, social background, symptoms, diagnosis, or preferences of the patients, nearly every patient was assigned serially as he came into the clinic to a new therapy group made up of ten to twelve fellow-applicants who had presented themselves over a span of time. Of eighty applicants, only fifteen were withheld from the study for administrative and clinical reasons, while another fifteen absented themselves from the clinic before diagnostic studies were completed. Fifty-six patients were introduced to the group treatment program. Each was studied in clinical interviews by one or two psychiatrists who filled out a standardized rating scale and by one or two psychologists who administered the Rorschach test. These evaluations were made at the beginning and after one year of treatment.

The therapy was relatively standardized, subject to the variations of five or six individual personalities who functioned as the group thera-

*This research was supported by the United States Public Health Service Mental Health Project Grant OM-340, National Institute of Mental Health.

pists. Each group met for one and one-half hours weekly over an extended period of time in an atmosphere in which the therapist encouraged the full verbalization of all thoughts and feelings present in the patients while confining his remarks to the clarification and investigation of the interplay of forces within the group, i.e. the tendencies toward group disruption and group cohesion as they expressed themselves in the content of the sessions.

Range of Age and Diagnosis

Five of our patients were under 21 years of age and 5 over 50 while 30 patients ranged between the ages of 26 and 38. Twenty-three patients were diagnosed as character disorders, 16 showed chronic psychoneuroses and 13 patients presented borderline and frankly psychotic reactions.

Patient Selection

Only patients with the grossest of behavioral or social disruption were excluded, since in our experience, formal diagnosis, the type of symptoms, or psychopathology, or the estimated ego strength have no correlation whatsoever with the suitability of the patients for group psychotherapy. In fact, it was discovered that many borderline and severe character disorders continued and did well in the group while many mild neurotics dropped out.

Yet a high degree of predictability of group participation and group continuation can be made on the basis of Ryan's use of the Rorschach.[4,5] Assessed clinically, the important factors are: first, the patient's capacity to wait with his problem; second, to relate to other people hopefully; and third, to feel he is primarily responsible for his own well-being. With regard to the first factor, the role of recent stress in the precipitation of the patient's referral to treatment is crucial in assessing whether he would continue, since patients in crisis cannot endure the additional stresses and frustrations of the group situation. Second, when the "capacity to relate" or "need for approval of others" is prominent, as it is among even some quite disturbed impulsive or paranoid patients, it favors continuation in group therapy despite much anxiety and much conscious rebellion against membership. The third ego factor seems more complex and involves a balance or consonance between the patient's degree of intra-psychic disturbance and his level of self-estimation as to his responsibility for his disturbance. When these two characteristics were in consonance—for example, when the patient showed severe intra-psychic impairment and also displayed a serious disturbance in his self-esteem—he was more likely to adapt well to the group as a needed source of real help with his self-recognized problem. In contrast, patients who deny or project their problems primarily and see themselves relatively immune from personal responsibility and involvement cannot long endure the pressure of group exposure.

This cluster of ego traits does not seem directly related to traditional concepts of ego dysfunction or defenses but rather, in sum, seems to be an ability to become comfortably and helpfully interdependent with others. The therapy group is a situation of mutual dependency and mutual work, a situation in which the members must share, be willing both to give and take, be able to wait, receive and give help. This ability we have termed "capacity for mutual dependence," a factor which predicted 86% of the group continuers in these studies.

Therapy

Although the skillful handling of his group by the individual group therapist has undoubtedly some bearing on the dropout of patients from his group, these studies as well as many others have shown a consistent and crucial loss of slightly over one-third of the total number of patients within the first eight sessions. The most effective way to avoid this is to foster an interested and caring relationship with one member of the clinic staff prior to group therapy, and to maintain this relationship at least through the first two months of his group experience. It is a rare patient who survives the immediate plunge into group therapy after one single diagnostic interview with a stranger, even though that stranger may be the group therapist himself. Accordingly, the patient has two or three separate psychotherapeutic and psychodiagnostic hours with his individual clinic psychiatrist, apart from his group therapist, during which time the psychiatrist establishes a warm and trusting relationship while clarifying the patient's leading maladaptations and preparing him for group referral. The patient is offered further individually requested private sessions with his initial physician to discuss his resistance to and anxiety concerning the group. The prototype of this type of relationship might be that of the general physician who refers his patient to the specialist for surgery but maintains an interested and helpful contact with his patient during the surgical procedure and continues his interest in the patient following the treatment. This "backstopping of the group therapy process in the beginning of treatment has resulted in the continuation of many frightened and dubious patients, and seems to us to be an essential for the successful operation of the group therapy program.

RESULTS

Eight patients refused to participate in the treatment, and 12 more dropped out after less than ten sessions; yet after twelve months, 50 per cent of the cases remained in group therapy. Favorable results had occurred in over 60 per cent of these remaining patients, both in basic personality traits as well as in marked benefits in the areas of symptoms and social interaction. Although the loss to treatment of the total number of applicants was considerable, it does not vary from other clinics proceeding along more traditional lines nor do the results vary from accepted results in other situations.[6]

TOTAL CLIMATE OF THE CLINICAL STAFF

Although the crucial influence of group disruptive forces has been well studied in the subcultures within a mental hospital ward and other therapeutic settings, it is often ignored in the practice of the everyday operation of a clinic, and perhaps without appreciably deleterious effects to the treatment of the patients as long as their treatment program is one of many individual relationships in the same building. However, just as individual uncovering psychotherapy stirs and focuses the therapist's own unconscious reactions, the wholesale use of group psychotherapy in a clinic seems to actuate latent and very powerful group dynamics among the staff. Not only is the staff more interdependent because of the nature of the work, but the specific conscious interest in group processes tends to give a different cast and tone to the staff meeting and other formal and informal operations of the clinic. There seem to be mobilized within the staff the very processes seen in patients, posing as a new problem in clinic administration. Both group disruptive and group cohesive forces could be actively demonstrated in the staff of these projects and were critical in the handling of the entire project in order to maintain its success.

There was a definite relationship between continuation in group and the specific individual diagnostician who had performed the initial study and made the assignment to group. Specifically from 50 to 80 per cent of the patients of most diagnosticians continued in group therapy, but this figure was only 20 per cent for two of the staff. These same two diagnosticians were consciously aware of their dissatisfaction with various aspects of the administration of the program although totally unaware of the probable events in which they were unconsciously communicating some distrust or dissatisfaction to their patients, and indirectly affecting the entire operation of the clinic. Tense and painful staff meetings occurred during a span of time, and the tensions were resolved only when the persons concerned expressed their feelings to a sufficient degree for frank discussion, leading to their eventual withdrawal from the program for other, less conflictual pursuits. The remaining professional staff was more strengthened by these discussions which were vital to the success of the entire program. Much as Freud admonished analysts to continue their own self-analysis, so also should group therapists be involved in a group for progress and satisfaction in their work.

REFERENCES

1. RYAN, W., AND BURDON, A.: Patients Who Adapt to Group Psychotherapy, Proceedings of the III World Congress of Psychiatry, Montreal, 1961.
2. ——, AND ——: Broadest Practical Effective Application of Group Psychotherapy in a Community Outpatient Psychiatric Clinic, Annual Meeting, American Psychiatric Association, Chicago, May, 1961.
3. ——, AND ——: Group Psychotherapy as a Primary Treatment Method in an Outpatient Setting, DePaul Hospital Lecture, 1961.
4. RYAN, W.: Capacity for Mutual Dependence and Involvement in Group Psychotherapy, Ph.D. Dissertation, Boston University, 1958.
5. ——: Predicting Continuation in Group Psychotherapy with the Rorschach, Annual Meeting, American Psychological Association, Chicago, 1960.
6. FRANK, J. D.: Persuasion and Healing; A Comparative Study of Psychotherapy. Baltimore, Johns Hopkins Press, 1961.

Group Psychotherapy with the Alcoholic

by Hugh Mullan, M.D.

G ROUP PSYCHOTHERAPY, in the form of a face-to-face analytic and at the same time supportive treatment, appears to be a psychological method suitable for the treatment of alcoholics. Men and women, similar in symptom and coping mechanisms, under proper leadership, easily meet together to talk about their problems, the latest promising drug and job possibilities. For the alcoholic, meeting with other patients similarly troubled is less threatening than the one-to-one contact with the individual therapist or psychoanalyst.[1,2] In the group setting as compared to the individual session the patient quickly and easily experiences a sense of belonging and of identification. While this coming-together must be viewed as a kind of *quasi*-group cohesiveness, based as it is solely upon similar experiences of alcoholism, the therapist can grasp this opportunity to bring the group together and to maintain it initially.

However, it is well to emphasize at the start, that this seemingly conducive incentive for group therapy, based upon mutual identification and interest, expressed so readily by the deceptively gregarious alcoholic, *always* backfires, and acts later on as *a resistance* to more certain and deeper involvement.[3] While it is true that the compulsive drinker joins readily with his fellow group member and the therapist it does not necessarily follow that treatment ensues.

This chapter is devoted to a description of group psychotherapy with the alcoholic, the group psychotherapist, and the necessary steps that he must take to bring about group psychotherapy with the alcoholic patient.

THE GROUP PSYCHOTHERAPIST WITH THE ALCOHOLIC

The alcoholic, as all attest, is no easy patient to treat.[4] Frequent alcoholic lapses, broken appointments, abrupt departures, antisocial and bizarre escapades, countless evening and week-end telephone calls, forced involvements with neighbors, friends and relatives, endless excuses and neglected promises all adversely affect the group therapist. But this is not all. The leader, in sharing the therapeutic responsibility with the group, feels keenly for them when a disturbed patient unwarrantedly attacks or deserts his group.

Singular devotion to, sympathy for and understanding of the alcoholic must replace a technical, objective and a contrived accepting attitude.[5] Many writers have emphasized the therapist's need to be empathic and yet non-accepting of the alcoholic's continuous tendency to act-out.[6] While the therapist must be secure enough within himself to withstand frustration and anxiety he must also have the realistic expectation that the alcoholic will stop drinking and gradually assume responsibility for himself and for the other group members.

In addition the therapist must be well trained and experienced in group psychotherapy,[7] deeply concerned with the alcoholic's plight, aware of the social, cultural and physical aspects of alcoholism,[8,9] flexible in his ability to make use of the many therapeutic treatment methods,[10] and conversant with and able to call upon and use all means and institutions concerned with the rehabilitation of the alcoholic.

INITIAL CONTACT, ACCOMMODATION, AND ORIENTATION OF THE ALCOHOLIC PATIENT

Almost all group psychotherapy with the alcoholic must offer a general rehabilitation program which is most conveniently found in the alcohol treatment center. Physical, spiritual and social lacks must be acknowledged and supplemented while at the same time the patient's psychological needs are being met by his treatment group.

Clinic or office personnel must understand and accept the alcoholic's characteristic behavior. Because he is overly sensitive to rejection the alcoholic responds to expectations or criticism strongly and may withdraw from ever attempting treatment. The worker or nurse who is conversant with and values group psychotherapy paves the way for this reluctant patient to enter and remain in his therapy group.

Few patients are more confused and unmotivated toward group psychotherapy than the alcoholic. Under pressure from his exasperated spouse, about to lose his job, or be picked up for the 20th time by the police, he views treatment as wholly medical, psychotherapy as a form of counseling and education, and group psychotherapy as a "class."

In view of the importance of *continuous contact* and capitalizing on the unmotivated alcoholic's presence, regardless of his reason, daily appointments are scheduled. He is immediately admitted to an orientation group, usually conducted by a physician, consisting of prospective patients, their interested relatives and very close friends. These five to ten "class room" sessions, not to be confused with later group psychotherapy, use ingenious teaching devices to confront the members with the total problem of alcoholism and at the same time suggest a general rehabilitation program.[11]

SELECTION, PREPARATION AND GROUP INTRODUCTION OF THE ALCOHOLIC

Ultimate group participation is dependent upon the degree of motivation, usually found wanting in the alcoholic. The quick selection indices listed, seem preferable to prolonged psychometric probings which often discourage and defeat the alcoholic:

(1) Present or past acceptance of Alcoholics Anonymous, antabuse therapy, physical medication, hospitalization and pastoral, marital or vocational counseling.

(2) Present or past acceptance of individual or group psychotherapies.

(3) Evidence of faithfulness to appointments and to the orientation sessions.

(4) The presence of some capacity for insight and of psychodynamic interplay between the patient and therapist during interviews and orientation.

In similar practical fashion patients are not likely to benefit from the group experience, when they give evidence of:

(1) Overtly psychotic or severely disturbed behavior.

(2) A marked inability to relate to the admissions worker, the group psychotherapist and others.

The group psychotherapist sees the patient immediately and commences an indefinite number of preparatory sessions which have five general functions: (1) Appraisal of history, determination of the diagnosis, prognosis and group suitability, (2) Beginning establishment of the transference, (3) Confrontation of the patient with the "Idea of Group," (4) Undermining resistance, and (5) Orientation toward full group participation.[7]

Some group psychotherapists suggest immediate group placement. For example Fox states in part, ". . . So helpful is group therapy to the alcoholic, that it should be instituted as soon as possible, often on the very day of the first contact when resistance to this kind of help may be surprisingly low, perhaps because the alcoholic when coming off a prolonged drinking bender is so beaten down and his defenses so shattered that he hasn't the will to resist."[11] While admittedly the group therapist with the alcoholic as compared to other patients must be satisfied with a more superficial and tenuous relationship, individual sessions seem significant in deepening the therapist-patient relationship so that intense group interaction in the future will not cause the patient to drop out of therapy. In addition, preparatory sessions, although time consuming, allow for a greater number of patients actually to attempt intensive group psychotherapy.

As the steps of preparation are accomplished the group therapist begins to determine his ability actually to engage his patient. This occurs, from the therapist's standpoint, when he discovers that the patient is a unique individual and is much more than alcoholic. For the patient, engagement begins when he is able to respond with affect as he hesitatingly begins to investigate and evaluate himself.

Physical treatment, except in emergencies, and psychological testing should be instituted *after* the patient is established in his group. Confirming this practice Vogel states, "At first my rigid standards required careful screening, physical examination and psychometrics. However, between the initial interview and plans and appointments for these workups, many patients were lost to the ever-present competitor—alcohol. This has to some extent been eliminated by instituting therapy immediately, and assigning the patient to a group as soon as possible, with psychometric testing and other examination done concomitant with therapy."[12]

In a warm, accepting atmosphere, carefully oriented and individually prepared men and women, some recovered alcoholics and others actively drinking, meet twice weekly preferably, for 1½ to 2 hours. Late afternoon, evening and Saturday hours permit the alcoholic to regain or maintain his vocational responsibility. At times of psychic emergency individual hours should supplement the group sessions. Fees, if required, should be individualized, bearing realistically upon the patient's ability to pay. At first and for a while lapses are to be expected. Sanctions and rules must be practical and individualized, keeping in mind that the therapist's first responsibility is to the group and second to the patient. Very close and sympathetic cooperation among the staff members will offset the confused alcoholic's tendency to manipulate and turn one clinic member against the other.[13] Once he becomes a member of the therapy group, the patient is repeatedly told to take all matters up in *his* group first before going to other sources.

The Group Climate: The Alcoholic's Resistance to Therapy

For many months the alcoholic in the therapy group solely identifies himself as one who has a "drinking problem." He manifests certain "alcoholic" personality traits concisely described by Feibel as follows: "(1) Marked tendencies toward regression rather than repression; (2)

denial of unpleasant external and internal realities; (3) acting out of instinctual impulses with or without the help of alcohol; (4) blackouts; (5) dependency upon the environment; (6) strong social fears; (7) archaic superego structures where id impulses are turned destructively against the self in contrast to a less cruel superego that helps the ego defend itself against the instincts; (7) introjection and projection."[4]

As a result of these traits commonly held attitudes and behaviors emerge in the group and bring about an initial *quasi*-cohesion. At the same time, however, effective purposeful interaction is limited and, therefore, therapeutic group process all but comes to a standstill.[3] These attitudes may be described as follows:

Identification

"I am alcoholic, therefore, I belong in this group."

Alcoholic groups form a group identification quickly and easily. Members relate to one another as if they had enjoyed a long standing friendship. In this, however, they ignore all other aspects of their lives and relate to each other exclusively through their drinking and through those activities connected with their alcoholism. Dreams if reported are again related only to their alcoholism. At this time, genuine bindings between individuals mystify the new patient. He clings to the belief that the essential reason for being together is that he is alcoholic and it is only later that he feels the emerging responsibility for himself and others in the group.

Commitment to Fantasy

"I prefer *my* fantasy to reality."

The alcoholic lives in an inner world of fantasy. But as the emotional "give and take" in the group, the response to and analysis of behavior, dreams and fantasies begin to undermine this, anxiety mounts. The patient begins to commit himself to reality as he remains in his group without recourse to alcohol.

Misinterpretation of Therapy's Purpose

"This group is for education and socializing."

Society's approach to the alcoholic is one of education. It is hoped that an intellectual appreciation of the effects of alcoholism will inhibit drinking. To offset the new patient's understandable expectation about the group being a "class," the therapist must be clear as to the difference between orientation which is primarily didactic and therapy.[14] The poorly motivated alcoholic is in the treatment group to experience his life differently, to develop a responsibility for his immediate behavior and to understand this behavior. The therapist does not teach in the usual sense but encourages members to feel and express their feelings, thereby assuring evolving intimate relationships.

Unless the group therapist is alert extra-group gatherings will occur which act to increase resistance, deny anxiety and dilute the therapeutic experience. In alcoholic groups the use of the alternate session* is believed to be contra-indicated because it encourages aggressive and sexual acting-out.[7]

The Use Of Alcohol

"I need to drink because . . ."

There is no question that many alcoholics in treatment groups need to drink. Concerning this Fox states, ". . . Since he has become psychologically dependent on alcohol as his chief source of pleasure as well as his chief prop in meeting the day-to-day problems of living, sobriety throws him into depression and panic. . . . he finds himself with nothing to contribute and his self esteem is nil."[11] Drinking, however, by a group member regardless of its effect and meaning, retards therapy for all. The tense session which occurs at this time focuses jointly upon the members' inept and wasted lives and upon the rescuing of the inebriate.[15]

The group therapist realizes that unless the patient attains sobriety, psychotherapy for him is not possible.[6] Implementing the usual psychotherapeutic techniques, the concerned group psychotherapist counsels, sets limits and offers individual supplementary sessions. He refers the patient to Alcoholics Anonymous; to a vocational counselor; to a physician for possible medication and a physical check-up; to a hospital for physical rehabilitation or "drying-out"; and so forth.

The Avoidance of Responsibility

"I can't help it. It is the alcohol, not me. Don't you know that I am alcoholic?"

For a long time the responsibility that the alcoholic has for the day-to-day arguments, emotional flare-ups, and inadequate solutions in his treatment group are hotly denied. The alcoholic implies that he is in the grip of an uncontrollable force to which he compulsively responds in fixed ways. A homosexual patient approached another male group member; this so threatened the group member that he left therapy.

---

*A group session, regularly established and sanctioned by the therapist but one from which he absents himself.

When the aggressive male homosexual was questioned as to his behavior and feelings he angrily replied, "What did you expect? Don't you know that I am alcoholic and that all alcoholics are homosexual?"

In this milieu the group psychotherapist finds himself all but excluded. Although it is *his* group the early forces which bind the members together limit his function and prevent his participation. A group member openly gave voice to this need to separate out the non-alcoholic group leader from the others when she said, "If we know someone is alcoholic, we know *something* about him, his weaknesses and his vulnerability." And then turning to the therapist she added, "We don't know yours."[3] If psychotherapy is to ensue the group therapist must more and more become a part of the group he is conducting.

Modification In the Group Climate: The Therapist's Functions

Rather than rely solely upon interpretation and analysis the group psychotherapist must also affectively respond to the resistive alcoholic. When the patient is prone to drink, absent himself from treatment, and refuses to face his group responsibilities, four means are suggested for the group therapist's participation which in turn assures therapeutic group process.

The Therapist Responds Directly and Uniquely to Each Member

A timely expression of the group therapist's thoughts and feelings is critical if the alcoholic is to begin to experience himself as an individual. Emphasizing the uniqueness of the person, the therapist responds to each member differently. When the group brushes aside the fact that several members are absent by explaining that they are "at some bar getting stoned," the therapist, in contrast states, "I am concerned about George. I will call him." "I am sorry about Rose. However, I am at the end of my patience. I wonder why this is so? What goes on between Rose and me that I should feel so frustrated and hopeless?" This genuine interchange, identifying Rose and George as much more than alcoholic, in addition asks the group to assume some responsibility for what is transpiring in the therapeutic hours together.

The Therapist Expresses His Despair

Controversial though this point is, in order for the group therapist to reach the self-centered and alienated alcoholic this step, the therapist's expression of discomfort, disillusionment and even at times despair, is decisive. A direct expression of affect and ultimately concern helps the befuddled patient much more than the therapist's technical withholding of himself which further serves to discourage the alcoholic and separate him from others. The group therapist is first a human being with affect and needs and it is his very genuineness as a person which the alcoholic first encounters.

The Therapist Views the "Drinking Problem" Uniquely For Each Member

The group therapist and later the members pin-point the specific meaning for a patient's sudden binge, blackout or relapse. Responding to the inebriate, or better still, responding at the first sign of a pending period of inebriation, they symbolically confront the anxious patient with, "George is angry with us again," "Mary is out to frustrate her mother," "Robert is killing himself again. When will he stop?", "Lucille is successful once more. Now watch her mess it up again?" Highlighting the patient's *peculiar* use of alcohol, these responses individualize motivation for drinking and imply that there are other ways for each patient to handle his inner stress.

The Therapist Emphasizes the "New" and the "Now" in the Group Interaction

The alcoholic who habitually tends to deny and generalize must be made to experience the uniqueness of each treatment moment. When emotions are freely expressed, the therapist focusing upon latent themes allows the members to sense and understand themselves differently. During a heated intellectual and philosophical discussion the therapist intervened, "George, how do you really feel about Jim?" The spontaneous reply, "He gives me a pain in the ass!" served to impel the group into a consideration of feelings of inadequacy and homosexuality, hitherto carefully hidden.

REALISTIC AND PRACTICAL GOALS

The destructive pattern of life, characteristic of the alcoholic, is to be interrupted and replaced by more meaningful and responsible activity. Intermediate goals which insure the patient's availability for treatment—sobriety, regular group attendance, and physical health—must not be overlooked. The alcoholic is urged to respond to all unusual or fleeting feelings that he experiences in the group. In this way it is hoped that he may become aware of his responsibility to himself and to others. Moreover, satisfying and gainful employment is an aim not to be ignored in the alcoholic as it curtails acting-out, enhances his self esteem, and contributes to his and the group's morale.[3,13] As Martensen-Larsen points out, it is important "to enhance the patient's *own* potential so that he can gradually rely more upon himself."[16]

But this is only the beginning. The alcoholic must realize that even though now sober his problems are not resolved. Many who stop treatment at this point, accepting support from other groups, i.e., religious organizations, Alcoholics Anonymous and so forth, have achieved a limited and somewhat restrictive goal, a "transference-cure." Although this result should not be minimized it would be far better for the patient to be encouraged to continue or perhaps move into a heterogeneous therapy group where additional reconstruction may occur.[7] When the remitted alcoholic requests additional group or individual sessions they should be supplied, if at all possible. Ideally, termination occurs when the person is able to choose his way in life, responding to life's inconsistencies in a more or less creative fashion. The alcoholic *cannot* drink again, however, and the paradoxes which confront him must be met without recourse to alcohol.

REFERENCES

1. Fox, R., and Lyon, P.: Alcoholism, Its Scope, Cause and Treatment. New York, Random House, 1955, p. 179.
2. Gliedman, L. H.: Concurrent and combined group treatment of chronic alcoholics and their wives. Internat. J. Group Psychotherapy, 7: 414, 1957.
3. Mullan, H., and Sangiuliano, I.: Group Psychotherapy and the Alcoholic. 2. The Phenomenology of Early Group Interaction, Presented in part at the Fifth International Congress for Psychotherapy, Wien Austria (August 21-26) 1961.
4. Feibel, C.: The archaic personality structure of alcoholics and its implications for group psychotherapy. Internat. J. Group Psychotherapy, 10:39-45, 1960.
5. Moore, R. A.: Reaction formation as a counter-transference phenomenon in the treatment of alcoholism. Quart. J. Studies Alcohol, 22:481-486, 1961.
6. Tiebout, H. M.: Direct treatment of a symptom. In: Problems of Addiction and Habituation. New York, Grune and Stratton, 1958.
7. Mullan, H., and Rosenbaum, M.: Group Psychotherapy Theory and Practice. Glencoe, The Free Press of Glencoe, 1962.
8. Jellinek, E. M.: Alcoholism, a genus and some of its species. Canad. M.A.J., 83:1341-1346, 1960.
9. Bell, R. G.: A method of clinical orientation to alcohol addiction. Canad. M.A.J., 83:1346-1352, 1960.
10. Fox, R.: Basic attitude of the physician. In: The Treatment of Chronic Alcoholism, The Medical Clinics of North America. New York, W. B. Saunders Co., 1958, pp. 805-806.

11. ——: Group psychotherapy with alcoholics. Internat. J. Group Psychotherapy, 12:56-63, 1962.
12. VOGEL, S.: Some aspects of group psychotherapy with alcoholics. Internat. J. Group Psychotherapy, 7:302-309, 1957.
13. MULLAN, H., AND SANGIULIANO, I.: Group Psychotherapy and the Alcoholic. 1. Early Therapeutic Moves. Presented at the Third World Congress of Psychiatry, Montreal Canada (June 3-10) 1961.
14. ——, and ——: Group Psychotherapy With The Alcoholic, Summary of Work Shop 19 American Group Psychotherapy Association New York (Jan. 24-27) 1962.
15. LINDT, H.: The "rescue fantasy" in group treatment of alcoholics. Internat. J. Group Psychotherapy, 9:43-52, 1957.
16. MARTENSEN-LARSEN, O.: Group psychotherapy with alcoholics in private practice. Internat. J. Group Psychotherapy, 6:28-37, 1958.

PART VIII

INSTITUTIONAL AND COMMUNITY

Principles for Developing a Therapeutic Community

by ROBERT N. RAPAPORT, PH.D.

THE PARTICULAR TYPE of milieu therapy with which we are focally concerned in this paper is that of the "therapeutic community," which attempts to use *all* the elements of milieu therapy as a principal therapeutic approach. In the extreme case, as at Henderson (Belmont) Hospital, England, the total milieu utilization was the *exclusive* therapeutic approach. In most hospitals, however, it is linked to other therapies with varying degrees of emphasis given to it in the overall program.

Wherever it is used, with whatever degree of centrality as an instrument of therapy and with whatever specific goals for particular patients or groups of patients, there are certain principles of organization which might usefully be kept in mind. These principles pertain to social systems generally, but are expressed in terms that give them special relevance to the enterprises of developing more therapeutic social systems.[1]

PRINCIPLE A—THE FORMATION OF AN EFFECTIVE TREATMENT IDEOLOGY

Postulate 1. It is important to make explicit the ideas that are held by members of the group about how the milieu should be developed and used.

Every social system functions in part through a shared set of goals and ideas about the acceptable means for achieving these goals. Where there is uncertainty about what these goals are, there tends to develop conditions that detract from the capacity of a social system to provide a coherent and concerted force in the

---

[1] The principles and postulates developed here are adapted from the book by Robert N. Rapoport and others, Community as Doctor: New Perspectives on a Therapeutic Community, London (Tavistock) and Springfield, Ill., Thomas, 1960.

direction of any particular goals. Individuals may withdraw from involvement in the group's goals, or work at cross purposes to one another, or simply pursue different sets of goals that are allowed to exist through compartmentalization of activities within the system. Thus, while each individual may have ideas about how the environment may be used for therapy, the system as a whole cannot formulate a very concerted approach to the problem unless these are made explicit so that the work of arriving at consensus may proceed.

Postulate 2. A higher degree of consensus than is necessary in most hospitals is desirable among practitioners of milieu therapy.

We have evidence, both from the negative side (i.e., that dissensus works against the interests of providing a therapeutic milieu)[2] and the positive side (i.e., that consensus is helpful)[3] to indicate that there is special value not only

Postulate 3. The principles developed should be explicitly related to therapeutic goals as means toward these goals and not as ends in themselves.

In modern, innovating therapeutic communities—where there is still uncertain knowledge about what principles of social organization are most effective for the therapeutic effort, some principles will be chosen and embraced because of their intrinsic appeal. Thus, it may seem commendable to be "democratic," or "permissive" as good things in themselves, particularly if Postulates 1 and 2 are realized and the group gives a good deal of explicit, shared recognition of the value of these goals. To the extent that this involvement in means as ends in themselves occurs, staff members may actually exert influences that are antitherapeutic, though consistent with a generally held value. Conversely, behavior inconsistent with one of these intrinsic values might be therapeutic. For example, where being permissive may result in murder, suicide, destruction, breakdown and the like, it is clearly to be curbed in therapeutic communities—however valuable it may be as an ideal under some circumstances. The initial enthusiasm for such ideas as democratization and permissiveness came as the result of a reaction against the autocracy and suppressiveness of conventional mental hospitals. Being *more* democratic, *more* permissive and so on than these old-fashioned hospitals were was clearly desirable—not only from a humane point of view, but as an instrument of milieu therapy. However, if their instrumental value is distorted they may become entrenched, irrational shibboleths which themselves may have to be revised and replaced.

---

[2]Stanten, A. H. & M. S. Schwartz, The Mental Hospital, New York, Basic Books, 1954. Leighton, A. H., My Name is Legion, New York; Basic Books, 1958.
[3]Rapoport, R. N., ibid.

in working toward making the ideology explicit, but in working toward arriving at consensus about it. In other hospitals, where compartmentalization of care allows one ward to proceed in one way while another proceeds in another, one doctor to follow one set of therapeutic tactics while another pursues a contrasting set, the problem of consensus is not as critical. Consensus over more peripheral things—like the scheduling rather than the specific content of activities—is usually sufficient to allow the system to function effectively. However, where a system depends on welding disparate actions of individuals within the system into a concerted impact on its members, as does the therapeutic community, a large degree of consensus is indispensable.

Postulate 4. Continuous efforts must be made toward relating the abstract principles for organizing a therapeutic community to specific practices in the hospital.

One tendency in response to the wish to make the ideas of therapy more explicit and generally acceptable among the personnel is to make them more abstract. Being more democratic, for example, is something that can not only be espoused as something that sounds morally good and therapeutically effective but it is vague and general enough so that many people doing many different things may consider themselves to be sharing a democratic orientation. To give the idea operational effectiveness, it must not only be made explicit and agreed upon as an idea—but efforts must continually be made to relate the idea to behavioral referents in the life of the hospital. This is possible only through the continual and detailed discussion of concrete experiences, preferably experiences to which all or many of the group have actually been exposed. By doing this, misunderstandings and conflicts may be minimized to the extent that they occur as a result of diverse referents for the same term.

Postulate 5. The ideology should be internally logical as well as having the above-mentioned characteristics.

While each element of the therapeutic ideology can be plausible and of demonstrated therapeutic efficacy under certain conditions, unless the ideology as a whole is woven into an interrelated system its implementation will be open to confusion and conflict. An example of this would be in a situation where an alcoholic patient, democratically entrusted with the funds for the patients' entertainment committee is seen by another patient entering a bar. Two elements of the ideology of the therapeutic community that might occur to the patient could be on the one hand the ideal of permissiveness (according to which he would not take strenuous efforts to block the erring patient's course on the grounds that something might be learned from this piece of acting out) or, on the other hand, the ideal of reality confrontation in the interests of rehabilitation, according to which he would put pressure of varying degrees on the other to restrain himself and "face reality." The ideology should thus not merely be composed of a series of acceptable, explicit, well understood ideas—but it should be continuously examined for how these ideas relate to one another, and under what circumstances particular elements of the ideology take precedence over other, potentially contradictory ones.

Postulate 6. Ideological tenets may profitably be presented in concise, shorthand form, with enthusiasm and a sense of conviction.

Many observers of therapeutic communities have noted that one of the most impressive aspects of these innovating units is their enthusiasm, through which a sense of unity and purpose is welded. Slogans have always been rallying points for social groups and movements and this is a clear case where the promotion of a sense of certainty, definiteness and effectiveness is helpful to therapy, which depends on the impact of a unified group's efforts. Slogans like "freeing communications," "sharing responsibilty," "facing reality," are effective in mobilizing support—where such qualified statements as "we favor a good deal freer communication than the old-fashioned mental hospitals do, especially when it can be brought into supervised contexts and primarily verbal communication" would be less likely to, however much they represented a truer picture of the actual functioning of the therapeutic community. A hardened psychopath and a young psychiatrist might agree that "doctors do not know anything about the working class values" for long enough to begin to establish a relationship which might not even begin to form if all the implicit elements of differences in the sense in which each means this assertion were immediately to be made more explicit.

Postulate 7. Slogans that are used as shorthand devices for welding social solidarity must be recognized to be in fact subject to certain implicit qualifications.

Unless staff members retain an awareness that their shorthand statements of operating principles actually stand for far more complex propositions with numerous implicit qualifications, they may allow several anti-therapeutic trends to come into being. For example, patients may develop an unrealistic expectation of the therapeutic community which may lead to a sense of disappointment, or, stronger, a feeling of staff betrayal or hypocrisy when the experience occurs that makes an unexpressed qualification the effective basis for choice of staff action.

Postulate 8. The enthusiasm and positive involvement in ideological tenets should not close the minds of the staff to the need for constant critical evaluation and revision.

The ideologue, who see his system of ideas as absolute and not open to critical evaluation is inimical not only to science but to therapy. One of the fundamental principles of therapeutic community development is an appreciation of the fact that the term "therapeutic community" is to some extent a wish fulfillment. At best the "therapeuticness" of the attempt to use the community resources for milieu therapy is something that is in a constant state of becoming. The best of therapeutic communities is only partly effective. The ideology, must, therefore, be kept an open one—capable of rational reappraisal and, where appropriate, revision.

PRINCIPLE B—THE SOCIAL ORGANIZATION OF STAFF ROLES SHOULD BE STUDIED AS PART OF THE WORK OF THE THERAPEUTIC COMMUNITY

Postulate 9. Sources of role conflict based on discrepancies of expectation must be made explicit if they are to be effectively dealt with.

Personnel in innovating therapeutic communities are particularly susceptible to role conflicts based on discrepancies between the new, ideal principles and the established conventional ones.

Every social system has ideal-real discrepancies that can affect the morale and performance of its members. This is especially true in innovating organizations where the ideals are formulated before the practical wherewithal is worked through—particularly in the area of role definitions. Nurses, for example, may be expected to keep the wards spotlessly clean in accordance with their training and with the prevailing expectations for members of their profession, while in the therapeutic community context it may be felt that greater attention should be given to understanding patients' behavior, even if this entails the sacrifice of emphasis on cleanliness and orderliness. Making these discrepancies in role expectations explicit usually helps in dealing with them.

Postulate 10. Making discrepancies explicit is a necessary but not sufficient condition for dealing with role conflict.

There are various ways of dealing with discrepancies once they are recognized. They may be neutralized through some kind of scheduling of activities (with conformity to one set of norms relegated to one time period and conformity to the other to another time period), or insulation (e.g. where one type of norms is rationalized as belonging to one part of the hospital and the other set to another part), or by structural changes (e.g. changes in the formal system of expectations or changes in the innovating therapeutic community ideology to bring the two more into harmony.)

Postulate 11. Where discrepancies are recognized and where none of the above devices for neutralizing their efforts may be developed, explicit recognition should be given to the fact that individuals within the innovating system will have their performance conditioned by the presence of the contradicting set of norms.

Where the individuals in the therapeutic community are subject to conflicting role expectations and where these cannot be neutralized, unless recognition is given to their dilemmas, they may react with a sense of guilt or failure, or they may deny the difficulties but act out their consequences through denial, withdrawal or involvement and other maladaptive mechanisms seen from the point of view of the functioning of the organization.

Postulate 12. Efforts should be made to institutionalize and perpetuate new role types adapted to the requirements of the therapeutic community.

One reaction to the deficiencies of conventional role expectations from the viewpoint of the requirements of the therapeutic community is to recruit untrained staff, using them in a relatively transient way, and to stress their value in providing a "natural," "spontaneous" milieu—in contrast to the "rigid," "institutional" or "disciplinary" traditional regime. Whatever the merits of this device, it would seem that the best long run effects for the profession as a whole would be accomplished through attempts to define the attributes of the new role and to train people to propagate the new approach within the profession rather than to allow those experienced in the new approach to disperse with little effect on the mainstream of training and institutionalization of therapeutic staff practices.

PRINCIPLE C—THE STRUCTURING OF SOCIAL ROLES FOR PATIENTS
SHOULD RECEIVE COMPARABLE ATTENTION IN ITS ORDER OF
COMPLEXITY TO THE STAFF ROLE SYSTEM

Postulate 13. The effectiveness of the therapeutic community is a function of the variety of relationships it provides its patients.

In contrast to the classical psychoanalytic relationship, where the analyst tries to remain as neutrally defined as possible so that a variety of patients can project a variety of relationship tendencies into the situation, the therapeutic community depends on generating relationships that actually resemble those which patients have in the outside world and thus reflect their typical problems in these relationships. Thus, to reconstitute something like replicas of their net-works of troubled relationships, patients will benefit by having available people of different ages, sexes and interpersonal tendencies.

Postulate 14. Even granting that patient participation in one another's therapy is potentially of great, perhaps unique advantage—it must be recognized that this undertaking is fraught with hazards.

The advantages in using patients as allies in therapy have been brought out well by enthusiasts for the therapeutic community approach. They live together around the clock, they share many values and communication patterns that sep-arate them as a group from the staff, they are often gifted and insightful diag-nosticians, they often are more influential figures in affecting one another's atti-tudes and perceptions than staff members could be. On the other hand, research as well as defensive reaction to the idea of turning patients loose on one another as therapists has indicated that the problems of using patients in this capacity are complex. They can have a contratherapeutic influence as well as the reverse—influencing their fellows against participating in the therapeutic situation, re-enforcing distorted perceptions of reality, providing noxious elements in the rela-tionship, etc. Patients, on becoming "little therapists," may use their new skills and language aggressively, not only with one another but with the uninitiated members of their families outside the supervised context of the treatment institu-tion. In general, it seems advisable to be alert for the differences in patients' ca-pacities for therapeutic alliance at different points in their careers, and to provide supervision for the extended use of patients as therapeutic auxiliaries under all conditions, and finally, to caution patients about the harmful as well as beneficial potentialities of the "therapeutic mode" of interaction if indiscriminately used.

Postulate 15. Permissiveness, in its extreme form, can pose problems for patient care different from but comparable in seriousness to rigid coercion.

This point has been discussed to some extent under some of the postulates on ideology. It would seem that extreme permissiveness is not only potentially fright-ening and harmful to many patients and to others involved with them in the therapeutic community, but impracticable administratively. A recognition of the general limits of permissiveness in the particular context seems essential. In addi-tion, there should be an explicit acknowledgement of the conditions under which staff will intervene or interrupt the practices of permissiveness whatever their customary limits, in favor of other supervening principles of therapy.

Postulate 16. In addition to the internal problems posed by a poorly limited and inexplicitly qualified system of permissiveness, such a system poses problems of discontinuity between the kind of environment patients experience within the hospital and the kind to which they must adjust outside.

Neither the extremely repressive milieu nor the extremely permissive one pre-pares the patient for coping with the normal stresses of life outside the hospital. Every patient experiences secondary problems of social adjustment entailed in having to make the transition from hospital life to life outside. To the extent that there is a great gap in the type of experience engendered in the therapeutic community and that prevailing outside the hospital, these secondary stresses may effectively contravene the benefits of therapy.

Postulate 17. In general, to the extent that a therapeutic community functions according to values discrepant from those in the patients' normal social environments outside the hospital, it should provide structured experiences to ease the transition.

Permissiveness is only one of several values characteristic of many therapeutic communities that are at variance with those prevailing outside. Indeed, if the inside community were to be identical with that in which the patients developed their disorders, there is little likelihood that it could be therapeutic. However, the types and degrees of differences to be recommended will vary from patient to patient and it is inadequate to assume a blanket solution of either viewing the hospital as a microcosm of the outside world or as entirely different. The congruences and incongruences should be a continual topic of study, and structural transitional experiences introduced into the patients' treatment career as appropriate.

Postulate 18. Periodic collective disturbances are characteristic of therapeutic communities, making both patients and staff behave in ways variant to their preferred and characteristic modes.

Because of their tendencies toward permissive policies and the "freeing of communications," therapeutic communities tend to allow expressive trends to develop to an unusual degree. The interlocking group structures and general fluidity of role definitions further accentuate this tendency, providing elements of emotional contagion. Therapeutic communities high on all these factors—communication, permissiveness, group activities (especially with shifting, interlocking group membership), and role interchangeability—will be especially prone to cyclical collective disturbance.

Postulate 19. Collective disturbances among patients are neither intrinsically good nor intrinsically bad for therapy. They provide certain forces that can be harmful when operating dysfunctionally, or that can provide unusually potent forces for therapy under optimal conditions.

The general tendency in hospital practice has been to regard collective disturbances as intrinsically harmful and to be avoided. In our studies of Belmont Hospital, we have accumulated considerable evidence to support a more qualified view. If these disturbances are allowed to occur without control and without understanding of their dynamics, they do indeed entail impressive casualties. Some patients become seriously disturbed, others take their discharges prematurely, staff morale and role performance may be adversely affected, and the therapeutic community may get into trouble with its external relationships. On the other hand, if optimally managed—which would include the possibility for individuals to leave the system temporarily when they found the stresses too great and then return when they and the system were able to manage it—these "oscillations in social organization" may have potent therapeutic value. They mobilize a sense of involvement, put guilt feelings to work functionally, and have other characteristics of a therapeutically effective nature. These findings are consistent with the more general viewpoints of the group of social psychiatric theorists who are impressed with the maturational potentials of crises of various kinds (cf. Erich Lindemann, Gerald Caplan, James Tyhurst, Irving Janis, Grete Bibring, etc.)

Ultimately, an effectively functioning dynamic therapeutic community will harness oscillatory forces in its social organization to maximum advantage—controlling intake, discharge, build-up and dissipation of tensions so as to inter-digitate optimally the requirements of the social system as a whole and those of individual patients within it.

Postulate 20. Democratization of patient-staff role relationships, like permissiveness, is desirable—but in modified and qualified forms.

Some enthusiasts for the development of therapeutic communities, in their reaction against the extreme autocracy of the custodial system, have seemed to imply that the most desirable form of a therapeutic milieu involves the complete flattening of the authority structure.

The actual degree of leveling and diffusion of authority functions in any particular therapeutic community varies—but the postulate with which we are here concerned stresses the need to recognize *limits* of democratization. Complete diffusion of authority is not possible within the medical or other authorized care aegis, because responsibility remains lodged in the staff and not in the patients. Particularly at times of crisis, those responsible for the maintenance of the institution and for the provision of legitimate therapy within it must assert their authority. Unless the limits are recognized in defining patient roles, there may ensue a sense of staff "hypocrisy" or inconsistency which may be inimical to the goals of developing a therapeutic milieu.

Postulate 21. The goal of individuation of patient care is not inconsistent with the goal of developing a coherent therapeutic ideology and an organized system of social roles.

There may be a tendency in working toward the development of therapeutic community—with its stress on democratization, communal living and so on—to assume that individual care is a sign of "favoritism," that it stimulates malfunctional rivalries, or that it works against the goals of unifying the social environment into a well-organized and coherent system of influences. Even viewing the therapeutic community as a single treatment instrument, it is possible to consider it as composed of differentiated parts. The different experiences provided in the therapeutic community are distinguished by their coherent organization and purpose in the different activities provided. Modern therapeutic communities are giving attention to providing different kinds of experiences to different patients at different points in their treatment careers—while at the same time attending to making the hospital community as a whole meaningful in terms of its own social organization and for each individual patient within it.

PRINCIPLE D—THE CULTIVATION AND EFFECTIVE USE OF A NUMBER OF KINDS OF EXTERNAL RELATIONSHIPS ARE IMPORTANT FOR THE INTERNAL FUNCTIONING OF THERAPEUTIC COMMUNITIES

Postulate 22. Recognition should be given to the pitfalls of maintaining a feeling of great opposition to the ways of traditional hospital practitioners.

As the therapeutic milieu approach becomes more generally acceptable in psychiatry, this postulate becomes less salient to innovators for therapeutic communities. In earlier experiments, the innovations of therapeutic communities represented not only departures from traditional modes of organizing hospital care, but tended to involve strong elements of protest against the inequities of such care. Because of the threatening potential of the innovations and the critical attitudes of the innovators, traditional practitioners have tended to react reciprocally, criticizing milieu therapy innovators. This has had positive functions for the development of internal cohesion of the innovating groups, and provided external targets for the expression of hostility. However, the pitfalls of this situation ought to be recognized. External opposition affects the recruitment of high calibre staff from the relevant professions; it affects the degree to which the new procedures will find broad acceptance; and it affects the kinds of attitudes engendered in patients toward external authority figures. One of the goals of therapy in the therapeutic community, as in other psychotherapies, is to mitigate the tendency of patients to project malevolence unreasonably into authority figures. By re-enforcing such tendencies, an innovating therapeutic community that uses external opposition as a convenient locus of scapegoats for deflecting internal hostilities is making short-term gains at the possible expense of long-term benefits to patients.

Postulate 23. Another kind of external relationship that might be profitably attended to by those interested in the therapeutic community approach is that embodied in the family relationships of patients.

Family members have acted as significant forces in most patients' lives, and in most cases they continue to exert important influences on them and on their potentials for functioning outside the hospital. To the extent that the goal of therapeutic communities is to cultivate an understanding of the forces that have formative influences on patients' personalities and that underly their contemporary behavior, it is important to seek information from family members. Patients' own perceptions of themselves in the context of their family relationships are important kinds of therapeutic information and need dealing within their own terms. However, familial information may supplement this in important ways—both for the intra-psychic treatment of patients and in terms of their rehabilitation. To the extent that family members provide a crucial part of the social environment to which patients must adjust subsequent to discharge from the hospital, it is important to assess and if possible to influence them directly as well as indirectly through the patient himself.

Postulate 24. It is important to recognize that familial involvements in patients' careers are complex, so that the involvement of family members in the therapeutic program ought to be done within the context of a differentiated set of goals.

The practitioner of the therapeutic milieu approach, feeling the importance of familial factors in the diagnosis, treatment and rehabilitation of his patients, and being willing to enlarge his scope of therapeutic responsibility beyond the individual patient, may tend to use the blanket ideal of "bringing the family into the treatment," as a universally applicable pre-requisite for his patients' therapy. This attitude, like some of the other ideological simplifications mentioned above, needs qualification if it is to be optimally employed. The first such qualification has to do with the goals of involving family members. The goals of learning more about the patient's early history and behavioral patterns from family members is a different one from the goal of changing family members so as to be better able to absorb a patient (perhaps a chronically disabled one) back into the family with minimal ensuing repercussions either for the ex-patient or for other family members. While a certain amount of preliminary work may have to be done—e.g. in general family discussion groups—to determine which constellations of patient-in-family may be most usefully approached with one set of goals and which with another set—provision should be made for dealing differently with situations that have different goals.

Postulate 25. The goals adopted for a particular patient in reference to his family will depend on part on factors extrinsic as well as those intrinsic to the hospital.

After the first step of formulating goals appropriate for the situation of any particular patient as he is seen in the hospital and as his family situation becomes known to the hospital personnel is made—a further step is necessary to determine the potentialities of those external to the hospital for participation in the ideal social psychiatric plan. Even if it is seen as desirable, for example, to work toward helping the mother of the above mentioned type of patient as well as the patient himself (or, in a more complex situation, to work for the mental health of a married patient through improving the functioning of his marital unit rather than through working to dissolve it so that he can pursue his individual psychological goals) extrinsic factors may interfere with the plan. The other family members may live at too great a distance, be too alienated from the therapeutic situation to wish to participate, be too difficult to influence even if they do agree to participate, etc. The ideal goal, must, therefore, be modified by a consideration of the impingement of extramural factors on the situation in focus.

Postulate 26. In assessing patients' families' assets and liabilities for the therapeutic enterprise the concept of "fit" might usefully supplement more individually-centered concepts like "need." This should assist the therapist in working out a consensus about goals of family therapy and in harnessing family assets in the therapeutic process.

The concept of "fit" is especially useful in assessing the asset-liability balances in any given patient's configuration of personal and familial factors. Better functioning may be achieved through improving different elements of the way the patient and other family members fit together. Changes in cultural norms or values and changes in behavioral patterns in role performance may be as effective in improving family functioning in a given situation as attempts to change the individual patient's personality or the fit between his personality and that of other family members. Even where basic personality change is a goal, greater therapeutic success may be realized if fit in this dimension is the target of the treatment.

Postulate 27. The problem of therapeutic technique with families can be considered separately from the above considerations.

Experimentation with the treatment of individuals-in-their-family contexts is underway on numerous fronts. The adaptation of particular forms of therapy to the therapeutic community approach will vary according to the preferences and styles of particular practitioners. Within the therapeutic community at Belmont, for example, where there was universal acceptance of the importance of the family in diagnosis, treatment and rehabilitation, each of the four doctors preferred a different technique. One dealt privately with family members and patient, sometimes introducing other staff members or other patients as he saw fit; another brought patients into group therapy sessions but did not see them privately; a third insisted that the strategic family member (e.g. spouse) entered the unit also as a patient, but receive "community" treatment like other patients, not necessarily in the same group therapy sessions as the spouse; while the fourth dealt with family members of many patients outside the regular therapeutic community regimen but all together in a large group called the "family group."

On further study it will probably emerge that particular physicians' styles aside, each of these strategies is most effective for particular kinds of problem situations as outlined above. The introduction of a family member into the hospital as a patient in his own right has certain advantages in terms of distributing the onus of receiving treatment within the family, but it has the disadvantage that most hospitals are not set up to accommodate family living in anything approximating their normal manner. To the extent that the replication of external patterns is important in the strategy of therapeutic community treatment and rehabilitation, this would seem an important consideration. Aside from building hospital accommodations that might meet this set of problems, and aside from working out how the development of internal sub-systems like families within the larger therapeutic community would affect the character of the overall system, it would seem that the trend in future social psychiatric work along these lines would emphasize the reaching out from the hospital into the community to deal with families in their own home settings. Increased fluidity of transition between hospital and family setting—for one or any combination of members would seem the ideal image for future cultivation in this sphere of therapy.

PRINCIPLE E—THERE ARE ADVANTAGES TO MAINTAINING A CONCEPTUAL DISTINCTION BETWEEN TREATMENT AND REHABILITATION, EVEN IN THERAPEUTIC COMMUNITIES WHERE THE GOALS OF TREATMENT AND REHABILITATION ARE SO CLOSELY INTERTWINED

Postulate 28. The distinction between the goals of social adaptation (rehabilitation) and personality change (treatment) may help to clarify changing requirements of patients at different therapeutic stages.

Traditionally, the separation of treatment goals and measures from those of rehabilitation has had harmful consequences for patients. Aside from separating, and sometimes setting at odds, the activities of different specialists to the detriment of the patient, this separation allowed a tendency to develop measures that might have helped individuals out of their social context but which could not produce persisting results in their ordinary world of social reality. One reaction to these undesirable features of many conventional therapeutic practices has been the merging of the goals, with the implication that they are inextricably joined —that they do, or should amount to the same thing. Good treatment, it is said, *is* good rehabilitation, as the modern socially oriented psychiatrist treats with reference to adjusting the patient to his social context and not to some abstract set of ideals. Our own research however indicates that this tendency in thinking, if carried too far, can set up another kind of problem—namely a blurring of thinking and strategies in situations where it is advantageous to consider these goals as conceptually distinct, however intertwined they may be in ultimate reality or in particular therapeutic experience. Emphasis on the inextricable nature of treatment and rehabilitation in a therapeutic community might, for example, lead to the exclusive adoption of "realistic" workshops, like those of the patient's outside world. Patients who could not adjust to the requirements of participation in these shops would be considered as incapable of being treated in this context. A better way of conceptualizing the problem of the place of workshops in therapy would seem to be based on the conceptual distinction between treatment and rehabilitation. Patients might need "treatment" (i.e. participation in a special kind of occupational set-up with expectations very different from those of the outside world,) until he is ready intra-personally to participate in the rehabilitation experiences of the more industrial-like workshops.

The therapeutic program could then be planned for each patient in terms of stages which are conceptualized as pathways toward the goals of therapy. Recognition could be given to the different requirements of different patients at different times. Different groups, role relationships or prescribed activities can then be assigned as appropriate for the patient as part of his overall therapeutic career.

Postulate 30. All the distinctions recommended above can lead to a harmful set of consequences unless welded into a coherent set of experiences through giving constant attention to integrative activities.

PERSPECTIVES

Social scientists, in studying hospitals, tend to analyze the situation observed in terms of abstract dimensions such as authority structure, ideology and so on—and to talk such processes as multiple subordination, covert disagreement, and oscillations in social organization. Psychiatrists, on the other hand, tend to ask questions like: how big should the unit be, should we mix different types of patients (e.g. psychotics, psychopaths and neurotics), how long should patients be treated, and so on. There is a feeling that social science should be useful in answering practical questions as well as providing interesting ethnographic documentation and illuminating abstract conceptual issues. A major contemporary problem is how this can be best accomplished. One line of work that seems especially promising for the implementation of existing ideas as well as for the generation of new perspectives is that known as "action research." This kind of research is best done through the collaboration of psychiatrist and social scientist under less insulated and fragmentary relationships than in much of their collaborative efforts to date. The essential purpose of action research in this context would be to begin with propositions already expounded on the basis of accomplished research—propositions like those indicated above—and to apply them in the particular situation at hand. The application, with whatever modifications are considered appropriate through joint formulations of psychiatrist and social scientist, is then studied to determine its effectiveness. This kind of study is different from ordinary evaluation studies in that the effort is to understand process as well as effect, and to develop successive reformulations that will bring about increasingly improved results with the framework of a single undertaking. Thus, there is a joint period of translation of postulates into action implications in a given setting, a period of action implementation with accompanying study of the processes and effects of the action, a period of joint reformulation and then to a revised action program, etc., as long as is necessary or possible in the particular situation.

The action-research approach requires very special kinds of professionals, both on the psychiatric and the social science side. The social scientist must be ready to feed back his formulations on a schedule geared to clinical requirements and to participate in the task of drawing implications from his work; the psychiatrist must be prepared to accept criticism from a relatively uninvolved collaborator without feeling excessively threatened and thus prone to defensive reactions that might discourage the participation of high calibre social researchers and distort his own capacity to use the research. When these conditions are realized, a sense of partnership, of joint exploration and joint creativity potentially entailed in this kind of work are exceedingly valuable and of great promise for the field of social psychiatry as a whole.

REFERENCES

CAPLAN, G.: An Approach to Community Mental Health. New York, Grune and Stratton, 1961.

CAUDILL, W.: The Psychiatric Hospital as a Small Society. Cambridge, Harvard University Press, 1958.

GREENBLATT, M., LEVINSON, D., AND WILLIAMS, R.: The Patient And the Mental Hospital. Glencoe, Illinois, The Free Press, 1957.

JANIS, I.: Psychological Stress. New York, Wiley, 1958.

JONES, M.: The Therapeutic Community, New York, Basic Books, 1953.

KLEIN, D., AND LINDEMANN, E.: Preventive intervention in individual and family crises situations. In: Caplan, G. (ed.) Prevention of Mental Disorders in Children. New York, Basic Books, 1961.

LEIGHTON, A. H.: My Name is Legion. New York, Basic Books, 1958.

RAPOPORT, R.: Community as Doctor, London: Tavistock Publications and Springfield, Illinois, Charles C Thomas, 1960. In collaboration with Rhona Rapoport and Irving Rosow. Introduction by Maxwell Jones.

RAPOPORT, R.: A Social Scientist Looks at the Therapeutic Community: Suggestions for Developing Action Research. In: forthcoming Proceedings of the World Congress of Psychiatry, Montreal, 1961.

SCHWARTZ, M., et al.: Social Perspectives on Mental Patient Care. New York, Basic Books, in press.

TYHURST, J.: Individual reactions to community disaster. Am. J. Psychiat., 107: 764-769, 1951.

A Psychiatric Crisis Ward

by EDWARD STAINBROOK, PH.D., M.D.

THE TERM "CRISIS" has long denoted a decisive change in a disease process for better or worse. We speak easily also of critical life-situations and of psychological crises in the lives of persons. Such personal crises are engendered by complex but highly individualized patterns of determinants arising in the body, in the self and in the persons, things and social institutions in the ambient community. Such experiences of threatening helplessness, incapacity, inadequacy, debasement or coercion may be resolved by the individual through some degree of mastery and a resulting restoration to the *status pro ante* of most of his character and situational resources. Indeed, he may achieve also some new learning and an increased psychological adequacy. Frequently, however, the resolution by the person of a life-crisis may be expressed as a more or less acute adaptational failure. This failure-reaction to crisis is character-ized by a sometimes shifting but always totally involved patterning of deviance in biological, psychological and social action.

In our society, the sick role in one of its possible action-patterns within or without a hospital organization is used as a socially provided resource for the reduction of stress and the maintenance and facilitation of body and self integrity. If the psychiatric hospital is the social organizational context in which the person-in-crisis seeks to participate as a patient, then the hospital should be prepared not only to bring its specialized helping personnel individually to the patient's aid, but it should also become for the patient a restitutive and supporting social organization fulfilling temporarily certain basic social needs. In other words, the rational treatment of any illness demands not only an aggregate of skilled and knowing helping individuals, but also the therapeutic use of what can be a very versatile social institution, namely, the human-group organization of the hospital itself.

These considerations about the values and the treatment of behavioral distress and deviation underlay the conception of a ward within the psychiatric division of a large metropolitan public general hospital designed to provide a few-days' to a few-weeks' intensive help for persons in a critical life-situation and thus avoid state hospitalization. Additionally, there was an increasing necessity to provide immediate, short-term aid and then to end, in many instances, the treatment relationship when compensation has been reestablished—even though such a therapeutic activity and attitude is doubly demanding and uninviting to the resident psychiatrist who implements so many of the teaching and training clinics. This is so, first, because the professional model motivating the most interested identification is that of the psychoanalyst. Second, the assured management of the brief, intensive therapeutic encounter requires mature skill and experience.

Some general ecological concerns about behavioral deviance also motivated us in our thinking about the sociological use of the ward-group. In times of the rapid influx of population into a large urban area, such as Los Angeles, the social organization of the city is unable to "process" adequately all the humanity which comes to it. The result is that many people are neither adequately related to informational sources about the life around them, nor are they able to contact and mobilize the social resources potentially available to them. In the first instance of informational and communicative inadequacy, the cognitive inference about surrounding persons and events may become quite distorted. When lack of access to social participation occurs, feelings of deprivation, helplessness and impotent isolation may be experienced.

Very many of the almost 9,000 admissions each year to the psychiatric division of the Los Angeles County General Hospital and of a greater number of persons who are seen either in the out-patient clinic or in the pre-admitting clinic are recent migrants to Los Angeles. Many are completely alone and unrelated to any immediately available person or human group. Or they are in a critical situation because they have just lost the significant relationship which had sustained them.

The crisis ward, as do many other wards of the hospital, temporarily provides repair of the social isolation, furnishes some immediate satisfactions arising from individuals and from the group, and creates, however tenuously and ambivalently, a reference group which the patient may use, even if only partially, as he participates in a day plan. Alternatively he may use it for support only in fantasy and memory recall when he is no longer in the hospital but has the assurance of being able, if necessary, to return.

The utilization of the ward as a "retreat" from an acutely distressing present, motivated by needs for regression and for avoidance and withdrawal is, of course, desired to a variable extent by most people in crisis. The ward policy and expectancy, however, is that all patients will participate immediately in the daily therapeutically structured activities of the situation. In the first day or two of entrance into the ward society, the patient may be allowed to be alone and to withdraw or sleep at times when an essential group or individual encounter is not arranged for him. In essence, however, we say implicitly to the newly admitted patient, "we understand how stressed you feel, and for a day or two we want simply to help you restore yourself and to feel psychologically stronger. As soon as you feel able, we shall try to understand together how it is with you and your situation and how you can come to a more adequate sense of your own abilities to master your circumstances." From the beginning, therefore, although we accept with empathy and unstinted support the patient's need to be taken care of, we also from the beginning insist that as soon as the patient can, he shall begin, in the therapeutic process, to use his own resources as much as possible in an active collaboration with the personal relationships, the professional functions and the technical and social resources which constitute the ward society. Both implicitly and explicitly, the perception of the hospital merely as a "place to rest for a few days" is consistently negated.

The ages of patients in the ward-group may at any one time range from 14 to 70 years. There are many essential sociological differences from a family in this relatively fortuitous, temporary and constantly changing group of patients and personnel. Nevertheless, the ready transference perceptions and responses initially learned in the original socialization in becoming an individual in the basic human group of the family are evoked immediately in patients, and in personnel as well, by a wide spectrum of family—reminiscent roles and counter-roles. Such a variety of possible role-persons makes it highly likely that the most distressing interpersonal problems of the incoming patient will be experienced and, hopefully, observed in the here-and-now of the ward society. Then, to a limited but maximally exploited extent, the therapeutic action-plans executed in group and individual psychotherapy and in the continuing transactions with nursing personnel are directed, in a varying pattern for each patient, to tension-transformations through thought, talk and action, to personal experience with an empathetic, supporting and esteeming other person, and to any self-reflection and reconceptualizing of self and of others that seems possible.

A significant factor determining the motivations and the treatment conceptions of the ward personnel is the recognition by them that the existing therapeutic action of the crisis ward is planned by choice and did not evolve as an expedient adjustment to necessity forced by a lack of resources or by an absence of therapeutic imagination and vitality.

An additional decision to emphasize the therapeutic importance of the personnel and of the social organization of the ward is the exclusion of electro-convulsive procedures and of any other so-called physical therapy from the treatment resources. Pharmacologic alteration of behavior is attempted only with the objective of reducing the emotionally-engendered generalization of perception and response in order to restore some measure of the patient's characteristic capacity to discriminate cognitively internal and external objects, persons, actions and feelings. Neither drug-induced tranquility nor euphoria is sought as an end in itself.

Every hospital service such as we are describing will be influenced by some purely local considerations. One influence in our immediate situation is our goal, over the past few years, to arrange for an ever-increasing number of voluntary referrals from the large urban-serving "receiving" section of our psychiatric hospital serving the Los Angeles area. However, the admitting and evaluation wards of our hospital are adapted functionally to the 72-hour observation limit which the California State Welfare Code imposes upon us. Increasingly, we are trying to reduce to a minimum the number of such 72-hour admissions in order to avoid as much legal detention process as possible for psychiatric patients.

We found, however, that partly because of an inadequate referral experience and an insufficient working through of the anxiety and other problems of the patient and of his social situation, many persons entering our hospital voluntarily did not for many reasons voluntarily enter a state hospital; but, about 65 per cent did so. Many of the rest were discharged by us to outpatient clinics or to private psychiatric hospitals.

During the first three months of its operation, most of the voluntary patients who had previously entered the admitting-evaluating wards come to the crisis ward. Among voluntary patients having this experience, the highest percentage who went on to a state hospital was 28 per cent in contrast to the 65 per cent established previously. This percentage has continuously declined to less than 3 per cent in recent months. Part of this decline, however, is due to the adaptation of the intake service of the hospital to the clearer definition of the goals and functions of the crisis ward. Voluntary patients for whom on the basis of past history and present situation an admission to the state hospital seems at intake evaluation to be the most rational decision are no longer admitted to the crisis ward. From this first three months' experience, nevertheless, it was quite demonstrable that for the voluntarily entering patients who were explicitly prepared to accept state hospital entrance, the imposition of a limited experience of three weeks or less in the crisis ward dramatically and significantly reduced the number who would have gone on to a state hospital. This is another confirmation from actual hospital action-research for the established hypothesis that "splinting them where they lie" is valid also in psychiatry.

For a characteristic recent month, the crisis ward admitted 42 persons, 18 male and 24 female. Fifty per cent of the males admitted were between the ages of 18 and 25, while 50 per cent of the females admitted represented an older age range between 26 and 35 years. The general diagnostic categories were represented in percentages of approximately 45 per cent psychoneurotic reactions, 35 per cent psychotic reactions, almost exclusively schizophrenic, and 20 per cent character disorders. Thirteen of the 42 patients admitted in the month remained in the hospital from at least 8 to 14 days. Fifteen others stayed from 15 to 21 days. Seven patients were discharged within one week and five patients remained longer than the three weeks' ostensible limit.

With reference to final disposition for the month's total admissions, three of the patients continued hospital treatment on our own longer-term treatment wards. Two patients were signed out as leaving against medical advice, meaning, in these instances, failure to return after being out on pass. Five returned to the hospital for a variable period of time on a day plan. Seven were referred to our own or some other outpatient continuation. The rest were discharged without any formal referral to psychiatric treatment sources.

TECHNIQUES OF THERAPY

All of the people, personnel and patients, comprising the ward society meet together immediately after breakfast for the first hour of every weekday. The group is moderated usually by the senior psychiatrist and the interaction is designed for the reporting, primarily by patients, of attitudes, perceptions and feelings related to the present life experience. In addition to the energy transformations involved in the behavior of talking and being in the group, the exchange of information facilitates a less idiosyncratically distorted person-construction of each other by the group members and makes possible a quick learning about the role-related conditions of participating in the ward group. Other important transactions, such as the recognition of individual differences as well as similarities, occur. Since the smaller therapeutic groups, limited to 7 or 8 patients and providing for much closer social contact, convene right after the total group, the first large meeting stimulates much of the motivation for the usual high-level participation and commitment to the therapeutic tasks that characterize most of the small group interaction.

The three small groups meeting each day are created from the total patient society on the basis of a brief psychological test, "The Fundamental Interpersonal Relations Orientation Behavior Schedule." Patients about whom it is inferred from test and other clinical information that they are more self-reflective and concerned about exploring personal feelings, problems and past experiences and are aiming at a more comfortable adjustment with themselves are assigned to a therapeutic group directed by the senior psychiatrist. The psychologist moderates the group of patients who are more openly aggressive and antagonistic and who are primarily concerned about working out their relationships with other people, while one of the resident psychiatrists works with the rest of the patients.

One or two interns and nurses also "sit in" with each group as part of the teaching and training function of the hospital. At some time later in the day each patient has an encounter of variable time duration with an individual therapist, who may be the senior psychiatrist, a resident psychiatrist, the psychologist, or one of the four medical interns assigned to the crisis ward, among other duties in the psychiatric hospital, for periods of three weeks.

Some of the patients also see during the day the psychiatric social worker, who, however, spends most of her time with the significant other persons in the patients' lives. Increasingly, an attempt is made to see the family, including the patient, as a group as well as to deal with groups of relatives.

In order to structure more definitely the social articulation of patients with each other and with the organizational resources of the ward, a patient government program is constantly maintained. In a rapidly changing ward such as ours, a formal organization of administrative participation by patients not only provides for a democratically determined constructive channeling of opposition and resentment, but also assures nuclear stability of the patient society. The delegation of ward government decisions reinforces daily the motivation of the patient group to assume collective responsibility for much of the on-going social behavior of the ward, not the least of which is the supporting introduction of new members into the group and the minimizing of the disorganizing effects of the departure of old members.

The educational exploitation of the crisis ward is organized at various levels of professional maturity and for various role groups. The residency education and training program utilizes a three-month assignment of the resident in his first year and in his third year to the crisis ward. The first-year resident has the experience of learning early in his training that time-limited help given in a critical period can be most effective for the patient and highly rewarding to the therapist. The third-year resident, if he has not had a previous crisis ward experience, is even more surprised and rewarded by his direct therapeutic experience and has the additional opportunity to supervise the psychotherapeutic learning of the interns on the ward.

Nurses and nursing students intimately participate also in learning how to be restorative, communication-catalyzing and reassuring other persons for people in distress. They also come to learn increasingly how to give patients the experience the patient needs at that particular time with another person. And they also learn to know when, by a formulation suggested in the margins of an interpersonal happening, they can help a patient label, reconceptualize and reflect upon his experiences.

Throughout the present year, about 50 non-psychiatric physicians have been attending a two-hour weekly session in the hospital at which patients from the crisis ward are interviewed both by the physicians as well as by the teaching staff of the Department of Psychiatry of the University of Southern California. Determinants of the patients' problems as well as methods of treatment are discussed. As part of practical training in the management of the patient in crisis, some of these general practitioners and non-psychiatric physicians, who are also attending staff members in other departments of the hospital, are now actively treating within the psychiatric hospital some of the crisis ward patients.

The State Hospital Consultant Team as an Educational Instrument*

by Robert L. Stewart, M.D., Elizabeth Jacob, M.A., Harold Koenig, M.D., Ruth Koenig, M.D., Warren G. McPherson, M.D., Arthur A. Miller, M.D., Philip F. D. Seitz, M.D. and Dorothy Stock, Ph.D.

THE TEAM APPROACH has won a secure place in the treatment of psychiatric patients. The use of the team as an educational and training device, however, has been little explored. In this report we shall describe the use of a coordinated commuting psychiatric team to provide on-the-job training for the professional staff of a state hospital remote from urban psychiatric centers. Some of the training problems encountered are no different from those met in a psychiatric residency program; some problems are characteristic of state hospitals generally; and still others arise out of the sociologic characteristics of a specific hospital. The coordinated consultant team has certain advantages in solving some of these problems, and is a potentially valuable tool for the training of existing professional staffs in remote state hospitals.

Five psychoanalysts, a neurologist, a psychologist, and a psychiatric social worker, together with an administrative assistant and a secretary, constitute the consultant team described in this report. This team works in close collaboration with the Illinois State Psychiatric Institute (ISPI), to which it is administratively responsible. It is also sponsored by the Chicago Institute for Psychoanalysis. The team was organized after one of its members was asked to give a series of lectures at various state hospitals. Dissatisfied because of the impossibility of achieving meaningful, continuous contact with the staffs of several hospitals, he proposed to organize a team which would concentrate its efforts on a single hospital. The East Moline State Hospital was selected for the project because at

*The Consultant team wishes to acknowledge the invaluable assistance and support of Drs. Jules Masserman and Robert C. Drye, past and present Directors of Education, Illinois State Psychiatric Institute. This project was supported in part by Research Grant 17-100 from the Illinois Research and Training Authority.

that time it had no regular training and consultation program, it is too far from Chicago to attract consultants from there, and yet it is reasonably accessible from Chicago by rail and air.

To care for its two thousand patients, the East Moline State Hospital had a medical staff of twelve physicians, all of whom were born in other countries and none of whom spoke English as his native language. They came from many parts of the world—the Philippines, Poland, Lithuania, Greece, Germany, Yugoslavia, Mexico, Cuba, Colombia. With the exception of the superintendent, none was trained in psychiatry. A few had been specialists in other fields such as ophthalmology and surgery. Most had come to the United States to escape from political oppression, and several had left flourishing practices in their native lands. All were faced with making a new start in a strange country, learning a new and difficult language, and coping with unfamiliar ideas and customs. They were working in a state hospital not by choice but because it offered the only medical jobs available to them.

By contrast, the other departments of the hospital, such as psychology, social service, nursing, and activity therapies, were for the most part made up of non-foreigners. The psychology and social service staffs took the leadership in psychiatric matters, since they were better trained in these than the physicians had been. The official line of decision making, with the physician responsible for all matters of patient care, was recognized nominally, although in practice the doctor was unable to take actual professional leadership. The physician tended to see his job simply as caring for the physical needs of his patients, leaving the psychiatric matters to the other disciplines.

The primary aims of the consulting team, then, were to provide the medical staff with sufficient technical knowledge to carry out their jobs as psychiatrists, and concomitantly to give them a solid professional identification. The physicians on the consulting team, therefore, worked almost exclusively with the doctors. They did not give formal lectures, but instead conducted seminars, staff conferences, worked with patients on the wards, and supervised assigned preceptees. The consultant team's psychologist and psychiatric social worker worked with their respective departments. As was expected, the delicate unspoken balance between the various professional divisions of the hospital was soon upset, and more and more of the staff demanded special training. Two more psychiatrists with special interests were added to the consulting team to meet those demands. At the present time, almost all divisions of the professional staff are engaged in some training program with a consultant.

The original team (there have been additions to the team during the project, but no one has dropped out) was made up of persons who had worked together in the past and who shared the same points of views about psychiatry and other matters. The three psychiatrists of the original team had worked together in a university department of psychiatry, and working in the new team offered them an opportunity for continued personal and professional relationships.* The other members also had worked with one or all of the psychiatrists. It was possible, therefore, to recruit a consultant team in which the interpersonal relationships were based on prior friendship, mutual respect, and a common theoretic orientation.

The team operates by sending a psychiatrist to the hospital a full day each week. The neurologist, psychologist, and social worker each make one trip a month to the hospital. On returning from the hospital each person writes a detailed, ear-to-the-ground report of the events of the day, which is then sent to all other members of the team. In addition, the coordinator of the team telephones each member before and after his trip to alert him to problems which might need special attention and to learn of any developments requiring immediate action. All members of the team meet for a monthly breakfast and at that time discuss matters of general policy and any other details which require group attention. Occasionally the team meets with representatives of ISPI and of the Institute for Psychoanalysis for long term planning.

A number of educational problems have come into focus during the more than two years of the team's operations. The medical staff of the hospital is a heterogeneous group of mature men and women whose personal and professional interests lie elsewhere than in psychiatry and who find themselves in a state hospital only because of political accident. Some of them have been discouraged about making a new start in life, and most have regarded their jobs in the state hospital system as only a temporary haven. Many have been deeply concerned about relatives and friends left behind. For these reasons there is often little or no incentive to learn a new and difficult specialty. Much of their available energy is spent in learning English, and in studying for state boards and the American Medical Qualifying Examination. Attending a full day of teaching conferences seems to them at times just one more thing to be put up with. In the early months of the project the daily routine of the staff seemed to be regulated more by the noon whistle than by professional requirements, a reflection of their deep sense of personal dislocation and professional insecurity in the face of too great demands. Some of the

---

*Margaret Mead, in a personal communication, pointed out that this may be one of the more important rewards for the members of a consultant team. She suggests that new teams might be recruited from graduates of the same medical school, or from contemporaries of the same residency program, etc.

physicians, however, displayed an admirable professionalism which compensated for lack of motivation to learn psychiatry and for the various other pulls which overtly and covertly interfere with the learning process.

One practice of the hospital which added to motivational difficulties was that of giving each physician an unbalanced and often stultifying job assignment. It was perfectly possible for a doctor to see none but long term patients, and rarely have an opportunity to deal with challenging problems of diagnosis and treatment of more acute cases. Or, a physician might be given the job of exterminating cockroaches and of doing two thousand physical examinations, and yet have no psychiatric patients of his own. To compensate for this unbalanced professional diet, and also to foster some healthy intra-staff competition, the consultant team encouraged the recent initiation of a unit system which in effect divides the hospital into three coordinate teams, each with its own personnel and its own complete set of services.

Another difficulty which arose in part from the ambiguous role of the physician and his difficulty in assuming actual leadership was the tendency of the staff to use the consultant team as intermediaries with the administrators of the hospital and with other departments. The use of the coordinated team has unique advantages in dealing with this problem, in that every such attempt immediately becomes apparent to all the consultants. The consultants, however, were themselves at times tempted to intervene in administrative matters, using the rationalization that it was necessary "for the good of the training program." That proved uniformly to be a mistake.

Initially the hospital regarded the consultant team with understandable suspicion. Many on the staff felt that a group of big-city psychoanalysts would have little understanding of the problems confronting state hospital psychiatrists. Psychoanalysts, they said, were too accustomed to dealing with the "wealthy neurotic." They expected that the team would quickly lose interest in their problems and the project would fade away as other projects had done in the past. But the staff and the consultant team both found that they could learn from each other. To the psychoanalyst, state hospital psychiatry offers a fascinating opportunity to make basic observations from his own frame of reference which he is seldom able to make in office practice. To the state hospital physician, it was reassuring to find that there exists a frame of reference which gives meaning to the puzzling and anxiety-provoking manifestations of mental illness. Needless to say, this two-way learning process has not always proceeded smoothly, and the consultants must be on guard at all times against "the pedagogic analogue of countertransference."*

---

*Maurice Levine, personal communication.

Problems thus far discussed are some which have their roots in the organization of a particular hospital. Perhaps in this group also should be included the problem of language. The physicians are required by the hospital to study English—at best a difficult language which few non-English speakers completely master. Lack of ease in English causes the doctor to want to avoid close relationships with his patients (one must also look elsewhere for other causes of this difficulty). Surprisingly enough, the doctor's struggles with English rarely seem to cause much trouble for his patients. There is a tendency for those who speak the same language to form cliques within the staff, within which that language is used. A compensatory force is to be seen in the pride which some of the foreign-born doctors take in forgetting their native tongues, even in the privacy of their homes. Whether or not insisting on the exclusive use of English is good, so far as the training goals of the project are concerned, is an unanswered question. An experiment to be tried in the future is the use of textbooks and articles in the native languages of the doctors, although the discussions would of necessity be conducted in English.

Complaints about difficulty with English are almost always a rationalization. This is driven home in those instances in which a doctor has a patient who comes from his own country. Given the opportunity to talk with the patient in his own language, it quickly becomes apparent that the real difficulty in learning and practicing psychiatry lies elsewhere, for the doctor may then reveal all too clearly a lack of understanding of the psychologic problem confronting him.

One of the cornerstones of the team's training policy is that each doctor should have at least two patients in supervised psychotherapy. We have felt that, while he could not be expected to treat more than a very small number of his patients with psychotherapy, he would learn much which would be immediately, although indirectly, helpful to all his patients. This aspect of the program has been disappointing, for only a few doctors have shown genuine interest in psychotherapy. (Those who have, however, are gradually becoming the professional leaders of the hospital.) There are several possible reasons for this disinterest. One is that traditionally in this hospital psychotherapy is done by the non-medical disciplines and the physician gives medications. This is a powerful tradition. Hand in hand with that factor is the fear of the psychotic patient which the beginner in psychiatry is likely to feel. This has been successfully met by working with the doctor and his patient on the wards. The structure of the team and its plan of working means, however, that individual supervisory sessions are a month apart, making it difficult for the team to offer optimal support in what could be a chaotic situation. Although the doctors are free to call their preceptors by long distance telephone, they have not made much use of this extra channel of communication and support. A phenomenon perhaps parallel with the rejection of psychotherapy is the absence of any tendency for the doctor to use supervision to discuss his personal problems—the "couch diving" familiar to all supervisors of psychiatric residents.

Still other difficulties, which overlap some of those already discussed, arise from the problems inherent in training any person in psychiatry, and as such they are not peculiar to a state hospital, although they might exist there in an exaggerated form. Psychiatric educators are aware, for instance, that a good deal of unlearning goes into the making of a good psychiatrist. To give but one example, the principle of parsimony applies axiomatically in most specialties, but it has a limited and special application in psychiatry. The physiology-oriented doctor is suspicious, therefore, of dynamic psychiatry, its all-but-unintelligible jargon, and the ease with which it deals with multiple etiological factors. The consultant team has been consistently psychoanalytic in its theoretic orientation, and has, for instance, taught an object-relations (more accurately, an object-cathexis) theory of psychosis in preference to other possible theories. This has been only moderately fruitful with some of the physicians, but others have been able to grasp the basic principles and to apply them successfully in their daily work.

Does the use of the coordinated team such as described in this report have any particular advantages in teaching state hospital psychiatry? We believe that it does. First of all, many psychiatrists who consult in state hospitals complain of a feeling of isolation. They might teach one afternoon a week for many years, and yet never feel that they have been integrated into the workings of the hospital. They may never meet their fellow consultants who are grappling with the same problems. The co-ordinated team does away with that source of frustration. It also makes it easier to plan an educational program on a more comprehensive scale than might otherwise be possible. This requires, of course, the full use of all available channels of communication. Not the least of the advantages of the team is that the members can buoy each other up in moments of discouragement, and help one another to spot "countertransference" reactions. For the hospital, this means a consistent, comprehensively designed program of training. In effect, the consultant team becomes a small faculty for the hospital.

The commuting consultant team approach also has its disadvantages. For one, even a single trip a month requires an emotional and sometimes physical investment which is difficult to maintain over a period of several years. One of the consultants travels almost five hundred miles each way. It was found at the beginning of the project that the trip to the hospital the night before, a full day of teaching and consulting, often with only a short break for lunch, the return trip home, and the uncertainty of weather and its effects upon air lines schedules were all an enormous drain on the consultant's emotional and physical resources. Added to this was the irrational feeling of each consultant that somehow the responsibility for two thousand patients rested squarely on the shoulders of the team. As the project has progressed, however, it has been possible for each consultant to see his proper role as a consultant and teacher, rather than therapist, greatly reducing that source of strain.

At this time, a team of consultants* from the hospital's nearby communities has been organized and is preparing to replace the Chicago team. The local team works side-by-side with the commuting team and is similarly responsible to ISPI. The new team will continue to provide teaching and consultation to East Moline after the Chicago team moves on to another hospital.

The results of this project, as we see them at present, are encouraging. The doctors have gained much in diagnostic skill and sensitivity, and they are becoming leaders of their own professional staff not only in name but also in fact. Some who left the program in its early stages are now seeking residency training in psychiatry with the help of the team. The physicians are tending to stay longer in their jobs in the hospital, and some are coming to regard state hospital psychiatry as a possible satisfying career. The morale and professional standards of the entire staff have been elevated, and patient care has improved. In addition, the staff has begun to take more interest in their own self-education; for example, they have formed a new inter-departmental journal club and participate actively in a number of special research projects. The present writers continue to hope, therefore, that the coordinated consultant team approach may provide one of the many needed answers to the training and educational problems of state hospitals generally.

REFERENCES

1. BELKNAP, K.: Human Problems of a State Mental Hospital. New York, McGraw-Hill, 1956.
2. CRAWSHAW, R.: Reading List on Psychiatric Teams. Canada's Mental Health. Spec. Supplement, 1960.
3. GAP Report Number 51: Toward Therapeutic Care. A Guide for Those Who Work with the Mentally Ill. Formulated for the Committee on Psychiatric Nursing. New York, Group for the Advancement of Psychiatry, 1961.

*Drs. Orlando Cabrera, Roland Erikson, Alice Harpring and Werner Hollander (Coordinator).

4. HUTT, M. L., MENNINGER, W. C., AND O'KEEFE, D. E.: The neuropsychiatric team in the U.S. army. Mental Hygiene, 31:103-119, 1947.
5. JONES, M., et al.: The Therapeutic Community—A New Treatment Method in Psychiatry. New York, Basic Books, 1953.
6. LINN, L.: A Handbook of Hospital Psychiatry—A Practical Guide to Therapy. New York, Int. Univ. Press, 1955.
7. SEITZ, P. F. D., et al.: A coordinated consultant team for remote state hospitals. Arch. Gen. Psychiat., in press.
8. STANTON, A. H., AND SCHWARTZ, M. S.: The Mental Hospital—A Study of Institutional Participation in Psychiatric Illness and Treatment. New York, Basic Books, 1954.
9. MASSERMAN, J. H.: Residency training for institutional service. Am. J. Psychiat., in press.

An Organization of Ex-Patients for Follow-Up Therapy

by JACOB H. FRIEDMAN, M.D.

THE PRESENT POLICY of the mental hospital is to discharge patients as soon as possible; therefore, the problem of preventing rehospitalization has assumed major importance. The ex-patient can be placed in a foster home, sent to a day or night hospital, be referred to a sheltered workshop, attend a mental hygiene clinic or a State hospital after-care clinic, or see a private psychiatrist. But another useful method of preventing a patient's return to the mental hospital is the ex-patients' organization or club, which also can serve as a means for follow-up therapy. Although the first organization in the United States of ex-patients of a psychiatric hospital was established in 1934, there are still only seventy ex-patients' clubs, as of 1959, throughout the country.[1] The total membership is less than two thousand active members,[1] which is less than 1 per cent of the patients released from mental hospitals each year. It is understandable that many ex-patients wish to forget their hospital experience as quickly as possible and therefore are reluctant to join an organization which reminds them of a form of hospitalization which still carries a stigma for themselves and their relatives. It is also difficult to have ex-patients join or remain in an ex-patients' group because of diverse educational status, occupation, religion, and social interest. Frequently, patients change residences and the club locality then becomes inconveniently situated. All these factors limit the formation of ex-patients' organizations. However, the function of mental hospitals should be not only to treat underlying mental illness, but also to inculcate the concept that each ex-patient can help others as well as prevent a recurrence or relapse in his own condition.

The impetus for organizations of ex-patients must originate from the hospital milieu and the enthusiasm of the hospital staff. This was first accomplished in the U.S. by the Wender Welfare League,[2,3] voluntarily founded in 1934 by thirty former patients of a forty-one bed endowed psychiatric hospital, the Hastings Hillside Hospital, Hastings-on-Hudson, New York. Only ex-patients and their immediate relatives were eligible for membership, with the exception of a few doctors, nurses, an occupational therapist, and members of the hospital staff. The success of this League was favored by the favorable milieu of the former Hastings Hillside Hospital, which constantly stressed the worth of the individual. The Director represented the good omnipotent father, but each patient was required to assume responsibility when able to undertake it. Common participation in menial but necessary tasks tended to eliminate snobbish or superior attitudes. In individual psychotherapy each patient became aware of his unconscious conflicts, his sexual immaturity, and his inadequate, hostile, helpless or dependent patterns. The dynamics of group psychotherapy[4,5] through intellectualization, patient-to-patient transference, catharsis, and group interaction, helped the patients to understand family living and to work through their early infantile frustrations and inadequacies. A positive group transference was established, similar to the positive transference in individual psychotherapy, vestiges of which can last for a lifetime. Members of the Wender Welfare League, the name of which was changed to the League For Mental Health, Inc. in April 1936, would visit the hospital and provide bi-weekly entertainment and refreshments for the patients. The members of the League had an intimate knowledge of the hospital and its needs, and thus the money raised was spent wisely in providing additional hospital facilities and comforts. An annual field day was held at the hospital in which patients and ex-patients participated. By revisiting the hospital, the ex-patients helped encourage those at the hospital in realizing that they too could become well. In 1939 the Hastings Hillside Hospital moved its quarters to Glen Oaks, L. I., and its name was changed to Hillside Hospital.

Although now no longer connected with Hillside Hospital, the League For Mental Health continued its activities. Regular monthly meetings were held in midtown New York City and about one hundred fifty members would attend a meeting which was partly devoted to business, followed by entertainment and refreshments. A four page bulletin was published by the members for distribution to the membership. The more enthusiastic members were active on committees which planned and initiated various projects. The League established and operated a thrift shop to rehabilitate ex-patients not working for the first few months in order to have them face economic reality. In 1944 it initiated the first evening mental hygiene clinic at Beth Israel Hospital, New York City, enabling people of low economic status to obtain psychiatric treatment while continuing their daily work. In 1945 it created a hospitalization fund which subsidized private institutional psychiatric care for people who required intensive and individual treatment, available at that time only in costly private hospitals. In 1952 it operated a subsidized psychotherapy plan and consultation service. A selected group of patients received treatment from a panel of psychiatrists at a minimum fee, one-half of which was paid by the patient and one-half by the League, the patients continuing with their normal occupations and being treated in the offices of the psychiatrists. In 1956 it established the "Dr. Louis Wender Psychophysiologic Research Laboratory" at the Abraham Jacobi Hospital associated with the Albert Einstein College of Medicine. Recently the League has initiated a Research Laboratory at the Psychiatric Department of the Hadassah Medical School, Hebrew University in Israel. In 1941 the League changed its constitution so that those interested in the field of mental health could join its organization. There is, at present, a membership of over five hundred. Although a number of the original members have died, the main work of the organization is still carried on by a group of early participants. The League has always depended on membership dues and financed its projects chiefly from contributions from members and fund-raising activities, since it is not subsidized by any individual or foundation. Volunteers do all the work, the only operating costs being printing, mailing, office rent, and meeting room expenses. Many discharged patients stated that the League helped in their adjustment during the difficult transitional period when they needed to recover fully their normal standing in society by receiving encouragement and sympathetic companionship. Furthermore, through these person-to-person contacts, each ex-patient was an active participant in allaying the stigma of having had a mental illness.

Since I have followed personally seventy-three ex-patients who have been active in the League, I am able to submit the following results: fifty-five patients continued in a recovered state, being symptom free and functioning well socially and economically. Seven died, their deaths having no connection with their functional illness. Seven have endogenous depressions which recur from time to time, but I believe the duration and intensity of their depressions are diminished by their attendance and activity in the League. Four patients are considered to have had a relapse of their illness. A great number of patients who were formerly active in the League left after they moved out of the City or because they married and their spouses were not too interested in having them continue as members. Nevertheless, many are still on the mailing list and help financially support the League's undertakings.

To illustrate the manner in which the League has helped the patients in their therapeutic process, abstracts of three severe cases are given.

Case 1. C.H. was hospitalized at Hastings Hillside Hospital in April, 1936 because of anxiety symptoms. Since he had to return to his business, he left the hospital in June 1937, much improved but not considered recovered. He saw the writer in psychotherapy for a period of a year because he was lackadaisical about his work, was subject to spells of vomiting and was unable to establish a satisfactory relationship with his business partner as a carry-over from his poor relationship with his alcoholic father. In the League, being on committees and working with others, he was able to achieve rapport with everyone, on the basis that all the members were former patients at Hastings Hillside Hospital, and had a common positive transference towards its Director, Dr. Louis Wender. With the League as a stepping stone in the process of maturing, the patient terminated his partnership, obtained a job as a clerk, and graduated from night high school. He then opened his own stationery store, became financially quite successful, married and now has two children.

Case 2. D.R. was seen by the writer in 1946 because she suffered from obsessive ideas in relation to death wishes against her only daughter and future son-in-law. She recovered after electroshock therapy on an outpatient basis. After her daughter's birth in 1928, she had her first attack in which she was hospitalized at Hastings Hillside Hospital. She had another attack in 1943 when her only son was taken into the military service, but she again recovered after electroshock treatment and several months of psychotherapy. She was one of the founders of the League, held many offices, and continues to be an active member. Her compulsive and aggressive traits were sublimated in volunteer secretarial work and fund raising functions for the League, which lessened her social isolation, increased her awareness of other people and raised her self-esteem. Her husband, who had borne the brunt of her symptoms during her periods of illness, joined her in these activities. In 1959 this patient, at the age of 66 years, developed diabetes and an intercurrent depression, but after electroshock treatment and diabetic therapy, she again became active in the League, and resumed her role as a successful housewife and an asset to her community, despite her obsessive-compulsive traits and her three periods of depression.

Case 3. J.K., with a history of two previous hospitalizations for manic-depressive psychosis, was admitted to Hillside Hospital in November 1941 for a year. He lost his professional civil service position, but became a member of the League For Mental Health. Through its subsidized psychotherapy fund, the League partially paid for his treatments with a private psychiatrist for 41 visits. In the absence of other opportunities, he was able to accept a menial position as a delivery man in a food market, although he held an M.A. degree. In the interim, his wife became psychotic, but he refused to certify her as there would be no one to take care of his home and two children. He continued to attend League meetings and did clerical work during one of the League's ventures in fund-raising, on the basis of which he was able to obtain a clerical position in industry. His wife's condition became worse so that she had to be sent to a State hospital, where she died after a lobotomy. With the support of the League and Dr. Wender, he continued to work, reared his children, and had no recurrence of his manic-depressive attacks. He recently confided to the writer that he would like to remarry since his children are grown and on their own.

CONCLUSIONS

An organization of ex-patients of a mental hospital* can organize programs whereby patients are visited at the hospital in order to bolster their morale and provide small incidental comforts. These ex-patients' clubs can serve as a social medium and as a liaison with the psychiatrists and social workers. The members of these clubs can demonstrate to the community that it is no stigma to have had a mental illness, and that one can recover from such illness through mutual effort. Fund-raising for worthy projects in relation to mental health can also be accomplished by these ex-patients' organizations.

REFERENCES

1. OLSHANSKY, S.: Social life. Ment. Hyg., 46:361-369, 1962.
2. FRIEDMAN, J. H.: An organization of ex-patients of a psychiatric hospital. Ment. Hyg., 23:414-420, 1939.
3. ———: An organization of ex-patients of a psychiatric hospital (twenty-five years of service). Dis. Nerv. Syst., 22:645-648, 1961.
4. WENDER, L.: Dynamics of group psychotherapy and its application. J. Nerv. & Ment. Dis., 84: 54-60, 1936.
5. ———: Group psychotherapy: a study of its application. Psychiat. Quart., 14: 708-18, 1940.
6. WECHSLER, H.: The self-help organization in the mental health field: Recovery, Inc., a case study. J. Nerv. & Ment. Dis., 130:297-314, 1960.
7. FISHER, S. H., AND BEARD, J. H.: Fountain House: A Psychiatric Rehabilitation Program. Masserman, Jules H., Ed. Current Psychiatric Therapies, Vol. II. New York, Grune & Stratton, 1962, pp. 211-218.

---

*Recovery, Inc.,[6] Fountain House[7] and The Bridge (Hilda and Israel Strauss League of the Hillside Hospital) are other such organizations.

PART IX

FORENSIC CONSIDERATIONS

Privileged Communication and Right of Privacy in Diagnosis and Therapy

by Ralph Slovenko, Ll.B. and Gene L. Usdin, M.D.

P RESENT-DAY medical privilege laws offer only a modicum of assurance that communications in psychotherapy are protected from disclosure, and the fact that many of the problems of psychiatry are virginal insofar as these laws are concerned adds to the uncertainty of the protection that they afford. With lawsuits becoming a national pastime, there is every reason to believe that hitherto disregarded potentials of litigation concerning privileged communication and confidentiality will arise with increased frequency.

Privilege: Its Meaning

Pretrial discovery and proof at a trial are governed by procedural rules called rules of evidence. One group of these rules is known as "privileges," which permit the exclusion of evidence, although relevant, on the theory that the matter is not as great as some other social value served by suppressing the evidence.[1] A privilege of non-disclosure applies in all states to communications (and observations) by a client to his attorney, to communications of husband and wife, and in some jurisdictions to communications by a penitent to his priest, by a client to his accountant, and by an informer to a newspaper reporter or to the government. While about thirty-six American states have a physician-patient privilege,[2] these statutes are so riddled with qualifications and exceptions that they do not adequately meet the needs of patients in psychotherapy.[3]

Psychiatrists, being licensed in the practice of medicine, are included within the riddled statutory privilege accorded to "physicians." Georgia in 1959 and Connecticut in 1961 enacted a specific privilege for communications between psychiatrist and patient, but these statutes, too, fail to cover many problems peculiar to psychotherapy.[4] Psychiatrists and others have pointed out the great social harm that may be done to count-less numbers of patients, ex-patients and future patients by even a rare subpoena of a psychiatrist to testify. Freud expressed the need for con-fidentiality thus: "The whole undertaking becomes lost labour if a single concession is made to secrecy."[5]

Contrary to the belief of many psychiatrists, privilege (when it exists) belongs to the patient, not to the physician. The psychiatrist therefore can be compelled to testify when his patient or ex-patient so desires. The patient is given legal control over his destiny, irrespective of other fac-tors.[6] The patient may believe, quite unrealistically, that testimony of his psychotherapist may aid his legal position. A patient's waiver of the privilege may conceivably be a self-destructive technique; it may be an expression of hostility toward the psychiatrist; or it may be an attempted repetition of an early power struggle. An attempt even to clarify to a patient why it would be inadvisable to call upon the therapist to testify can be markedly prejudicial to effective therapy, especially when it comes at an inappropriate stage in treatment.

PROBLEMS OF PRIVILEGE

The ordinary medical statute, and classical psychoanalysis, envisions a one-to-one physician-patient relationship. Yet a one-to-one psycho-therapeutic relationship is not always justified as a matter of treatment. Child therapy can never be a strictly two-person arrangement. It is in-creasingly accepted that the one-to-one psychotherapeutic relationship alone, analytically oriented or otherwise, does not meet the needs of the schizophrenic inpatient. The family unit and the therapeutic team have vital roles to play. However, the law has traditionally taken the position that disclosure to a person not included within the statute terminates the privilege. The law equates a disclosure to a third person with a general publication to the world. Hence, the logic has it that since "the world knows about it, why should not the court?"

With this as a background, let us consider various situations and prob-lems that arise in the practice of psychiatry.

Domestic Cases

One area where the privilege is frequently asserted is in domestic matters, among which are cases of divorce, "alienation of affections," and custody of children.

(1) Where there is no privilege, psychiatrists in contested divorce cases could be asked to testify regarding the "fault" (e.g., adultery or brutality or criminality) of the patient-spouse. Patients involved in

marital infidelity or sexual deviation may fear litigation and consequently might not speak as freely if they suspected that the psychiatrist could be compelled to testify. It is to be recalled that most states penalize as criminal practically all sex activity other than the most conventional heterosexual act; hence, almost any clinical details of sexual material could conceivably be the start of criminal action as well as divorce proceeding against the patient.[7]

By the time spouses turn to a psychiatrist for help in working out marital difficulties, the marriage is often already in severe trouble. There are times when psychotherapy does not avert divorce, but rather ends in it. Many marriages are contracted out of neurotic purposes, and with the cure of the neurosis, separation and divorce may be a healthy solution. Those states which have lax divorce laws (such as divorce on the basis of a short period of living separate and apart) avoid allegations of fault, but in other states, where a petitioner is put to proof of fault in order to dissolve the marriage, the testimony of the psychiatrist who has treated one of the spouses would be highly pertinent (the law here out of pragmatic considerations labels one spouse as being "bad" or at "fault" and does not consider the neurotic interaction and mutual provocation which takes place between the partners).

A psychiatrist during the course of therapy may see both spouses as patients, either separately or jointly. Usually treatment of husband and wife is conducted independently by two therapists, but there are situations, such as preparatory interviews to analysis, and marital maladjustment and family problems which are not to be psychoanalyzed, in which both spouses are seen effectively by the same therapist. In such cases the legal question arises whether or not the psychiatrist can testify on behalf of the spouse who wants him to testify. The opponent spouse can apparently claim privilege as to communications obtained from him and observations made of him by the psychiatrist. Yet, by seeing the opponent spouse in therapy, the psychiatrist will naturally be affected in his evaluation and testimony on behalf of the proponent spouse.[8] No medical statute expressly covers the problem.

(2) Where there is no privilege, psychiatrists can be called upon in "alienation of affections" cases to testify whether or not a third person alienated the patient-spouse's affections away from the other spouse. In a case in Illinois, which at the time had no medical statute, counsel for Mr. X sought to question his wife's psychiatrist concerning information she had revealed during psychiatric consultations.[9] The Illinois trial court excused the psychiatrist from testifying. The decision, however, is generally considered without justification in law, as Illinois had no medical statute. In legal circles, it is generally considered that had the case

been appealed to a higher court, the psychiatrist would have been instructed to testify or would have faced punitive action for contempt. The fact that a trial judge and a witness take the law into their own hands is cause for concern. Rights which exist *sub rosa* do not lend dignity to the law. Yet, rather than reveal confidences, many psychiatrists claim that they would risk contempt charges.

(3) Statistically, about 40 per cent of the 400,000 divorces granted in this country each year involve children. Where there is no privilege, a psychiatrist who treats a child, or one of the spouses, may be subpoenaed to testify in a case involving custody of the child.

In child therapy especially, psychiatrists are likely to involve other members of the family in the treatment process. "Environmental manipulation" may be essential in the treatment of children. As the parents in this situation are strictly speaking not "patients," there is little assurance that the privilege under the orthodox law will be held applicable. Although there was no general publication to the world, a third person —someone other than the physician and patient—received the information and, in the eyes of the law, confidentiality has been "profaned." Under the Connecticut statute enacted in 1961, unlike under other statutes, the patient has a privilege to prevent a witness from disclosing communications between members of the patient's family and the psychiatrist.

In child custody actions, one spouse may contend that the other spouse is mentally ill and therefore incompetent to have custody.[10] Expert testimony regarding relative degrees of incompetency of the parents in borderline situations could place the psychiatrist in an omniscient, and undesirable, role. In this situation testimony could be compelled from the psychiatrist which might influence the legal decision in a way contrary to health. The psychiatrist may be required to reveal material contrary to present cultural standards but not necessarily contradictory to good parenthood.

The fact of psychiatric treatment of itself is sometimes utilized as a bargaining device against the patient-spouse in reaching a property and custody settlement. A patient-spouse, particularly one who is seeking custody of the children, is quite often willing to give in and make little or no demands, even though the conduct of the other has been outrageous. The threat of revelation of the history of psychiatric treatment, should the case be contested, often results in the patient-spouse conceding to an unfavorable agreement. Individuals are sensitive to such exposure. When divorce and custody cases are contested, attempts are made to use a history of psychiatric treatment to imply that the patient-spouse was at fault, hence not entitled to alimony or to custody of the children. The traditional medical privilege protects the content but not the fact of treatment visits.

Personal Injury Cases

In suits for personal injuries, the privilege is considered waived by the patient by virtue of his instituting the litigation. As one legal scholar has stated, the patient cannot make the medical statute both a sword and a shield.[11] The confidence of the medical consultation is considered no longer necessary, because, in bringing suit, the patient makes his physical or mental health a matter of public record. Furthermore, it is said that a good-faith claimant suing for personal injuries would not object to the testimony of any physician who examined or treated him, but rather would want the physician to testify.

The psychiatrist is sought to testify about "psychological trauma" or predisposed factors or pre-existing illness. However, therapy may be jeopardized by testimony of the treating psychiatrist; as a result, rightful causes of action may go by the board when therapy is considered more important by the patient than the outcome of the litigation. Yet, there is another way. Other evidence is usually available. Medical evidence no longer depends only upon the subpoena of the attending or treating physician. Modern court technique may make use of a non-treating medical expert. Under the Federal Rules of Civil Procedure and in states that have adopted similar rules, the trial court may order examination by a physician of a person whose mental or physical condition is in controversy.[12] The rule does not invade the confidentiality of communication. The patient is aware that he is not in a confidential relationship with the examining physician, and he retains his privilege regarding communications with his treating physician. The promise of confidentiality is essential for therapy, but not for diagnosis. It is true that cooperation with the examining psychiatrist will lead to a more reliable report. The party usually cooperates with the appointed physician; if he does not, this will come out at the trial and work to his prejudice. The psychiatrist's report will include the fact of non-cooperation. It is true that the testimony of the treating physician might be very valuable, but in considerable measure the second-best evidence of the appointed examining physician is usually adequate. There is no need to say that suit for personal injuries waives the medical privilege. Confidentiality of the treatment relationship is still essential, even though, in bringing suit, the patient makes his health a matter of public record. From the viewpoint of therapy, it would seem desirable to retain the privilege for the treating physician even in suits claiming damages for mental anguish. At the extreme, the patient might be penalized by dismissal of the case, that is, by presuming fraud on the part of the patient unless he himself waives the privilege. An automatic waiver or exception to the privilege, on the other hand, would allow opposing counsel, over the patient's objection, to put the attending psychiatrist on the stand and to require him to disclose confidences.

Will Cases

In will contest cases, the testamentary capacity of the patient is often under inquiry.[13] The rule in many jurisdictions is that death terminates the privilege. Thus, a legatee to a will in testamentary actions, or a beneficiary of a life insurance policy, cannot claim the privilege of the deceased patient, and the physician cannot insist on remaining silent.[14] As previously mentioned, the privilege belongs to the patient and not to the physician. As a result, the psychiatrist may be placed in the position of revealing scandalous conduct not only of the testator but also of family members.

Some law firms, at the time of preparation of a will, assemble proof that might be needed in the event of a will contest. Statements are taken from law witnesses who can establish, if any issue is later raised, that the testator was of sound mind. However, if a psychiatrist is called in to examine the testator, and a will contest should later occur, the argument would inevitably then be made that there must have been grave misgivings about the testator's mental competency, otherwise a psychiatrist would not have been called in.[15] To avoid suspicion, law firms can make it a matter of ordinary routine by regularly resorting to psychiatric evaluation even though the testator clearly has capacity to make a valid will.

Actions on Life and Accident Insurance Policies

Suits involving life and accident insurance policies often concern the truth of the insured's representations as to his health. Here, the insurer may desire to introduce testimony of the insured's physician to show fraud on the part of the insured in making his application. The medical privilege may be circumvented quite easily by the insurer by inserting in the application a provision whereby the insured waives his right to the privilege, for both himself and his beneficiary. As death usually terminates the privilege, a psychiatrist or any physician can be compelled to testify regarding a suicide which might affect payment of an insurance policy.

Personnel Screening

The law's requirement that communications relate to treatment leaves unprotected those made to a psychiatrist involved in screening persons who may be seeking employment, insurance or school admission. Furthermore, as in the case of insurance companies, business firms frequently insert in applications for employment a provision calling for waiver to the privilege, thereby opening the courtroom door to the treating physician.

Hospital Records

Mental illness, especially hospitalization in a mental institution, carries a stigma. Once a person has a record of having been in a mental hospital, the public at large, both formally in terms of employment and other restrictions, and informally in terms of day-to-day social treatment, considers him to be set apart. Public disclosure of hospitalization does not allow the patient any easy return to the community. The protection of secrecy afforded by the law in many jurisdictions leaves much to be desired.

The hospital setting is a situation where a one-to-one psychotherapeutic relationship is impossible. Indeed, every attendant and nurse in a psychotherapeutic hospital is urged to be more than attendant or nurse—to be also a therapist. Hospital records are inevitably passed into the hands of nurses, social workers and clerks. Furthermore, treatment in a hospital requires an organized effort on the part of all members as a therapeutic team, and they must be given such information as will make their efforts meaningful and helpful. Since so many people know about the patient and have the information, courts in many states take the position that the medical privilege does not protect the record from subpoena.

In view of their possible use in court, it is important to note that hospital records are all too frequently poorly kept, due to the overload of patients, shortness of time for adequate recording, or negligence of the physician. Staff members often do not feel sufficiently confident to record, or they are too busy to record anything but acts of disobedience. Furthermore, apart from considerations of time, able psychiatrists may purposefully keep information in the record to a minimum to prevent sadistic members on the staff, attendants or nurses, from using the information to torment the patient (although an institution with such a staff is obviously not much of a hospital). As a result, physicians and other staff members when called to court have often found themselves squirming in the witness chair trying to justify or excuse an awkward, irresponsible or inadequate recording in the hospital record, on which the legal profession perhaps unduly places great value.[16] Impressions derived from reading case summaries or test reports are often misleading.

Some states have provided by special statute that hospital records are privileged from public scrutiny. For example, Louisiana's statute provides: "The charts, records, reports, documents and other memoranda prepared by physicians, surgeons, psychiatrists, nurses, and employees in the public hospitals of Louisiana, public mental health centers and public schools for the mentally deficient to record or indicate the past or present condition, sickness or disease, physical or mental, of the patients treated in the hospitals are exempt [from public scrutiny], except when the condition of a patient admitted to a general hospital is due to an accident, poisoning, negligence or presumable negligence resulting in any injury, assault or any act of violence or a violation of the law".[17] The records of "public mental health centers" are considered to include records of guidance centers, mental health treatment centers, evaluation centers, and centers for the treatment of alcoholics.

Although statutes may provide for hospital records, applications for employment, insurance or school often question the applicant about previous hospitalization or treatment for mental illness. Honesty begets a truthful answer on the part of the applicant. Some may consider that such inquiry constitutes an undue invasion of an individual's right of privacy. However, the courts generally hold that a false answer constitutes misrepresentation. This is another example of the stigma of treatment for mental illness. The result is that many persons defer treatment, much to their detriment. It has been suggested that patients should receive legislative protection against injury of this type.

When information is withheld as confidential, health agencies and others complain that they cannot obtain necessary information to institute preventive health or disease control measures. In certain research, identification of the patient is unnecessary (for example, number of cases of hepatitis), but other research cannot be accomplished without names of patients and other information (for example, follow-up studies of children seen in guidance clinics). To remedy this situation somewhat, seven states have passed laws protecting members of committees and hospital groups engaged in special studies of morbidity and mortality.[18] In general, the statutes provide that all information used in the course of medical study shall be confidential; that such information shall not be admissible as evidence; and that the furnishing of such information shall not subject any person or institution to damages. [19] The statutes in effect provide that disclosures made for scientific studies are not to be considered a public disclosure which would terminate the privilege.

While the hospital record and the records of physicians or health officers are generally kept confidential, the judicial record on commitment is traditionally considered a public record and in the absence of express legislation the hearing and the resulting records are available to one and all. It is to be noted that in this country court commitment is the procedure most commonly used in the admission of patients to mental hospitals.[20] The model Draft Act Governing Hospitalization of the Mentally Ill, adopted, however, in only a few states, makes confidential the records of courts, health officers, and hospitals involved in the commitment process.[21] There is precedent for maintaining the secrecy of judicial commitment records; adoption records and juvenile records are kept private.

In those states which join hospitalization (commitment) and incompetency (interdiction) proceedings, further difficulties arise. For example, when a patient, even when discharged, proposes to sell property, prospective purchasers and title companies would have a legitimate interest in inquiring as to the patient's status (that is, whether he is on conditional release and whether the incompetency has been judicially removed). Otherwise, the purchaser's title to the property would be voidable. The Draft Act recommends complete separation of hospitalization and incompetency proceedings. It provides in effect that a person is not deprived of his right to sell or buy property, execute documents, enter into contracts, or vote because he has been hospitalized as mentally ill. A person requiring treatment in a hospital is not necessarily incapable of exercising these various rights.

Yet there are problems even when a person is not adjudicated incompetent by virtue of commitment. During the course of hospitalization, or afterwards, it may be essential to institute incompetency proceedings for the appointment of a guardian (curator). In doing so, attorneys often communicate with the hospital seeking evidence to justify the proceedings. More often than not, the proceeding is in the interest of the patient or ex-patient. It seeks to appoint someone to manage the patient's affairs, which the patient may be unable to do while hospitalized or afterwards. Not all incompetency proceedings, as the myth would have it, are maliciously instituted by members of the family to rob the patient. However, the patient on occasion does not consent to release of information; he does not want to be tagged an incompetent. The result is a begging of the question: incompetency proceedings are instituted because it is felt that the patient does not have the legal capacity to consent, yet hospital cooperation is refused because the patient declines to consent.[22]

Office and Clinic Records

When it exists, the privilege protects the doctor's notes, memos, appointment books, financial records, et cetera, but, as the privilege belongs to the patient, he may waive the privilege and compel their disclosure in the courtroom, just as they may be subpoenaed in states where there is no law granting privilege.

There is considerable discussion in the literature on the medical doctor's duty out of the courtroom to tell the "truth" to a patient about his illness. Hospitals encounter similar requests by patients for a copy of their records, purely for their own information. Yet there are circumstances under which the hospital or doctor cannot, for the patient's own good, tell him the "whole truth." The paranoid patient is the type of psychiatric patient that most frequently requests a copy of his record; compliance with the request would further aggravate his mental condition. While a doctor is ethically bound to do whatever is best for his patient and to avoid doing him harm, there is little or no legal authority bearing upon the right to withhold information from a patient. A patient goes to a physician for information, which he may need in planning out his life (e.g., making a will or disposing of his property). Diagnosis implies prognosis, and there are times when the information works to the detriment of the patient, as illustrated in the film "The Last Weekend," where relying on an erroneous diagnosis of a fatal disease, Alec Guinness goes out to a luxurious resort for a last fling, and is ironically killed in an automobile accident. It ought further to be considered that physicians make diagnoses with an eye toward disposition (one diagnosis is made for the court, another for Blue Cross, and so on). The Judicial Council of the AMA advises (presumably considering physical illnesses) that the decision in a non-court situation to give the contents of a report to a patient rests with the doctor who knows all the circumstances involved in the situation; but in pretrial discovery or in a courtroom, on the basis of a subpoena, the patient may require production of the records when they are pertinent to litigation.[23]

Medical records of a private physician are considered his property, but they are subject to "a limited property right" on the part of his patients with respect to the information which they contain. The patient can therefore demand disclosure, not only to himself, but also, for example, to an insurance company. Psychiatrists would argue that a different principle is needed for patients in therapy. A psychiatric record, unlike an x-ray, might reasonably be said to be the entire work product of the therapist. There is also the pragmatic consideration that psychiatric records can readily be destroyed or they may be prepared in a way unintelligible to others.

Ownership of records of patients seen in guidance centers, etc., presents a special problem. On the termination of the psychiatrist's employment with the center, the question arises as to the proper custodian of the records developed during the term of employment.[24] It has been urged that psychiatric records are the property of the psychiatrist preparing them and are not subject to "transfer" to another psychiatrist coming to the center, or to a court or social agency, unless the records were prepared in the first instance by the request of such other person or body. This argument presupposes that the center and the replacing psychiatrist will not maintain the confidentiality of the records. As we see guidance clinics in operation, physicians go and come, but the records remain; otherwise the clinic would be very much damaged by the departure of a physician. The records remain where they have always been; they are not "transferred." Patients usually return to a clinic irrespective of the presence of a particular physician. Also, taking a page from the law on self-incrimination, we might note that it has been many times held that "quasi public records" as well as "public records" are deemed to belong to the government, and the recordkeeper therefore may not object to their introduction as evidence.[25]

Psychologists, Social Workers and Counselors

Professional practitioners of psychotherapy are almost as varied as the range of persons they seek to help. The largest group of professionals trained to conduct psychotherapy are psychiatrists, numbering about thirteen thousand in this country, and they are supplemented by well over four thousand clinical psychologists and five thousand social workers. Clinical psychologists and psychiatric social workers are members of treatment teams in hospitals and clinics under psychiatric supervision, but they also practice independently in social agencies, family agencies, marriage counseling centers, and so on, and as private practitioners. In addition, a wide variety of counselors and guides (such as marriage counselors, rehabilitation and vocational counselors, parole officers, group workers, and clergymen) may use psychotherapeutic principles with their clientele. The different disciplines tend to describe their activities in different terms, as, for example, medical and quasi-medical practitioners "treat" patients, psychiatric social workers do "case work" with clients, clergymen offer "pastoral counseling", and group workers do "group work."

The medical privilege covers only the physician (the psychiatric and non-psychiatric physician). The protection afforded when other members of the treatment team are involved is nil except that a few states relatively recently have adopted special statutes granting the privilege to psychologists.[26] The attorney-client privilege covers the attorney's agent,[27] but in most states the physician's agent, the nurse, is not generally included within the medical privilege, unless expressly provided by statute.[28] Likewise, psychologists, social workers, counselors and stenographers may not come within the scope of the medical privilege, even when working under psychiatric supervision. Communications to these persons may be compelled in court. This is important to the psychiatrist, who often relies on such persons.

Personnel in probation departments, welfare offices, social agencies, and child guidance clinics frequently have access to case files. Can they be trusted with confidential information? Will they gossip about what they learn from case records? If as a matter of common practice confidentiality is maintained, ought not the law allow a privilege even though there is not a one-to-one relationship? Experiences in hospitals and prisons generally have confirmed the trustworthiness of non-clinical employees (career correctional workers and welfare workers) regarding the confidential material in the case history when the importance of confidentiality has been fully explained to them. Likewise, experiences with teachers also have confirmed that with very infrequent exceptions they are, when properly prepared, as respecting of confidential material as are clinicians, lawyers, or other professional people.[29] Actually, there is no better use for case histories, so costly in their preparation, than that their findings be used by those who are involved responsibly in the care or treatment of the patient. In institutions, basic psychotherapeutic help is provided by the ordinary staff member who spends many hours with the patient or inmate, rather than by the specialist who sees him occasionally and then only briefly. The Connecticut privilege, enacted in 1961, covers communications between any persons who participate, under the supervision of the psychiatrist, in the accomplishment of the objectives of diagnosis or treatment. Other statutes, as stated, do not protect disclosures to non-psychiatric treatment personnel.

Social workers have particular problems regarding adoption and custody reports. The parent adversely affected by the report naturally wants to know the evidence. Yet, disclosure may jeopardize the relationship with the parent for further casework. Also, if reports are disclosed, no one may reveal anything to social workers. Since there is no privilege, social workers in some places resort to subterfuge. Two types of records are made.

Group Therapy

Patients in group therapy have transference between themselves, but legally, and strictly speaking, patients *inter se* do not constitute a physician-patient relationship. Hence, it would seem that the medical privilege does not protect against disclosure in court by a member of the group. The privilege exempts only the physician from testifying. To borrow a leaf from the husband-wife privilege, we learn that conversations held in the presence of children and other members of the family are not privileged.[30] Privileges, being derogations from the general law, are narrowly construed by the courts. The law has traditionally considered privileged communications as involving a dyadic relationship: in the case of the medical privilege, a licensed physician and a patient. It is necessary to reformulate the medical privilege in view of group therapy.[31] Given the shortage of psychotherapists, apart from the intrinsic value of group therapy, some therapists even predict a time in the near future when patients will be treated primarily in group situations.[32]

Military Cases

A privilege is not recognized in military law for communications made to medical officers and civilian physicians, although military law does recognize the privilege relationships of attorney-client, husband-wife, and priest-penitent.[33] With a disruption of the inductee's dependency equilibrium, it would appear that the need for a psychotherapy privilege exists to as great a degree in military as in civilian life. Servicemen, away from their homes, look to someone to whom they can entrust their problems and fears. They may turn to a psychiatrist as well as to a priest. In combat, the need for comfort and guidance is even more pronounced.

It might be noted that psychoneurotic and psychotic tendencies are no longer sufficient reason for draft exemption, unless it has incapacitated the individual in civilian life. The revised rules are in contrast to those applied during World War II, when more stringent requirements of emotional stability were in force. It is reported that elaborate psychiatric examinations of inductees are no longer conducted,[34] and as a result, there may be more servicemen needing psychotherapy. Today, then, with greater public acceptance of psychiatry and with more persons seeking psychiatric assistance, there is an increased need for psychiatric services in the military, and a privilege to encourage its use.[35]

There are, of course, cases of neurotic individuals in the military where psychotherapy is contraindicated, just as in the outside world.

There are many persons who enlist in the military service to satisfy infantile dependency needs. They are, as Erich Fromm would put it, escaping from freedom. In these cases, therapy is often inadvisable. The professional serviceman is often best left alone, leaving his compensatory system undisturbed. Homosexuals, we might mention, although they are not officially accepted in the armed forces, are found there in goodly numbers. Treatment is not sought or is ineffective where the homosexual is content with his way of life; indeed, the majority of homosexuals defend their form of sexual activity as perfectly normal (one aspect of homosexuality that is often ignored is the extreme dependency shown by homosexuals or by persons having considerable latent homosexuality). Be this as it may, psychiatry has a vital role to play in the military, particularly for the inductee.

Public Security

There are times when revelation may be necessary for the protection of society. This thorny problem was brought to the fore when two National Security Agency employees, Vernon F. Mitchell and William H. Martin defected to the Soviet Union. The psychiatrist, who had seen Mitchell, turned over his records and testified before a secret session of the House Un-American Activities Committee. He stated: "I believe a man loses his right to privileged communication if he defects. Furthermore, if the national security is threatened, I believe the rights of the Government far exceed the rights of individuals." The psychiatrist disclosed problems of family, religion and sex. He was taken to task by a number of general practitioners and psychiatrists.[36]

It is always debatable whether a disclosure can be construed as benefitting the patient or the community. However, revelation of information which is of no benefit to the patient or the community demanded by subpoena is subject to criticism, but disclosure of information without legal compulsion (as apparently happened in the Mitchell situation) is deplorable.[67] The State can ferret out its evidence, and ought to be put to its proof, without impinging on confidential relationships, such as the attorney-client, husband-wife, priest-penitent, as well as the physician-patient relationship.[38]

FBI Director Hoover at one time urged all physicians to report to the Bureau any facts relating to espionage, sabotage or subversive activity coming to their attention. Psychiatrists generally criticized the American Medical Association for cooperating with the federal police and for going even further by urging its members to help catch even the petty thief. Guttmacher attacked this suggestion with wry humor: "It is not too fantastic to predict that before long the physician's inner examining room may resemble a rural post office with its walls plastered with the mugs of wanted felons."[39]

Criminal Cases

Criminal cases are one aspect of the public security problem. A patient in therapy may have committed or may be planning to commit a crime, for example, abortion or adultery. In such cases, the psychiatrist will be in possession of highly incriminating evidence.

Psychoneurotic persons, who constitute the majority of patients in office psychotherapy, try to adapt themselves to the way of society. In general, patients in therapy are not characterized by antisocial activity or by striking inability to pursue ordinary goals. Usually the patient in psychotherapy suffers from an overly strict conscience. The criminal on the other hand has a conscience, if it can be called that, which sets few limits on his behavior. When the exceptional case of a criminal in therapy arises, psychotherapy might provide the best possibility of having the individual return to lawful and gainful pursuits. Thus, without the need of tax-supported incarceration, the goal of rehabilitation might be achieved.[40]

Lunacy Commissions

Psychiatrists and psychologists serve on lunacy commissions as officers or agents of the court,[41] and hence, not being the accused's physician, there is no privilege. Nevertheless, surreptitious psychiatric interrogation of persons accused of crime is condemned, although such persons are not "patients" and revelations are not for the purpose of therapy. Confessions elicited with the aid of hypnosis, narcosis, or other forms of partial removal of inhibitions, especially when induced by the administration of drugs, have uniformly been struck down.[42] It is contrary to medical ethics, as well as against the law, for the police to resort to the relationship of physician and patient to obtain a confession from the accused.[43] Psychiatrists examining persons on court order are cautioned to point out to the examinee that communications are not privileged, notwithstanding the possible loss thereby of valuable information.

The Connecticut statute provides that communications to a psychiatrist in the course of a psychiatric examination ordered by the court are without privilege only on issues involving the person's mental condition (that is, the psychiatrist may testify as to the accused's insanity at the time of the offense or at the time of trial, but he may not report, for example, on the validity of an alibi.)[44] It has been suggested in some quarters that even though the psychiatrist in these cases is an examining rather than a treating physician, there should be a complete privilege, otherwise there can be no effective examination, unless the psychiatrist in one way or another deludes the examinee into believing that there will be confidentiality.[45] The examiner, it is said, cannot take the absurd position of warning the accused not to give him his confidence and then expect to receive information. A complete privilege, however, would preclude cross-examination at the trial and the psychiatrist's report would sound woefully oracular, and would be ineffective.

Presentence Report

The confidentiality of a presentence investigation report of a probation department is a matter which is receiving increased attention.[46] These reports to the court often play a very influential role in the type and the length of sentence given. The issue here is not the right of the defendant to have information withheld from the court, but rather the right of the court to withhold information from the convicted defendant. The District Court of Appeal of Florida recently had an opportunity to indicate, for the first time in the jurisdiction, the status of a presentence investigation report.[47] Counsel for the defendant argued that the right to see a presentence report is basic and fundamental and that to deny him this right is to allow hearsay evidence to stand against him, depriving him of cross-examination and confrontation of witnesses. The court, however, concluded that a presentence report should be treated as a confidential compilation of information for the use of the sentencing judge, and not as a public document, and hence the defendant is not entitled to access thereto. "To strip a presentence investigation report of its confidentiality," the court observed, "would be to divert it also of its importance and value to the sentencing judge, because there might be lacking the frankness and completeness of disclosures made in confidence." Most judges feel that strict adherence to confidentiality in the use of the presentence report has made it possible for the probation officer to obtain for the court a much more accurate picture of the defendant that could be obtained if it were known that the contents of the report were going to be divulged to others. However, there is a sizeable body of opinion which feels very strongly that no presentence report should be so confidential that the defendant should not be given an opportunity to reply to any information entered in it. It would be of considerable assistance to the probation service to have this problem of confidentiality thoroughly considered in an effort to reach some sort of agreement on criteria.[48]

Prison Psychiatry

The use of psychotherapy in prison is so minimal that it hardly merits discussion. Indeed, the majority of jails and prisons, as presently constructed, and as overcrowded as they are, do not even have a suitable place in which to hold sessions. The dining room may not be available until well after the evening meal. The chapel is usually unavailable, but even when it is, smoking is not permitted, and the religious atmosphere is always there. Security precautions forbid meetings in the visiting room at most hours of the day. Attendants feel that their authority over the place is threatened by the therapist, and they resist, actively or passively. In the future, jails and prisons hopefully will change to accommodate advances in penology. In the meantime, consider the privilege of confidentiality in prison psychiatry, as theoretical as it may be.

MacCormick, a prison administrator and criminologist, has said of the prison psychiatrist's obligation of confidentiality: "Giving parole boards access to what is dug up in individual and group therapy would be opening a veritable gold mine to them. But the shaft is sealed to them and to institution administrators, and must be sealed." He maintains, however, that a prison psychiatrist is duty bound to report knowledge of new crimes being planned by the patient.[49] Freedman's viewpoint seems well taken when he retorts: "It is my personal conviction that it is not the role of the psychiatrist to uncover such information under the guise of therapy, if he expects to expose it to the warden. I cannot help feeling that disclosure under these circumstances is a sort of 'psychic entrapment'. The physician ought either to warn his patient beforehand of the reservations he has concerning confidentiality or, having committed himself to secrecy, he should maintain it."[50]

Prisoners are usually distrusting souls. They feel there is no privacy or confidence, and so they do not even want to talk to a therapist, much less talk freely with him. The therapeutic situation hopefully will demonstrate to the prisoner that not all persons are to be mistrusted. Confidentiality is of utmost importance when treating individuals who are basically distrustful of others.

Execution of Sentence and Death Penalty

It appears that termination of the trial ends the defendant's protection by the rules of evidence. As noted, a presentence investigation report relied on by judges in the imposition of sentence is usually not made available to counsel for the defense, as it is considered that information would be unavailable if it were restricted to that given in open court by witnesses subject to cross-examination.

An Ohio court has recently ruled that the right of an imprisoned man to counsel does not extend to psychological tests which an attorney would have an unchallenged right to obtain prior to trial.[51]

The imposition of the death penalty is an even more striking example of the principle. The prevailing law in this country on the death penalty is that an insane person, for one reason or another, may not be executed.[52] In the majority of states, the issue of post-conviction insanity may be raised only by the warden (or sheriff) having custody of the prisoner. The United States Supreme Court stated in *Solesbee v. Balkcom*[53] that the manner of procedural effectuation of exemption for insanity is a matter of grace, not of right, and hence the state is under no obligation to provide a hearing. In the *Solesbee* case, the warden refused to allow an outside psychiatrist to examine the prisoner on death's row and refused to allow counsel to inspect the prison's psychiatric records. Thus, the execution of the capital penalty lies very much in the attitude of the warden toward the penalty. A convict, waiting on death's row often for years until legal maneuvers are exhausted, is quite likely to have become psychotic, but the application of the exemption rule usually depends upon the pleasure of the warden.

Waiver of Privilege

It has been suggested that privilege should belong to the physician rather than to the patient. When an individual waives a privilege such as the attorney-client privilege, or the privilege against self-incrimination, the decision is made with full awareness of the material which will be disclosed.[54] But, in psychotherapy it may be detrimental for the patient to see, e.g., the report of projective tests which he has taken and the results of which he has not seen. When the patient waives the psychotherapy privilege, he does not know what he is waiving. It may be harmful to reveal to the patient that he is schizophrenic (whatever that might mean).[55]

The issue is whether the law should allow an individual to make an irrational decision. One clergyman, when threatened by a call to the stand upon waiver of the priest-penitent privilege, said: "It is impossible to see how anyone could or would waive his privilege of confidence in a clergyman unless he is under some kind of pressure and falls into the trap of 'selling his soul for a mess of pottage'."[56]

Competency of Testimony

Incompetency of testimony renders entirely moot the need for privileges, which are needed only to exclude competent evidence. The fundamental test of admissibility of evidence is competency, that is, its trust-worthiness.

On the basis of certain data, hereinafter set out, one might suggest that, even though the patient waives privilege and asks the psychiatrist to make disclosure, the testimony is inadmissible on grounds of incompetency. In effect, the charge is that all psychiatric testimony, especially that of the treating physician, is incompetent for courtroom purposes and of no value. Let us take note of the data:

For one thing, it is said that a therapist cannot within any reasonable degree of accuracy present to the court in a few minutes material that has been produced in years of therapy. At staff conferences, attended by persons experienced in the field, it takes considerable time to present a case report. In the courtroom, the psychiatrist faces a jury reluctant to accept psychiatric theories and unable to evaluate the testimony, particularly when it must be done in summary fashion. Indeed, non-psychiatric physicians complain that psychiatrists talk in gobbledygook and have developed a private jargon of their own, a tower of Babel, resulting in a communication gap between psychiatrists and other physicians.

Second, it is said that "the art of psychiatry outweighs the science." At the 1962 American Psychiatric Association meeting, Dr. Robert Stotler and Dr. Robert H. Geertsma of UCLA related the results of an experiment showing that expert psychiatrists can differ widely in their clinical evaluation of a single case. The two California researchers pointed out that psychiatrists were unable to agree on the diagnosis, prognosis, etiology and other aspects of a case which all had observed equally. Psychiatrists, it is said, make their diagnoses in form of camouflaged social value judgments. It has been suggested that a new system of psychiatric classification is needed, based on the patient's reaction to the therapeutic situation rather than on the standard (and inadequate) clinical nosology. Some say consequently that as long as psychiatry is so much an art and there is so much confusion, psychiatric testimony lacks value for the court.[57]

Third, it might be said that data from free association, fantasies, or memories are not reliable for use in court as they represent the way the person experienced an event, and not necessarily how the event occurred. They are not "facts." Psychic reality is not the same thing as actual reality. In fantasy life, a patient may tell of hidden treasures; its correspondence in reality is not of crucial importance in treatment. A classic example is Freud's case of the young girl whose fantasied sexual traumatic relationship with her father affected her personality, although her father had had no overt sexual contact with the child. As the material revealed in psychotherapy does not deal with reality of the outer world, it would make poor, even prejudicial evidence. The material is often of childhood fantasies and not germane to current activities of the patient.[58] A 13-year-old girl in our culture who claims that she is having sexual relations with every male member of the family is sick whether or not it is the fact of the matter. The therapist is not compelled to check on the outer reality. Furthermore, the therapist does not cross-question his patient. In therapy, the important thing is how the patient looks at herself and the world. But, in the courtroom, in a criminal case, e.g., involving incest or contributing to the delinquency of a minor, it makes a world of difference whether the allegation is in the realm of fantasy or reality. Reik states that psychoanalysis has no contribution to make to evidence of guilt, as it is concerned with mental reality rather than material reality.[59]

There are times when the psychotherapist deliberately participates in the psychosis of a patient by entering the fantasy and from that position attempting to pry the patient loose from his psychosis (John Rosen and Milton Wexler are among the notable exponents of this practice). The procedure, however, has been reported to get out of control. Lindner reported that, as one patient was losing his delusion, larger and larger areas of Lindner's mind were being taken over by the fantasy.[60] Countertransference and identification with the patient results in a loss of objectivity.

Our reply, in brief, to the suggestion of incompetency of psychiatric testimony:

(1) It is a mistake to restrict the above observation, on the need to summarize, to the psychiatric witness. Every person asked to testify wonders, "How can I possibly report what happened in so short a time?". The practical administration of justice sets limits on the detail which can be required of the testimony of any witness. The court, unlike the scientist, is hampered by limitations of time. It is, therefore, incumbent upon every witness to present his testimony clearly and concisely. It is the task of every expert witness to distill in a few minutes information and knowledge acquired over the years. Indeed, one might say that this is the heart and substance of an expert witness. It is interesting to note, however, that when the psychiatrist avoids his jargon and uses the language of the law, he is admonished not to talk like a lawyer.[61]

(2) As far as the "art of psychiatry outweighing the science" goes, let us refer to one judge who analyzed the value of evidence and the adversary courtroom procedure in this way: "All the witnesses are lying, and everybody knows it, but somehow justice comes out of it." The judge, of course, did not mean to say that witnesses are guilty of perjury, but rather that subjective elements (memory and perception,

feeling and will, attention and thought) are involved in the observation of "facts". In the courtroom, as in science and in every other mode of experience, subjective factors are operative and cannot be eliminated.[62] Furthermore, a single witness is not expected to carry the entire burden of proof. He is expected simply to further the inquiry.

(3) It is true that a psychotherapist does not make use of a corps of investigators; a psychotherapist is sedentary, he does not pursue his practice in the homes of his patients or in their places of business. External facts if obtained might in truth, blind him to the inner reality of the patient. Further, a search for evidence may jeopardize the therapist's confidential relationship with the patient. Yet, a psychotherapist is soon able to feel a difference in reports that have no basis in outer reality. Thus, a report of rape keeps changing when there is no correspondence with outer reality. The fact that Lindner was finaly able to write about the delusion as a delusion shows that he was able to get outside of it.

PROBLEMS OF THE RIGHT OF PRIVACY

Privileges, as pointed out, exempt certain confidential communications from the law's command to disclose. When the law does not require disclosure, an individual who breaches confidentiality out of the courtroom may be subjected to a suit for damages for an invasion of privacy (or for defamation). According to the AMA Law Department, one out of seven AMA members have been the target of a malpractice suit or claim.[63] Fortunately for psychiatrists, but unfortunately for patients who learn of breach of privacy, legal suits against psychiatrists for this or other grounds have not as yet occurred with the frequency that they could.[64] Psychiatrists are usually not sued for breach of privacy because patients do not want further to make their life a public spectacle or are not aware that they have a cause of action.

Social Affairs and Corridor Conversation

The First Amendment of the Constitution, protecting free speech, ordains that we are a "public opinion" state. We talk freely about politics, and also about our activities, and we love to gossip. Work constitutes a major part of our life, and many of us find little else to talk about. It is not surprising then to find a tendency among psychotherapists to discuss their patients outside the office, at home, at the club, and at cocktail parties. Sometimes, patients' names are used, and ofttimes the discussion degenerates into mere chatter. Some serious difficulties, for example, have arisen in the treatment of patients in clinics as a result of open discussion of patients in hallways. As a result, patients overhearing the discussion become quite upset and threaten to terminate therapy. There is a clear violation of the patient's right of privacy when treatment material is not kept confidential.[65]

Jeopardy to Patients or Others

It sometimes happens, as pointed out above, that to keep the confidence may jeopardize the patient or society. There may be danger, for example, that the patient will commit suicide. There is danger in an epileptic patient driving a bus, unless his employer is notified. There is danger in an airplane pilot who should be grounded because of mental illness, but who, fearful of losing his job, does not tell his employer. There is harm to the family of a patient who is dissipating, without their knowledge, all of the family's funds and property.

Under the law there is no duty to come to the aid of third parties, but the psychiatrist may act in emergencies. The physician may reveal a confidence when it becomes necessary in order to protect the welfare of the patient or the community. In such situations, the revelation is made only to avert the catastrophe; as the revelation is with just cause, the psychiatrist would not be liable in damages for invasion of privacy.[66] The general public, prospective patients and patients in therapy will not lose faith in the psychiatrist as a keeper of secrets when in cases of emergency he acts contrary to strict and absolute confidentiality. Sooner or later, the patient frequently realizes that the psychiatrist has acted in his interest (which is just the contrary when an opposing party in litigation compels the psychiatrist to testify). However, situations of real emergencies necessitating disclosure are rare.

Child Treatment

"Environmental manipulation," as pointed out, may be essential in the treatment of children. With some children, it is particularly desirable to involve the child's parents in the treatment process. Therapeutic gains with the child himself will often be short-lived unless the parents are also able to change. A meaningful relationship with the psychiatrist often depends upon cooperation. The psychiatrist may find sensitive teachers who may be able, in consultation with the psychiatrist, to contribute effectively to the child's treatment through the teacher-pupil relationship.

The broad treatment approach, however, does not forsake the confidentality of the child's revelations. The psychiatrist, as a matter of good practice, makes clear to both the child and his parents the type of rapport he will have with each. Confidentiality, realistically speaking, is maintained. There is no publication to the world. The psychiatrist is in this situation working with persons who are directly responsible for the patient and who can assist in the treatment.

There are times, however, when it may be necessary to write off the parents. There are various situations: the parents and/or the child may or may not be in treatment. All physicians have encountered psychotic parents who deny treatment to an acutely ill child or who are devastating to the child.

It is reported that physical assaults on children may be "a more frequent cause of death than such well-recognized and thoroughly studied diseases as leukemia, cystic fibrosis and muscular dystrophy, and it may rank with automobile accidents."[67] The percentage of mental assaults can well be imagined to be multifold that number. There is growing support for a law requiring doctors and hospitals to report cases of suspected abuse of children.[68] It is felt by many physicians, however, that such a law would be useless without a clause protecting doctors and hospitals from retaliation by irate parents who are investigated.[69] It may occur, however, that abusive parents may not bring their child to therapy out of fear of a report, or they may take their child out of therapy should abuse be reported.

Political and Other Candidates

We often find individuals running for political office who are extremely sick. Our century has had its share of pathological individuals at the head of government. By running for public office, it might be suggested that an individual is no longer entitled to keep his life and motivations in private, out of the public gaze. It might be said that the community has a right to know. It will be recalled that Senator Wayne Morse, in the course of his fight against the confirmation of Clare Boothe Luce as Ambassador to Brazil, asked Mrs. Luce's doctor if she ever had been under psychiatric treatment. It is occasionally proposed that potential leaders can be scientifically chosen.[70] Seemingly, psychiatrists and psychologists would be first to shun such an omniscient and apparently anti-democratic role. Suppose, among other things, that the individual refuses to submit to examination. Mind-tapping, as Szasz has called it,[71] without consent and cooperation would be a clear violation of constitutional rights. Psychiatrists are already accused of presumptuous interference in political, social, and cultural matters which are not directly pertinent to their medical province, the relief of individual suffering.

Personality tests have inspired the wrath of, among others, Martin L. Gross, whose recent book "The Brain Watchers" has already received wide notice. Gross attacks personality tests on two grounds: first, that the "brain-watching" system is a violation of human rights; and second, that it fails to isolate the qualities which its practitioners (quite wrongly) suppose to be the best. This is apparently a reaction to an overemphasis in past years of the value of psychological testing. It is true that psychological testing leaves something to be desired in measuring an individual's coping mechanisms, therefore the difficulty in predicting performance; however, the fact remains that psychological testing can tell us a great deal about the individual's pathological conflicts.

Yet the uncompromising moralist will say that all individuals, irrespective of whether they are candidates for public office or applicants for employment of school admission, should not even be asked to submit to mind-tapping.[72] As Justice Brandeis put it, in another connection, there is a right "to be let alone." The social values here are claimed to outweigh the objective evidence. A judicial or political decision after all does not rest solely on scientific evidence. It is interesting to recall the 1946 California decision holding that Charlie Chaplin was the father of Miss Berry's child, notwithstanding findings of blood-grouping tests; Chaplin, out of social considerations, was held to bear a responsibility to the girl.

Teaching and Writing

Scientific teaching and writing post a unique and difficult problem for the psychiatrist. This is an area where psychiatrists are especially vulnerable to suit. Non-psychiatric physicians in this regard usually have no difficulty; the configuration of the body can be discussed without anyone recognizing the patient. Psychiatrists are obliged to disguise their clinical data to avoid the recognition of the patient even though it involves detriment to the scientific value of the material.[73] The psychiatrist, more than anyone else, runs the risk of being charged with professional indiscretion. The doctrine of privacy prohibits the public use of identifying characteristic of any individual unless his prior consent has been obtained. The law of privacy makes available significant protection to the patient against the disclosure of intimate facts of his life.

Campus Psychiatry

A number of universities have appointed psychiatrists as part of their health services to examine disciplinary cases and to counsel or treat students. Some colleges, it is believed, require a report on some non-referral as well as on referral students. Campus psychiatry is beset with many problems.

In cases of physical illness, a surgeon operates on a minor only with the consent of the parent (or guardian) except in emergencies. However, in psychotherapy, a minor for one reason or another may not wish that contact be made with his parents. The requirement that a college or a psychiatrist notify the parents of all minors who consult the psychiatrist would destroy service at once. As a consequence, university health services treat students as though they were adults. Although the parents may afford private treatment, university clinics treat students on a long-term basis at a nominal fee when they do not wish to contact their parents. Good practice would require that no one is told about treatment unless the student's permission is obtained or there is a problem involving suicide, potential homicide, or some kind of behavior which is going to handicap markedly the student or his parents. In any case, no action is taken without letting the student know, except in instances of acute psychoses or danger to life.[74]

Some university health services, quite appropriately, notify students of exceptions to confidentiality in the following manner: (1) when a student's mental condition is such that immediate action must be taken to protect the student or others from serious consequence of his illness; and (2) when a student is referred for evaluation and an opinion or recommendation is requested.[75] In the first situation, immediate voluntary or involuntary hospitalization may be arranged and in such cases the college administration and parents are notified as quickly as possible. Cases in the second exception are called administrative referrals and in such situations the student is informed initially that a report will be made to the referring individual or agency, but the actual interview itself remains confidential as far as content is concerned.

Thus, we see that the prevailing practice on notification of parents in the case of treatment of minors for mental illness is, curiously enough, just the opposite of the procedure generally followed, and approved by the law, in the case of treatment of minors for physical illness. In the former case, notification is made only in emergencies; in the latter case, lack of notification in emergencies is legally excused. Of course, the usual reason for the distinction is the element of time.

Communications Between Doctors and Treatment Centers

Proper and efficient care of patients often requires communications between various physicians and hospitals. However, a release of information to other doctors interested in the patient should be cleared, preferably in writing, with the patient. If not handled properly, the physician may be sued for breach of confidentiality.[76]

In the majority of states, hospital records are not as readily available to clinics as they should be, and vice versa, resulting in considerable delay and duplication of effort. There is also marked need for improvement in exchange of information among clinics treating various members of a family. A coordinated mental health program requires the development of a record system that places patient and family history at the finger tips of physicians, clinics and hospitals. A record system similar to medical records of the military has been suggested. Under such a system, records would go with the patient from the hospital to the clinic in his community. If commitment is again necessary or there is a transfer between hospitals, the record would go along with the patient.[77]

The trend, however slow, is toward interrelated medical centers and central medical records. The trend is not only toward interrelated medical institutions, but also collaboration with nursing homes and other institutions. To what extent does a patient by undertaking treatment impliedly give permission to other physicians, and to researchers, recorders and others, to view the records? Apart from legal considerations, exchange and transfer of information should have the approval of the patient, otherwise the therapeutic relationship might be impaired. It is unlikely that a patient will protest a procedure designed to facilitate proper treatment.

Communications with Non-Medical Persons

When making application of one type or another, the patient may be asked and he may acknowledge that he is seeing or has seen a physician or psychiatrist.[78] As a result, the psychiatrist may receive requests for information from an employer, parole board, credit-rating organization, insurance company,[79] welfare department,[80] military,[81] schools or others. An insurance company inquires if the patient feels "insecure"; the football coach asks if the boy has "a sense of belonging"; the police want to know whether a driver's license should be taken away. The patient may regard the therapist as a potential spy or informer even though the information is furnished with his written consent. It is to be noted, as Hollender has pointed out, that the psychiatrist's traditional function has been oriented to treatment and not to public service; the physician's traditional job has been to treat the sick, not to prepare historical reports or explanatory documents.[82]

Fee Collection

In early law physicians could not maintain an action to recover fees for medical services. Fees were regarded as honorable, and not demandable of right. Times have changed. Patients sue now physicians for malpractice; physicians sue patients for payment of their bills. In some states the physician is allowed not only a cause of action, but also a ranking over other creditors.[83]

Yet, even in our "age of commercialism," the roles of creditor and debtor, issues of fairness of charges, promptness of payment—especially at times of emotional tension—are generally considered not to promote "warm human relations" or "mutual confidence." The psychiatrist is peculiarly sensitive about his standing in the community. He has special problems in enforcing his claim for payment of his bill; he is reluctant to engage the services of a bill-collecting agency or to bring the matter to court.

The Report of the Group for the Advancement of Psychiatry (GAP) states: "Psychiatrists are less likely to use such services since they tend to discuss financial matters with their patients more fully and reach agreements more often than do other physicians. While we will not argue the pros and cons of using such service, it should be pointed out that under some circumstances, when an account is turned over to an agency for collection, it may be a breach of the confidential relationship in that a patient should be able to control who knows he is in psychotherapy. This matter should be considered before such a step is taken."[84] However, it has traditionally been held in the law on privileges that confidentiality goes out the window in litigation between the parties.[85] Thus, when a patient sues a physician for malpractice, the physician may discuss diagnosis and treatment. By bringing suit, the patient waives his secrecy privilege. The same principle applies in a suit brought by the physician for the patient's failure to perform his obligation under the contract, to wit, to pay for services rendered. The fact that the privilege belongs to the patient does not prevent the physician from claiming payment in court for his services. The privilege precludes a third person from calling the physician as a witness against the patient; it is not applicable in suits between physician and patient (and similarly, between attorney and client).

Furthermore, it is to be noted that the medical privilege applies only to the communication itself, and not to the fact that a communication was made. Thus, under the orthodox medical privilege, the fact of the physician-patient relationship, that the person was under treatment, the number of visits, and the duration of treatment, are not privileged areas.[86] This may be all the information that may be needed to uphold a claim for payment. There may be no need to reveal the content of the sessions.

Be that as it may, the dynamics of behavior underlying failure to pay a bill surely are not to be ignored. Money has important meanings to everyone, on many different levels of psychic functioning. The pattern of giving and receiving money is symbolic of many interpersonal transactions. Lack of punctuality in the payment of fees may be a manifestation of temporary financial shortage, a problem in the patient related to money or to giving, an identification of money with "vulgarity," or an indication of resentment toward the therapist and of a desire to frustrate him. Likewise, counter-transference manifestations may reflect themselves in the therapist's attitude toward payment of fees. Conscious and unconscious conflicts may influence the therapist in determining his fee policy. Unlike most other medical specialities, as GAP points out, a fee in psychotherapy is usually agreed upon at the outset. A patient's disregard of a bill for a considerable period may indicate that the therapist himself is negligent in failing to bring to the patient's awareness possible avoidance of a responsibility which is part of the reality situation. Payment of fees is part of the reality situation which therapists supposedly impose on patients.

Combined Individual and Group Therapy

A patient who is in combined individual and group therapy may state that material discussed in the individual setting should not be brought to the group. This is, of course, a defensive mechanism on the part of the patient and a denial of the group process, but nonetheless it might be suggested that a breach of confidence would invade his right of privacy. As a matter of law, such a holding is unlikely. It might be said that the patient cannot complain when he voluntarily takes part in combined therapy, or it might be said that the therapist has in fact acted in his interest and there has been no damage.

Case Presentations

Patients treated by medical students, interns or residents are frequently presented at case conferences. Individuals beginning psychotherapy at an educational institution usually agree in advance to appear at a conference. Conferences are explained as a part of the educational program, designed to help the patient as well as the therapist. Presentation before a conference can be helpful not only for the training of the therapist, but also for the health of the patient. Conference presentation may result in a corrective emotional experience. The patient may derive a genuine sense of acceptability not only by the therapist but also by members of the group. In some institutions, a patient who is reluctant about appearing before a group, whether or not behind a one-way mirror, is not presented. The presentation of a patient behind a mirror, without his knowledge, might be said to violate his right of privacy.

A patient usually comes to the therapeutic situation with a fear that unauthorized persons may learn of his disclosure. This fear may be reduced by assurance that information given will not be passed on. The therapist must make good on this assertion. The maintenance of confidentiality, however, is a matter of considerable delicacy in view of the prevailing law on the medical privilege.

Connecticut in 1961 enacted a specific statute for the psychiatrist-patient relationship which has been recommended as a model for all states by GAP, following its abandonment of an earlier recommendation. The Connecticut statute is quite detailed in its provisions,[87] yet, as we have attempted to show, there are a number of situations which strictly speaking fall outside even its protection. Clauses might be added to the already complicated statute to cover these matters, but the fundamental solution must come by full and fair acceptance by the courts of the need of confidentiality even in the courtroom. Otherwise, the best of statutes will come to naught. The example that psychiatrists themselves show in maintaining the privacy of the patient might best convince the courts, and the general public, of the merit of a privilege. The fundamental guidepost is that no information about a patient should be released without authorization by the patient or his legally designated guardian.

A communication of whatever type is a bond between two people. The teller becomes part of the hearer's life, and vice versa. A relationship is established that is sacred in nature. A patient in psychotherapy especially expects an inviolable "a therapist who never tells anything", in fact as well as in law.

The problem in the law is where to draw the line separating the privileged from the unprivileged. The desideratum for all privileges, we would suggest, is that a communication made in reasonable confidence that it will not be disclosed, and in such circumstances that disclosure is shocking to the moral sense of the community, should not be disclosed in a judicial proceeding.[88] Many of the problems presented in this paper can fairly be resolved by the application of such an over-all principle. The alternative is cumbersome legislation to cover specifically every conceivable situation.

ACKNOWLEDGMENT

Thanks are due to Dr. Jay Katz of Yale University, Dr. Zigmond M. Lebensohn of Washington, D. C., and Dr. Philip Q. Roche of Conshohocken, Pennsylvania, for reading over the final draft and for their suggestions.

Notes and References

1. "The search for truth is the basic aim of our law. Truth, like motherhood, should be sacrosanct. Yet the law, in many of its rules of evidence, treats the search for truth in a cavalier fashion and as being far from sacred. Many rules of evidence result in the suppression rather than in the ascertainment of the truth. Nowhere is this better demonstrated than in the field of the testimonial privileges afforded several relationships. Every testimonial privilege afforded a party or witness necessarily and inevitably results in the suppression of material and relevant, and in some cases of basic, facts. Thus any testimonial privilege constitutes a legislatively created barrier to the search for truth. The public policy behind some of these privileges is so apparent and basic that it outweighs the public policy behind the unfettered search for the truth. But as to other testimonial privileges and public policy behind them is not so apparent or basic. The existence or continuance of such privileges presents a highly debatable and controversial question." Judge Peters, Book Review. Calif. L. Rev., 47:783, 1959.

   The following quotation from 8 Wigmore on Evidence (3rd ed.) §2192, pp. 64, 67, is an excellent statement of the law: "For more than three centuries it has now been recognized as a fundamental maxim that the public (in the words sanctioned by Lord Hardwicke) has a right to every man's evidence. When we come to examine the various claims of exemption, we start with the primary assumption that there is a general duty to give what testimony one is capable of giving, and that any exemptions which may exist are distinctly exceptional, being so many derogations from a positive general rule. . . . The investigation of truth and the enforcement of testimonial duty demand the restriction, not the expansion, of these privileges. They should be recognized only within the narrowest limits required by principle. Every step beyond these limits helps to provide, without any real necessity, an obstacle to the administration of justice."

   Opponents to privileges argue that privileges give first consideration to the individual client or patient, doctor or lawyer, as against the public interest or the welfare of the community as a whole. See, e.g., Baldwin, Confidentiality between physician and patient. Md. L. Rev., 22:181, 1962. But why identify a trial with the public interest and privileges with individual interest? It is just as logical to say that a trial concerns only the immediate litigants, and that a privilege concerns a broad class of persons (all patients and all clients).

2. Jurisdictions recognizing the physician-patient privilege are (with citation to statutes): Alaska (58-6-6), Ariz. (12-2235-36, 13-801-02), Ark. (28-607, 43-2004), Calif. (CCP §1881, Penal Code §1321), Colo. (153-1-7-1-8, 39-7-13), Dist. of Col. (14-308), Hawaii (222-20), Idaho (9-203, 19-2110), Ill. (51-5-1), Ind. (2-1714, 9-1602), Iowa (622.10, 782.1), Kan. (60-2805, 62-1413), Mich. (27.911, 28.945, 28.1045), Minn. (595.02), Miss. (§1697), Mo. (491.060), Mont. (93-701-4, 94-7209), Neb. (25-1206-07), Nev. (48.080), N.Y. (C.P.A. §352, 354), N.D. (31-0106-07), Ohio (2317.02, 2945.41), Okla. (12-385, 22-702), Ore. (44,040, 136.510), S.D. (34.3631, 36.0101-03), Utah (77-44-1,-2, 78-24-8), Wash. (5.60.060, 10.52.020, 10.58.010), Wis. (325.21), and Wyo. (1-139). Some other states have limited privileges, protecting only a narrow class of information. Kentucky (213.200) limits its privilege to vital statistics. Louisiana's privilege (15:

476) applies only in criminal cases. New Mexico (20-1-12) limits the privilege to cases of venereal disease and workmen's compensation claims. North Carolina (8-53) and Virginia (8-289-1) demand disclosure when it is necessary to "a proper administration of justice". Pennsylvania's privilege (28-328) extends only to information which tends to blacken the character of the patient. Virginia's privilege (8-289-1) is limited to civil cases. West Virginia's privilege (§4992) is available only before justices of the peace. Federal courts in civil cases adopt the rules of evidence of the state in which the trial is held: hence, the medical privilege exists in some federal courts and not in others; furthermore, in criminal cases, the privilege is disallowed in all federal courts. Jurisdictions without a physician-patient privilege are Ala., Conn., Del., Fla., Ga., Me., Md., Mass., N.H., N.J., R.I., S.C., Tenn., Texas, and Vt. Connecticut and Georgia recently enacted a special privilege for communications between psychiatrist and patient. See *infra* note 4.

3. As a result of adverse criticism, the physician-patient privilege, where it exists, has been narrowly construed by the courts. As one court put it, there has been "considerable criticism of physician-patient privilege statutes in recent years, on the ground that such statutes [have] but little justification for their existence and that they [are] often prejudicial to the cause of justice by the suppression of useful truth, 'the disclosure of which ordinarily [can] harm no one.'" Van Wie v. United States, 77 F. Supp. 22 (N.D. Iowa 1948). The legislative and jurisprudential restrictions on the medical privilege are enumerated in Slovenko, J. of La. State Med. Soc. 110:39, 1958.

4. The Georgia statute creates a privilege for "communication between psychiatrist and patient." The statute however sets out no guides, leaving the extent of protection to case-by-case determination by the courts. Ga. Code Ann. §38-418 (Supp. 1960). The GAP model statute proposed protection on the same basis as confidential communications between attorney and client (GAP Report No. 45, 1960), but it soon became clear that this proposal was inadequate, and in its stead GAP suggested the recently enacted Connecticut statute. The Connecticut statute is discussed in detail in Goldstein and Katz, Psychiatrist-Patient Privilege: The GAP Proposal and The Connecticut Statute, Am. J. of Psychiat. 118:733, 1962. The Connecticut statute is divided into three sections: the first creates the privilege; the second defines principal terms; the third sets out the conditions under which the privilege ends. Conn. Stat. Ann. §52-146a (Supp. 1961). The statute provides:

"§1. *Psychiatrist-Patient Privilege.* In civil and criminal cases, in proceedings preliminary thereto, and in legislative and administrative proceedings, a patient, or his authorized representative, has a privilege to refuse to disclose, and to prevent a witness from disclosing, communications relating to diagnosis or treatment of the patient's mental condition between patient and psychiatrist, or between members of the patient's family and the psychiatrist, or between any of the foregoing and such persons who participate, under the supervision of the psychiatrist, in the accomplishment of the objectives of diagnosis or treatment.

"§2. *Definitions.* As used in this act, 'patient' means a person who, for the purpose of securing diagnosis or treatment of his mental condition, consults a psychiatrist; 'psychiatrist' means a person licensed to practice medicine who devotes a substantial portion of his time to the practice of psychiatry, or a person reasonably believed by the patient to be so qualified; 'authorized representative' means a person empowered by the patient to assert the privilege and, until given permission by the patient to make disclosure, any person whose communications are made privileged by §1 of this act.

"§3. *Exceptions.* There is no privilege for any relevant communications under this act

"(a) when a psychiatrist, in the course of diagnosis or treatment of the patient, determines that the patient is in need of care and treatment in a hospital for mental illness;

"(b) if the judge finds that the patient, after having been informed that the communications would not be privileged, has made communications to a psychiatrist in the course of a psychiatric examination ordered by the court, *provided* that such communications shall be admissible only on issues involving the patient's mental condition;

"(c) in a civil proceeding in which the patient introduces his mental condition as an element of his claim or defense, or, after the patient's death, when said condition is introduced by any party claiming or defending through or as a beneficiary of the patient, if the judge finds that it is more important to the interests of justice that the communication be disclosed than that the relationship between patient and psychiatrist be protected."

A bill proposing privilege of communications between psychiatrists and their patients has been prepared for introduction at the 1963 session of the Maryland General Assembly. Item 117 before the 1961 Maryland Legislative Council. A Joint Committee is now working on a draft for a communication bill for Pennsylvania.

5. Freud, Collected Papers, vol. 2, p. 356 (Basic Books 1959).

6. In former times all personal rights were cast in terms of property rights.

7. Slovenko and Phillips, Psychosexuality and the Criminal Law, Vand L. Rev. 15:797, 1962. On occasion the physician is called upon to advise the single person about his sexual behavior. Without making a value judgment on premarital coitus, the fact remains that fornication may be a healthy milestone in the life of a person. Inasmuch as fornication by unmarried people is prohibited in all states except ten, the physician could theoretically be considered an accessory to the crime. There are also problems in giving advice to married couples (consider birth control advice). The privilege against self-incrimination of crime is available to the physician as well as to the patient.

8. See generally Brody, Simultaneous Psychotherapy of Married Couples, in Masserman, ed., Current Psychiatric Therapies, vol. 1, p. 139 (1961). In recent legislation, Louisiana has provided that whenever the parties to a separation or divorce proceeding effect a reconciliation prior to rendition of judgment, all pleadings and testimony can be separated from other court records and maintained in a confidential status. La. R.S. 13:4687 (Act 421 of 1962).

9. Binder v. Ruvell, Harry Fisher, Judge, Civil Docket 52C2535, Circuit Court of Cook County, Illinois, June 24, 1952, reported in A.M.A.J. 150:1241, 1952, and commented upon in Nw. U.L. Rev. 47:384, 1952.

10. Grosberg v. Grosberg, 269 Wis. 165, 68 N.W.2d 725 (1955) (child custody case in which testimony of a psychologist was used to establish the neurotic condition of the mother).

11. Chafee, Privileged Communications: Is Justice Served or Obstructed by Closing the Doctor's Mouth on the Witness Stand?, Yale L.J. 52:607, 1943.

12. Fed. R. Civ. P. 35; Ganes, The Clinical Psychologist as a Witness in Personal Injury Cases, Marq. L. Rev. 39:329, 1955; Hare. Medical Testimony: Doctors and Lawyers Cooperate, J. Am. Jud. Soc. 41:78, 1957.

13. Usdin, The Psychiatrist and Testamentary Capacity, Tul. L. Rev. 32:89, 1957.

14. Rhodes v. Metropolitan Life Ins. Co., 172 F.2d 183 (5th Cir. 1949). In some states, the heir can claim or waive the secrecy privilege. The Connecticut statute provides that when a deceased patient's mental condition is introduced by any party claiming or defending through or as a beneficiary of the patient, there is no privilege should the judge find "that it is more important to the interests of justice that the communication be disclosed than that the relationship between patient and psychiatrist be protected." Conn. Stat. Ann. §52-146a (Supp. 1961).

15. Proceedings of the Institute on Law and the Mind, p. 28 (U. of Wis. Extension Law Dept., 1961).

16. Radauskas, Kurland and Goldin, A Neglected Document—The Medical Record of the State Psychiatric Hospital Patient, Am. J. of Psychiat. 118:709, 1962. Consider the following court opinion of a hospital record: "There is good reason to treat a hospital record entry as trustworthy. Human life will often depend on the accuracy of the entry, and it is reasonable to presume that a hospital is staffed with personnel who competently perform their day to day tasks. To this extent at least, hospital records are deserving of a presumption of accuracy even more than other types of business entries." Thomas v. Hogan, 308 F.2d 355 (4th Cir. 1962).

17. La. R.S. 44:7(A).

18. Calif., Conn., Ill., Mich., Minn., S. Dak., and Neb.

19. Regulations of the Food & Drug Administration, effective October 1962, concerning investigational stage of new drugs, require complete records of the disposition of the drug and case histories of the patients, and that adequate reports be furnished to the sponsor, and that these records be open to inspection by the Food & Drug Administration on request. The records must include "characteristics of patients by age, sex and condition.

20. Ross, Commitment of the Mentally Ill: Problems of Law and Policy, Mich. L. Rev. 57:945, 1959; Slovenko and Super, Commitment Procedure in Louisiana, Tul. L. Rev. 35:705, 1961, and J. of La. State Med. Soc. 113:463, 1961. The new Ohio Mental Health Law provides that patient records, including hospital and court records, shall be kept confidential except under certain circumstances. An exception is made for court journal entries and docket entries, apparently for the benefit of those concerned with property and contract problems of patients since judicial hospitalization in Ohio still results in incompetency. Records may be disclosed upon consent of the patient and approval of the request by the hospital or court; when necessary in court proceedings; and when necessary to carry out the provisions of the mental health law. Ohio Rev. Code, chap. 5122, §§5122:31, 5122.36; Haines

and Myers, Hospitalization and Treatment of the Mentally Ill: Ohio's New Mental Health Law, Ohio State L.J. 22:659, 1961.

21. U. S. Public Health Service, Publication No. 51 (rev. ed. 1952). A brief summary of the act, by one of its authors, appears in Felix, R.: Hospitalization of the Mentally Ill, Am. J. of Psych. 107:712 (1951).

22. "Confidential medical information about a patient should not be released without the consent of the patient, if he is competent, or someone authorized to consent for him, if he is not competent, unless the disclosure is required by law or is vitally necessary for protection of the public interest. Where a court commits a patient to a mental hospital, authority to act for the patient will be granted either to a guardian appointed for that purpose or to a public official. This guardian or public official is subject to the control of the court. He is required to act in the best interest of the patient in all matters, including the release of information." AMA News, Sept. 17, 1962.

23. In the case of physical illness, the courts have held, for example, that an X-ray film belongs to the physician in the absence of a specific agreement to the contrary, but the patient may require the production of the X-ray in court. See McGarry v. Mercier Co., 272 Mich. 501, 262 N.W. 296 (1935). In Wallace v. University Hospitals of Cleveland, 171 Ohio St. 487, 172 N.E.2d 459 (1961), the Supreme Court of Ohio dismissed a former patient's suit for an injunction to compel a hospital to furnish him with a copy of his hospital record because, while the appeal was pending, the hospital furnished him with a photostatic copy of his record. As a consequence, the Court said, the case was moot and it felt bound to dismiss the case, which it did "reluctantly."

On whether a patient (treated for physical illness) is entitled to a copy of his medical report, the Judicial Council of the AMA states that, "Whether the contents of the medical report are to be given to the patient rests with the decision of the doctor who knows all the circumstances involved in the situation." The Judicial Council also points out that, "The records are medical and technical, personal and often informal. Standing alone they are meaningless to the patient but of value to the physician and perhaps to a succeeding physician. The patient, however, or one responsible for him, is entitled to know the nature of the illness and the general course or regimen of therapy employed by his physician. The extent to which the physician must advise his patient may be limited by the nature of the illness and the character of the patient. The physician in advising his patient must always act as he would wish to be treated were he in a like situation." AMA News, April 30, 1962. See also Physician's Legal Brief, Jan. 1963.

Records of a deceased physician cannot be sold because the information they contain is confidential (and therefore they are not inventoried as property in the estate of the physician). It is recommended that records of a deceased physician which might be pertinent to any litigation in which a patient may be involved should not be destroyed without prior notice to the patient. AMA News, Dec. 11, 1961, p. 14, col. 2.

24. Hospital records are exclusively the hospital's property. A few states apparently hold that clinical records are the property of the hospital and *also* the physician's property. Menninger, A Manual for Psychiatric Case Study, p. 35 (2d ed. 1962). In the Veterans Administration, the clinical records belong, not to the hospital, but to the Veterans Administration.

25. See Amato v. Porter, 157 F.2d 719 (10th Cir. 1946); Comment, Harv. L. Rev. 68:340, 1954. In a recent controversy in Wisconsin, Dr. Hertha Tarrasch, psychiatrist, claimed records and files relating to patients who availed themselves of psychiatric services offered at the Rock County Guidance Clinic upon a public basis. Dr. Tarrasch and social workers and psychologists under her direction and control compiled the records. Upon the termination of employment with Rock County, Dr. Tarrasch claimed the records, alleging (1) a proprietary interest in the records as constituting her work product and (2) a right to the records as being privileged confidential communications. The case was compromised. The parties agreed that the records and files would be placed under Dr. Tarrasch's exclusive control until 1970 but that their physical location would be determined by the court in its discretion.

26. Eleven states privilege the psychologist-client relationship, to wit, Ark., Cal., Colo., Ga., Ky., Mich., N.H., N.Y., Tenn., Utah, and Wash. The first psychologist-client privilege was enacted in 1948 in Kentucky. No jurisdictions privilege communications to social workers or marriage counselors as such.

    When specially protected, psychologists need not be concerned whether they fall under the medical statute as an agent of the physician. In recent years there has been an increase in the number of non-medical people engaged in psychotherapy, either privately or in an institutional setting or both. Psychologists, social workers, and even nurses conduct private or largely independent practices. See Jerome Frank, Persuasion and Healing (1961); Fischer, Nonmedical Psychotherapists, A.M.A. Archives of Gen. Psychiat. 5:7, 1961; Health Manpower Chart Book (1955).

27. Where there is no medical privilege, there is the important holding that the attorney-client privilege protects a report made by a doctor to the lawyer when the lawyer asked the patient to see the doctor. Lindsay v. Lipson, 116 N.W.2d 60 (Mich. 1962); City & County of San Francisco v. Superior Court, 231 P.2d 26 (Cal. 1951); Comment, Yale L.J. 71:1226, 1962.

28. First Trust Co. of St. Paul v. Kansas City Life Ins. Co., 79 F.2d 48 (8th Cir. 1935); Leusink v. O'Donnell, 255 Wis. 627, 39 N.W. 675 (1949). Physicians treating physical illnesses are frequently confronted with the situation where the patient is brought to the office by a housekeeper-companion who is present during the examination. In many states, courts hold that both the physician and third person can be called on to testify about the communications. Some states, however, hold that communications between the patient and physician are privileged when the third party is serving either as an assistant to the physician or as an interpreter between the physician and patient. Ostrowski v. Mockridge, 242 Minn. 265, 65 N.W.2d 185 (1954).

29. Fenton, Group Counseling—A Preface to Its Use in Correctional and Welfare Agencies (Institute for Study of Crime and Delinquency, Sacramento, Calif.); Fenton and Wallace, State Child Guidance Service in California Communities (1938).

30. Hopkins v. Grimshaw, 165 U.S. 342 (1897); Wolfe v. United States, 291 U.S. 7 (1934); 58 Am. Jur., Witnesses §381. Cf. Freeman v. Freeman, 238 Mass. 150, 130 N.E. 220 (1921) (discretion of judge to determine minor child's comprehension of parent's conversation).

Consider also the attorney-client privilege. If any of the attorney's or client's documents or verbal statements are disclosed to third parties (anyone other than the attorney or the client), then those documents or statements are no longer regarded as confidential. In the language of the old common law, the confidence has been "profaned" and the privilege terminated. Such "profanity" could occur either at the source or point of origin of the information, or it could take place later on. At common law the client's or attorney's necessity of having immediate office personnel permitted access to documents without destroying their confidential nature is accepted and approved.

The rulings on the medical privilege vary from state to state. Some courts allow the privilege when the third party is related to the holder of the privilege insofar as the testimony of the physician is concerned but not, oddly, as to the third party. The court in Denaro v. Prudential Ins. Co., 154 App. Div. 840, 139 N.Y.S. 758, 761 (1913) said: "[W]hen a physician enters a house for the purpose of attending a patient, he is called upon to make inquiries, not alone of the sick person, but of those who are about him and who are familiar with the facts, and communications necessary for the proper performance of the duties of a physician are not public, because made in the presence of his immediate family or those who are present because of the illness of the person. *Of course, the persons who are present are not denied the right to testify.* It is only the physician who is bound by the rule." (Emphasis added.)

31. Furthermore, in this day of highly sophisticated eavesdropping devices, it is practically impossible to assure privacy. Possibly the only way to be sure remarks remain private is not to make them. See Dash, Schwartz and Knowlton, The Eavesdroppers (1959).

32. Schecter, The Integration of Group Therapy with Individual Psychoanalysis, in Masserman, ed., Current Psychiatric Therapies, vol. 1, p. 145 (1961). "Group psychotherapy is booming." Time, Feb. 8, 1963, p. 38.

33. Oldham, Privileged Communications in Military Law, Military L. Rev. July 1959.

34. Perhaps this is a reaction to the earlier overemphasis on the importance of psychological testing. Too much was expected, yet now it is said that "the efforts to weed out personality risks from the armed forces during World War II was a complete fiasco." Review of Gross, The Brain Watchers, by Parkinson, Genius by the Yard, Sat. Rev., Oct. 13, 1962, p. 32.

35. See Glass, Artiss, Gibbs and Sweeney, The Current Status of Army Psychiatry, Am. J. of Psychiat. 117:673, 1961; Glass, Advances in Military Psychiatry, in Masserman, ed., Current Psychiatric Therapies, vol. 1, p. 159 (1961).

36. Washington Post Sept. 22, 1960, p. 1.

37. The report of the House Committee on Un-American Activities said Martin was "sexual abnormal: in fact, a masochist." It said Mitchell had "posed for nude color slides perched on a velvet-covered stool." AP News-Release, Aug. 14, 1962.

38. The image of the physician *qua* physician is little enhanced by divulgence of information. In the words of Dr. Victor W. Sidel:
". . . The doctor's duty to heal the sick . . . includes a duty to keep others from getting sick. Therefore, when he faces a food handler with

typhoid fever who refuses to recognize the danger of his disease to others, he sees no break in ethical principles in promptly reporting the danger to the appropriate authority. Again, the doctor's duty to the sick includes a duty to keep others from getting injured. When a patient, therefore, tells a physician that he plans to commit a crime of violence—for example, 'I'm going to murder the mayor at noon tomorrow'—the physician takes steps to see that the mayor is protected. Furthermore, such a patient is almost always really saying, 'I have a terrible urge (or very vivid fantasies involving the urge) to kill the mayor. Please protect me from my urge.' This is usually true also of the patient who tells the doctor that he plans to commit suicide. The doctor will not hesitate to make appropriate revelations to prevent violence, either self-inflicted or inflicted on others, because in so doing he is furthering his professional goals for his patient and for his community.

Sidel, Confidential Information and the Physician, New Eng. J. Med. 264: 1133, 1961; see also Sidel, Medical Ethics and the Cold War, Nation 191: 325, 1960.

39. Guttmacher, The Mind of the Murderer 215 (1960).

40. "[As a class], patients willing to express to psychiatrists their intention to commit crime are not ordinarily likely to carry out that intention. Instead, they are making a plea for help. The very making of such pleas affords the psychiatrist his unique opportunity to work with patients in an attempt to resolve their problems. Such resolutions would be impeded if patients were unable to speak freely for fear of possible disclosure at a later date in a legal proceeding." Goldstein and Katz, Psychiatrist-Patient Privilege: The GAP Proposal and the Connecticut Statute, Am. J. of Psychiat. 118: 733, 1962.

41. People v. Hawthorne, 293 Mich. 15, 291 N.W. 205 (1940); United States v. Chandler, 72 F. Supp. 230 (1947).

42. However, an old conviction was upheld when a drug administered to an addict in custody, to alleviate narcotic addiction withdrawal pains, rendered the arrested person talkative enough for production of a confession. Mueller, The Law Relating to Police Interrogation: Privileges and Limitations, in Sowie, ed., Police Power and Individual Freedom 131 (1962); Sheedy, Narcointerrogation of a Criminal Suspect, J. Crim. L., C. & P.S. 50:118, 1958.

43. In the case of Leyra v. Denno, 347 U.S. 556 (1954), the defendant, after being questioned by the state police for the greater part of four days concerning the murder of his aged parents, complained of an acutely painful attack of sinus. The police promised to get a doctor. They got a psychiatrist with a considerable knowledge of hypnosis. Instead of administering medical aid, the psychiatrist, working in a room which was wired, "by subtle and suggestive questions simply continued the police effort" to get the accused to admit guilt. The United States Supreme Court threw out the evidence.

In Oaks v. People, 371 P.2d 443 (Colo. 1962), it was held that a psychiatrist could not testify to what he had been told about the defendant, whom he examined for the state (before charges had been brought) on the basis that under the guise of psychiatric examination, the psychiatrist had obtained information on guilt.

In McDonough v. Director of Pataxent Institution, 183 A.2d 368 (Md. 1962), the defendant, a delinquent, refused a psychological examination on the basis of the Fifth Amendment, but the court found no violation of his constitutional rights.

44. *Supra* note 4. Compare People v. Bickley, 22 Cal. Rptr. 340 (1962), where the trial court allowed a psychiatrist to testify even after an insanity plea for an accused murderer had been withdrawn. The accused had not been compelled to give the psychiatrist any information but did so voluntarily. The California Supreme Court affirmed the trial court's ruling, holding that the accused's constitutional rights were not violated by allowing the psychiatrist's testimony, which was held relevant on the issue of penalty. The Court also ruled that the psychiatrist was qualified to testify that the accused had a character defect and was not susceptible to rehabilitation.

45. Haines, The Future of Court Psychiatry, vol. 2, no. 1 (1957), reprinted in Nice, ed., Criminal Psychology, p. 268 (1962).

46. Guttmacher, The Mind of the Murderer, chap. 19 (1960).

47. Morgan v. State, Fla. App., June 13, 1962.

48. Observation made by Louis J. Sharp, Chief, Division of Probation, Administrative Office of the United States Courts, at the Sentencing Institute and Joint Council for the Fifth Circuit, May 9, 1961. See 30 F.R.D. 185 (1962). Mr. Justice Black's opinion in Williams v. New York, 337 U.S. 241 (1948) seems to be authority for confidential treatment, although as noted there is controversy about the point. Sharp, The Confidential Nature of Presentence Reports, Catholic U. L. Rev. 5:127, 1955.

49. MacCormick, A Criminologist Looks at Privilege, Am. J. of Psychiat. 115: 1079, 1959.

50. *Ibid.* Our observations *supra* in the section on criminal cases on reporting of crimes is *a propos* here.

51. Holmes, The Sheppard Murder Case (1962).

52. Hazard and Louisell, Death, The State, and the Insane: Stay of Execution, U.C.L.A. L. Rev. 9:381, 1962.

53. 339 U.S. 9 (1950).

54. Silving, Testing of the Unconscious in Criminal Cases, Harv. L. Rev. 69: 683, 1956.

55. Hollender, The Psychiatrist and the Release of Patient Information, Am. J. of Psychiat. 116:828, 1960.

56. In the $1,000,000 Van Sant alienation-of-affections suit in 1961 in Delaware, which did not have a priest-penitent privilege, counsel made a motion asking that the Rev. Percy F. Rex be compelled to answer any and every question put to him. Rev. Rex, asking the court to be excused, said: "In all kinds of pastoral counselling the clergyman seeks information from all sides. His usefulness depends upon his impartiality and therefore he refrains from being judgmental, and seeks to reconcile the parties to each other and to the God of all mankind. To be forced to testify for public record in a court would tend to destroy his impartial position as a reconciler of person to person and persons to God."

　　Answer to Motion to Compel Answer, Civil Action No. 154, Superior Court, Wilmington, Del. The suit was finally settled out of court, and the Delaware Legislature shortly thereafter passed a privileged communication statute for clergymen.

57. Furthermore, it is often said: "Many medical men find it difficult to think and feel about psychiatrists as they do about other physicians. Psychiatry

appears to them strange, unfamiliar, and unlike other medical specialties." Bartemeier, American Medicine and the Development of Psychiatry, J.A.M.A. 163:95, 1957, quoted in Taylor, The Psychiatrist and the General Practitioner, A.M.A. Archives of Gen. Psychiat. 5:1, 1961. Sociologists make the claim that psychiatrists differ from their fellow physicians in "technical skills, conceptual systems, scientific orientation, historical background, and (attitudes toward) problems of confidentiality." Smith, Psychiatry in Medicine: Intra- or Interprofessional Relationships?, Am. J. Sociol. 63:285, 1959.

58. Slovenko, Psychiatry and a Second Look at the Medical Privilege, Wayne L. Rev. 6:175, 1960, revised version, Slovenko and Usdin, The Psychiatrist and Privileged Communication, A.M.A. Archives of Gen. Psychiat. 4:431, 1961.

59. Reik, The Unknown Murderer (1930), reprinted in part one of The Compulsion to Confess (1959).

60. 50-Minute Hour ("The Jet-Propelled Couch").

61. Commenting on the testimony presented in the case of Briscoe v. United States, 248 F.2d 640 (D.C. 1957), rev'd, 251 F.2d 386 (D.C. 1958), Watson observed: "[This case] involved a psychologist, a psychiatrist and a couple of lawyers, each of whom jumps their role. The judge talks like a psychiatrist; the psychologist talks like a lawyer; the psychiatrist jumps back and forth between both. The end result is that the only one who made the right diagnosis was the original policeman on the case and he, listening to the confession in a case of arson, said the man was nuts." Proceedings of the Institute on Law and the Mind, p. 77 (U. of Wis. Extension Law Dept., 1961).

62. Munsterberg in his *On the Witness Stand,* a work of note on the psychology of testimony, reports an automobile accident case wherein one witness testified that the road was dry and dusty while another witness stated that it had rained and the road was muddy. In another case, where it was essential to determine whether at a certain disturbance the number of guests in the auditorium was greater than the forty who had been invited to attend, Munsterberg reports that there were witnesses who insisted that there could not have been more than twenty persons present, and others who maintained that they saw more than a hundred. He points out that these were not cases of intentional deception or of mental disease. The witnesses were highly respectable persons who did not have the slightest interest in changing what they had observed. Moreover, these were cases in which every layman was prepared to give his impressions; these were not cases which demanded professional or technical knowledge. Munsterberg, On the Witness Stand (1927). See further Slovenko, The Opinion Rule and Wittgenstein's Tractatus, U. Miami L. Rev. 14:1, 1959.

63. Review of Medical Professional Liability Claims and Suits, J. of A.M.A., May 10, 1958, p. 227. According to a study of the California Medical Association, "The malpractice suit is a symptom of the breakdown in the doctor-patient relationship." Blum, Malpractice Suits—Why and How They Happen: A Summary of a Report to the Medical Review and Advisory Board of the California Medical Association, p. 4 (1958). It is also said that the courts are "tightening up" on the doctor's responsibility to his patient, Medical World News, Oct. 26, 1962, p. 37.

64. Legal suits in general are rare against psychiatrists. Bellamy, Malprac-

tice Risks Confronting the Psychiatrist: A Nationwide Fifteen-Year Study of Appellate Court Cases, 1946 to 1961, Am. J. of Psychiat. 118:769, 1962. Thus far anything goes on the couch; the ready defense: "That's my type of treatment." See Wittenberg, Common Sense About Psychoanalysis (1961).

65. The development of the law of privacy, which has been called the "right to be let alone," is often said to have come about largely because of one man's fury. The Boston socialite Samuel Warren became outraged at the depth of detail the local newspapers were printing about himself and his family in connection with the forthcoming marriage of his daughter. Warren felt that there ought to be a law against it. With his former law partner, Louis Brandeis, who was later to become one of the great justices of the Supreme Court, he turned out a challenging article which appeared in the Harvard Law Review in 1890. It laid the groundwork for the development of the law of privacy as we know it today. Hauser, The Right of Privacy, Sat. Rev., Nov. 11, 1961, p. 74.

66. In the case of A.B. v. C.D., 7 F. (Scott) 72 (1905), a physician who revealed to patient's spouse that the patient was suffering from a venereal disease was held not liable. Likewise, no liability was imposed on a physician who, after warning the patient to vacate a hotel, reported to the owner that his "guest" probably was afflicted with a "contagious disease." Simonsen v. Swenson, 104 Neb. 224, 177 N.W. 831 (1920). However, the Maryland court recently recognized "the right to redress for wrongful invasion of privacy" by unwarranted verbal disclosure of information which resulted in the patient's loss of employment. Carr v. Watkins, 227 Md. 578, 177 A.2d 841 (1962).

67. A.M.A. Journal quoted in Flato, Parents Who Beat Children, Sat. Eve. Post, Oct. 6, 1962, p. 30.

68. California at present is the only state that requires physicians and hospitals to report child abuse to law-enforcement agencies. The Children's Bureau has drafted a model law, based largely on the California statute, for submission to state legislatures.

69. "The key to solving the child-maltreatment problem," says St. Vincent's Dr. Fontana, "in the final analysis is in the hands of our lawmakers. Only they can protect the physician testifying in such cases from libel and malpractice charges. Only they can give the medical profession the means of preventing thousands of cases annually of permanent disability and death." Quoted in Flato, op. cit. supra note 67.

    Under the law, parents have an obligation to care for their young in sickness and health. An infant is made a ward of the court, invading the parents' custody, where the life or health of the child is endangered by the medical neglect of its parents, such as where the parents are members of a faith healing group and refuse to consent to a blood transfusion or a surgical operation for their child. See People v. Labrenz, 411 Ill. 618, 104 N.E.2d 769 (1952).

70. On testing of judges and jurors, see Frank, Courts on Trial 250 (1949); Forer, Psychiatric Evidence in the Recusation of Judges, Harv. L. Rev. 73: 1325, 1960; Redmount, Psychological Tests for Selecting Jurors, Kan. L. Rev. 5:391, 1957.

71. Szasz, Mind Tapping: Psychiatric Subversion of Constitutional Rights, Am. J. of Psychiat. 119:323, 1962.

72. In a recently enacted statute, Massachusetts prohibits an employer from establishing the polygraph examination as a condition of employment, or continued employment. One might speculate whether such a law is an unconstitutional limitation on the rights of employers. Some attorneys are skeptical about its constitutionality, but apparently a test case has not yet occurred. The General Counsel of the National Labor Relations Board has ruled that a company was within its rights to require applicants for employment to sign an agreement consenting to submit to polygraph examination as a condition of employment, or continued employment. Case No. SR-57, Aug. 6, 1959. See also Christal v. Police Commission, 33 Cal. App.2d 564 (police officer required to submit to polygraph examination when accused of attempting to commit a felony).

73. Consider one example of many, Wille's *Case Study of a Rapist: An Analysis of the Causation of Criminal Behavior*, J. of Social Therapy, vol. 7, no. 1, 1961. For the sake of preserving the anonymity of the persons involved, a good deal of the most vital data were deleted when Wille's article was arranged in its final form. Freud in his case history "Notes Upon a Case of Obsessional Neurosis" pointed out that it was not easy to compose, not only because of the inevitable compression, but also because of the need for greater discretion in print. The patient being well known in Vienna, it taxed his powers of presentation to the full. "How bungling are our attempts to reproduce an analysis; how pitifully we tear to pieces these great works of art Nature had created in the mental sphere." In his opening remarks Freud explained how it is that intimate secrets could be more easily mentioned than the trivial details of personality by which a person could be readily identified, and yet it is just these details that play an essential part in tracing the individual steps in an analysis. Freud, Collected Papers, vol. 3, p. 293 (Basic Books 1959); Jones, The Life and Work of Sigmund Freud, vol. 2, p. 262 (1955).

74. Farnsworth and Munter, The Role of the College Psychiatrist, in Blaine and McArthur, eds., Emotional Problems of the Student, p. 1 (1961); Peabody, Campus Psychiatry, in Masserman, ed., Current Psychiatric Therapies, vol. 1, p. 1 (1961).

75. Policy of Tulane University Health Center, publicized in student newspaper.

76. Berry v. Moench, 8 Utah 2d 191, 331 P.2d 814 (1958). In the case of Alexander v. Knight, 197 Pa. Super. 79, 177 A.2d 142 (1962), the court sharply rebuked a physician for giving a medical report on a patient, without consent, to another physician employed by attorneys who represented an opponent in the litigation. The court said: "We are of the opinion that members of a profession, especially the medical profession, stand in a confidential or fiduciary capacity as to their patients. They owe their patients more than just medical care for which payment is exacted; there is a duty to total care; that comprehends a duty to aid the patient in litigation, to render reports when necessary and to attend court when needed. That further includes a duty to refuse affirmative assistance to a patient's antagonist in litigation. The doctor, of course, owes a duty to conscience to speak the truth; he need, however, speak only at the proper time."

77. Davis and Silva, Proposal for a Statewide Mental Health Program (unpublished paper, Louisiana Department of Hospitals). A recent development in

the processing of records is the "Social Service Exchange," which acts as a clearing house for participating social agencies. GAP Report No. 45, Confidentiality and Privileged Communication in the Practice of Psychiatry (1960).

78. E.g., Hague v. Williams, 37 N.J. 328, 181 A.2d 345 (1962).

79. There is the requirement for medical certification of disability in order to qualify for workmen's compensation or other type of disability insurance benefits. The disabled patient finds it to his advantage to obtain such certification from his doctor.

80. Welfare departments question the physician about indigent patients that he has treated. The welfare authorities need a report to learn the extent of attention the patient requires. By requesting and accepting welfare medical care, it is considered that the patient waives his right to secrecy. However, there should be no disclosure of facts that might reflect on the patient's character. Physicians are cautioned to furnish information to organizations such as the Red Cross and the Cancer Society only upon written release from the patient. Eaton, When to Violate a Patient's Confidence, Medical Economics, Mar. 12, 1962, p. 147.

81. In one case the U.S. Air Force requested information from a physician concerning one of his patients whose work record in civilian life showed considerable absenteeism. Although superficially the cause could be ascribed to upper respiratory infections the physician knew the patient was an alcoholic. The physician wrote to the Air Force offering his opinion that the patient's poor work record was primarily due to alcoholism. After his discharge the patient sued the physician for breaching the physician-patient privilege. While saying that "a patient's illness has long been thought of as a protected professional confidence upon which every patient may rely," the court however found that the physician's "right, if not his duty, to his government to make a full disclosure of the facts superseded his duty to his patient to remain silent." However, this holding has been contested by medical authorities in other cases. Physician's Legal Brief, Aug. 1962, vol. 4, no. 8.

The medical privilege has been held inapplicable to investigations of the physician's books by the internal revenue. See Note, Syracuse L. Rev. 5:288, 1954.

82. Hollender, The Psychiatrist and the Release of Patient Information, Am. J. of Psychiat. 116:828, 1960. Szasz in a recent article discusses the matter of inquiries by psychoanalytic institutes to training analysts concerning analysands who are applying for admission to the institute. The institutes ask questions not only about the applicant's qualifications for analytic work, but also about his personality and his analysis. See Szasz, The Problem of Privacy in Training Analysis, Psychiatry 25:195, 1962.

83. La. Civil Code Art. 3191 (Slovenko ed.).

84. GAP Report No. 45, Confidentiality and Privileged Communication in the Practice of Psychiatry, p. 105 (1960).

85. In Yoder v. Smith, 112 N.W.2d 862 (Iowa 1962), a former patient had a good paying job, but was long past due on his bill, and showed no inclination to pay anything on the debt. The doctor resorted to a collection agency, which wrote the employer of the debtor for help in collecting the debt. The debtor thereupon sued, unsuccessfully, charging that his privacy

had been invaded. The court held that contacting the debtor's employer was a reasonable way for the creditor "to pursue his debtor and persuade payment, although the steps taken may result in some invasion of the debtor's privacy." In Patton v. Jacobs, 118 Ind. App. 358, 78 N.E.2d 789 (1948), the court denied a claim of invasion of privacy where a collection agency used by the physician notified the patient's employer of the bill owing the physician for medical services. However, unwarranted disclosure of indebtedness may be (and has been) treated as an invasion of privacy. See, e.g., Brents v. Morgan, 221 Ky. 765, 299 S.W. 967 (1927); Trammell v. Citizens News Co., 285 Ky. 529, 148 S.W.2d 708 (1941). It might be noted that the usual approach employed by collection agencies is "to instill anxiety and yet remain on friendly terms with the debtor." Black, Buy Now, Pay Later, p. 53 (1961).

See Crawfis, The Physician and Privileged Communications as They Relate to Mental State, Ohio State Med. J. 46:1082, 1950; Hassard, Privileged Communications: Physician-Patient Confidences in California, Calif. Med. 90:411, 1959. See also Wolberg, The Technique of Psychotherapy 663 (1954).

86. Compare United States v. Summe, 208 F. Supp. 925 (E.D. Ky. 1962), where an attorney, who had been called to appear at an investigation concerning the income tax returns of two of his clients, was asked certain questions concerning the preparation of the returns. The Court held that the investigating special agents did not have unlimited authority to examine the attorney but were, rather, limited to questions which did not violate the attorney-client privilege.

87. *Supra* note 4.

88. See the dictum by Judge Edgerton in Mullen v. United States, 263 F.2d 275, 281 (D.C. 1958).

Name Index*

(Principal References in *Italics*)

*Prepared with the aid of Savilla M. Laird.

320

Subject Index*

(Principal References in *Italics*)

* Prepared with the aid of Dr. Nelson Borelli.

325